# NUTRITIONAL HEALING

## AFTER THE WORK OF
## DR. MAX GERSON

Foreword by

Charlotte Gerson

---

A PATIENT
MANAGEMENT
HANDBOOK

# KATHRYN ALEXANDER

Copyright © 2015

All rights reserved. No part of this publication may be reproduced, stored in or introduced into a retrieval system, or transmitted in any form or by any means (electronic, mechanical, photocopying, recording or otherwise) without the prior written permission of both the copyright owner and the publisher of this book.

Book design & layout:  Kathryn Alexander
Cover photography:  Penny Riddoch    www.digitalphotodesigns.com

National Library of Australia
Cataloguing-in-Publication data:

Alexander, Kathryn, 1954- .
Nutritional healing, after the work of Dr. Max Gerson: a patient management handbook/Kathryn Alexander
Foreword by Charlotte Gerson

ISBN 978-0-9803762-3-4 (paperback)
Includes bibliographical references and index

Diet therapy
Immunologic diseases - Alternative treatment
Immunologic diseases - Diet therapy
Medicine, Chinese
Herbs - Therapeutic use

Other authors/contributors:
Gerson, Charlotte, writer of introduction

615.854

Disclaimer
*Nutritional Healing, after the work of Dr. Max Gerson: a patient management handbook* does not constitute medical advice. If you require advice on any medical or related matter, the author and publishers of *Nutritional Healing, after the work of Dr. Max Gerson: a patient management handbook* suggest you seek that advice from a qualified professional. As far as the law allows, all people connected with the writing, editing and publishing of this book disclaim all liability arising from the negligence of writer and publisher of *Nutritional Healing, after the work of Dr. Max Gerson: a patient management handbook*.

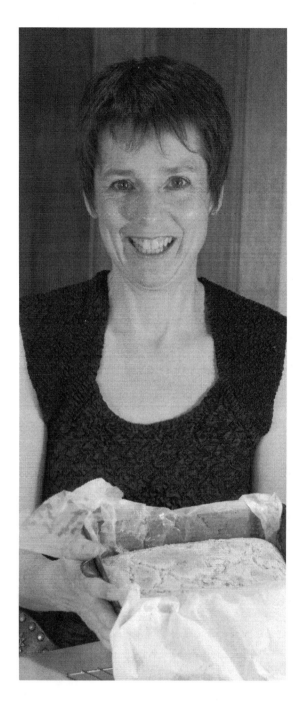

## Kathryn Alexander

D.Th.D., Adv. Dip. Naturopathy, Gerson Therapist

Kathryn is an internationally acknowledged expert in the field of detoxification and dietary healing, holding twenty years experience since qualifying as a dietary therapist in 1987, having studied under Dr. Lawrence Plaskett at the College of Dietary Therapy, London. Through her work with patients choosing the Gerson Therapy she has witnessed at first hand the fundamental role of specific dietary protocols in the healing of chronic disease.

Over the last ten years Kathryn has lectured widely in the UK, USA and Australia, developed training packages for both professionals and members of the public, and is the author of *Dietary Healing: the complete detox program.*

In 1999 Kathryn joined the board of directors of the Gerson Institute with responsibilities for research and development and practitioner training. She developed the training curriculum for the Gerson Therapy® and this current work *Nutritional Healing: a Patient Management Handbook* was produced both to facilitate training and to assist patients on the program.

Kathryn is also a recognised thought leader in the growing trend of the expert patient, where governments around the world are setting the trend toward the patient self-managing their chronic condition. As a consequence, a consumer-centric model of healthcare is now evolving in which patients seek to form partner-relationships with their primary health-care workers. This assists them in best practice management strategies that more closely reflect their own criteria for a best clinical outcome. Invariably strategies involve the combining of complementary and medical treatments, and medical professionals are increasingly required to have a working awareness of complementary protocols in treatment.

Kathryn is now based in Australia where her self-management courses have been well received by both professional and public sectors, with positive feedback from participants who are now equipped to either self-manage their own healing program and make informed decisions in treatment, or to case-manage those of their patients.

This handbook was developed by Kathryn Alexander to support her clients on the Gerson Therapy and emerged as a tool to assist in decision-making prior to and during the therapy. It is absolutely essential for anyone considering the therapy, and their informal helpers, to understand what is involved before embarking on the program. It is also essential that patients are able to communicate to other parties who may play a prominent role in their health care in a coherent manner in order to ensure appropriate decision-making within a meaningful context of their individual case.

The Gerson Therapy requires self-management and a successful outcome is not only dependent upon adequate knowledge of the program and the detoxification process by the client themselves, but also the development of a close working relationship with the practitioner. Although many people have undertaken the therapy on their own, it can be lonely and fraught with difficulties. Therefore, it is recommended that any patient embarking on the therapy seek assistance from health professionals and specialists with appropriate medical knowledge.

This handbook is a patient-practitioner management text, not a self-management manual. It is intended to form a bridge between the patient and practitioner, which will not only offer a clear understanding and sound basis of the therapy but also facilitate informed decision-making at critical points during the therapy, particularly when the patient needs to refer to different medical professionals involved in their overall case-management.

The information contained in this manual relating to all aspects of the nutritional healing therapy including dietary advice, indications, contra-indications, medical interventions, dosages of medications, is intended to be used in the context of appropriate medical knowledge and experience by the registered practitioner. This manual serves only as a guide to patient management in nutritional healing and does not constitute a means of determining appropriate medical treatment or intervention. The qualified practitioner should not rely upon this text as a sole means of treatment for any specific condition.

While every effort has been made to ensure that the information included in these pages is accurate, the author cannot make any guarantees nor can she assume any legal liability or responsibility for the accuracy, completeness, or usefulness of any information or process disclosed, or for any damage incurred directly or indirectly from the information contained herein.

Copyright© 2015 by Kathryn Alexander

# GERSON THERAPY®: THE BASICS

## by

### CHARLOTTE GERSON

In his last book, A Cancer Therapy, Results of 50 Cases, Dr. Gerson writes (p. 35): "In my opinion, cancer is not a problem of deficiencies in hormones, vitamins and enzymes. It is not a problem of allergies or infections, virus or others. It is not a poisoning through some metabolic or exogenous substance (carcinogen) [nor a genetic problem]. It is an accumulation of numerous damaging factors combined in causing the deterioration of the whole metabolism when the liver has been progressively impaired."

It is therefore unproductive to treat a single organ, search for a single cause, or use a method to extirpate or 'poison' a tumor. That is at best a temporary resolution.

The Gerson Therapy addresses all the above factors. By restoring the body's defences, with the immune system as one of the most important areas, by strengthening the liver in all its numerous functions, by intensively detoxifying all body systems, the Therapy addresses the basic causes of the body's breakdown: deficiency and toxicity.

With the hourly fresh juices, all food being produced by organic methods, the body is flooded with live, active nutrients, eliminating toxins and restoring cellular function. With the regular coffee enemas, the liver is relieved of its accumulation of poisons and can slowly resume its normal functions. Pain is usually overcome in short order making toxic pain control drugs superfluous, respiration and circulation is improved, tumors are promptly reduced and healing can begin.

It is important to note that 'a cure' is not obtained until all organ systems are fully restored to total function. Clearing the tumor is only the beginning, and the body will not able to maintain normal activity if the patient returns to an average diet just because the tumor is gone. The condition will shortly return until all the body's healing capacity is restored. For a terminal cancer patient, it takes two years of strict adherence to the Gerson Therapy to achieve the return to total health.

It goes without saying that the same basic principles apply to all other chronic, degenerative diseases including the killer heart and vascular diseases, diabetes, osteoporosis, chronic fatigue, rheumatoid arthritis and dozens more. Further, a somewhat less strict adherence to chemical-free (organic) salt-free vegetarian food is ideal for the prevention of all chronic 'modern' diseases, including depression, ADD (Attention deficit Disorder in children), even AIDS.

With the frightening increase of cancer in children, cancer incidence also in young people, and chronic disease in the population, the Gerson Therapy must be viewed as the preservation of the population for a healthy future. Health practitioners using nutrition will finally solve the problems orthodox medicine has been unable to alleviate with toxic drugs and/or surgery.

The present volume shows a deep understanding of the Gerson Therapy approach and philosophy and will represent the 'bible' of the nutritional healer of the future.

Charlotte Gerson, May 2001

# ACKNOWLEDGEMENTS

I would like to extend my thanks to both Charlotte Gerson and Beata Bishop who edited the original text for me and made many helpful contributions, back in 2001. My admiration goes to Charlotte for her tremendous vision and strength of purpose that has enabled her to ride the pressures of change and keep the therapy alive and intact. Charlotte was a wonderful mentor to me in my early years, and was always willingly on hand to help me with difficult cases. I also feel privileged to have the friendship of Beata. Through our exchanges I have come to respect and love her dearly for her values, tenacity, wise counsel and courage.

I also wish to acknowledge Dr. Melendez and Dr. Bravo, who not only taught me some of the vital principles of patient management, but inspired me through their compassion and dedication to reach for deeper understanding and commitment.

Thanks also go to all my patients for their great courage in deciding to take the reins of their health in their own hands by embarking on this extremely tasking healing program. I feel nothing short of admiration for all patients on this path, and only hope that we can measure up to them in providing all the support they need.

Kathryn Alexander  February 2015

# Contents

# Chapter 1

# DETOXIFICATION: A SCIENTIFIC APPROACH

*The in-text page references throughout this section are taken from "A Cancer Therapy, Results of Fifty Cases" by Dr. Max Gerson, unless otherwise stated.*

Detoxification, or the principle of using diet to effect cure, was an early feature of the naturopathic trends and treatments in Europe during the 19th and 20th centuries. Many famous names spring to mind when we are tracing the origins of detoxification, perhaps the earliest one being Professor Ehret who cured himself of Bright's disease (incurable glomerulonephritis) and went on to set up a sanatorium in Switzerland, later having clinics all over the world where he treated and cured incurables. All aspects of his dietary recommendations were tried and tested on himself and thousands of others.

Ehret published his book *Mucusless Diet Healing System* in 1914 and stated that the common fundamental cause of disease was internal mucus, generated by the tissues and organs in response to any type of injury (infection, trauma), and the eating of biologically unnatural foods and over-eating. "When the normal secretive organs become unable to cope with the disposal of the excess mucus, it will enter the bloodstream and cause heat, inflammation, pain and fever at such spots where the vessel system has contracted which could be due to a cold." Eventually this internal mucus or toxicity, would clog the tissues and arteries and harden. He maintained that the greater the degree of toxicity the more susceptible the individual became to bacterial and viral invasion and the less capable of fighting the infection.

His aim was therefore to:
- eliminate this disease-producing material; and
- to stop the source of it.

He advocated the mucus-less diet; the removal of all artificial foods, rich, fatty foods, milled grains, dairy and cooked foods. He discouraged the use of any dead foods, as they lacked enzymes. He proved that once the individual stopped eating these foods, then body would start to attack its "mucus" and "pus" and eliminate it. He basically advocated the raw food vegan diet.

Then we move on to Norman Walker. He became seriously ill through over-work and in 1910 established the Norwalk Laboratory of Nutritional Chemistry and Scientific Research in New York. He is famous for the Norwalk Juicer (still the finest juicing machine around) and his literature on juicing. He maintained that unless the patient was willing to take 2 litres of freshly prepared vegetable juice daily, then no reversal of health would occur.

Dr. Christopher is the next name that springs to mind. He was a famous American naturopath and herbalist, well known for his herbal recipes, his regenerative diet and three day cleansing plan. The aim of this plan is to replace the entire volume of toxic lymph with an equal amount of alkaline-forming vegetable/fruit juices. The patient fasts on a mono diet of juices (only one type of fruit or vegetable allowed) and then experiences the mucus release.

Dr Bernard Jensen, an equally celebrated naturopath is famous for his tissue cleansing through bowel management. The dietary protocol is similar and the end-result is a discharge of toxicity, through the colon, followed by healing. Dr. Jensen's method enjoyed some remarkable successes.

Next we move on to Dr. Max Gerson, who further developed the principles of detoxification and nutritional therapy for the treatment of chronic degenerative diseases, including cancer. He saw the liver as the primary organ of detoxification, and the support and regeneration of that organ took priority in his treatment. We reached the pinnacle of understanding with the work of this great man and since his death we have moved very little further forward, mostly hampered by the increasing toxicity in the environment and the deepening deficiencies in the food chain, resulting in a human population that has less resilience to disease than 50 years ago.

Many people now use Dr. Max Gerson's work as a benchmark in detoxification and nutritional therapy. He was able to collect scientific data from his work with patients suffering from terminal cancer, which supported his clinical observations and brought the principles of detoxification and healing into the 20th century scientific arena. It is through his work that we have begun to understand the criteria that must be met in order to initiate and sustain a healing by the body.

Dr. Gerson offered the world a simple basic framework with specific criteria. Any holistic therapy should aim to meet these criteria as fundamental laws of healing:

- detoxify the body, as healing cannot occur in a toxic environment;
- re-fill the cells with nutrients; and
- restore the immune system, so that the body can initiate a healing inflammation

It is possible through this framework to evaluate any supportive treatment in assessing how far, if at all, the treatment of choice is either going to assist or undermine the healing process. Once you have fully understood these criteria, you will become quite discriminative in your use of supportive treatments and in your ability to determine the progress of your patient and fine-tune the treatment.

There is an equation which you will find invaluable as you monitor your patients. The sole aim is to ensure that you bring your patient to a point where:

*The resistance of the body is greater than the resistance of the disease.*

By focusing on the healing process, through building the resistance of the person and reactivating the immune system, and focusing less on the disease process, you will not lose sight of the healing journey, of which remission is but a side-effect of the journey and not the end point of cure. As Dr. Gerson states "What is essential is not the growth itself or the visible symptoms; it is the damage of the whole metabolism, including the loss of defence, immunity and healing power." (p35) So the cancer or the disease is not the primary problem, but the condition of the patient that carries those risks. Generating an increase in the healing potential through the program will result in the removal of tumour/diseased tissue and the regeneration of new, healthy tissue.

There are several situations where you may find that the patient arrives with a great deal of tumour tissue in the body. In these cases the resistance of the tumour/disease appears stronger than the resistance of the body. We can never tell how these patients will respond to a detoxification therapy, but after the first 4-6 weeks it may be possible to make an evaluation. Invariably, these patients begin to respond, but we need to assess at all times if their response is sufficient to raise the resistance of the body/reactivate the immune system. Under certain circumstances we may choose to take steps to alleviate the burden on the body, if at all possible, through surgery, some radiotherapy or even light doses of chemotherapy. You must remember that any healing program, by default, is patient-centric and a rigid approach when the patient is not responding adequately may not be in the best interest of that patient.

The clarity with which Dr. Max Gerson approached the problem of healing and his precise methodology enabled him to leave a legacy that has stood the test of time and been validated from several standpoints in the scientific field. Dr. Gerson, like so many true healing physicians, was reviled by his colleagues.[1] Had he lived a little longer, he would have had the great satisfaction to have his observations and deductions acknowledged by the new scientific advancements, specifically in the field of NMRI (nucleic magnetic resonance imaging).

The philosophy embodying the work of Dr. Gerson, in the context of medical achievements/practices at that time, offers us a platform to move forward. It is edifying to see how modern technology corroborates and upholds much of Dr. Gerson's work.

The philosophy as applied by Dr. Gerson had a four-pronged approach:

- **Re-establishment of the oxidative metabolism.** The fundamental approach was the restoration of potassium (K) in the cells, along with the removal of sodium (Na) from the cells. He recognised that K was the key mineral in governing oxidation, energy production (ATP) - hence the metabolism of the whole cell. The potassium status affects every cell of every system in the body, including the immune system. As the restoration of metabolism was one of the principal keys to healing, this became a major challenge of the therapy.

- **Initiation and support of the healing inflammation.** This mechanism ensured parenteral digestion of the tumour tissue. This is a major determinant of progress and, once initiated, indicates an increasing resistance of the body and decreasing resistance of the tumour.

- **Elimination of the tumour tissue and toxicity (detoxification) by the liver.** Of critical importance was the capacity of the liver to detoxify. Dr. Gerson determined that if the rate of removal of toxicity from the cells exceeded the rate of elimination by the liver, then that patient would worsen and the liver would become more compromised. Assessing the capacity of the liver for detoxification, ensuring safe removal at the speed required in chronic disease, becomes a fundamental consideration of this therapy.

- **Restoration of tissues (structure and function).** Dr. Gerson ascertained that a period of restoration was essential for complete cure. He observed that even when the body had rid itself of all the tumoural masses and the patient felt that they were in the "clear", that without adequate restoration, then the chances of recurrence were greater (p16).

These four approaches to treatment are of equal importance. If a concerted effort is made on all four fronts, then indeed we can achieve cure. If say, however, just the first two approaches are taken, then we may secure control of the disease, but not cure. So supplying the body with good nutrition without securing elimination by the liver may only lead to a marginal improvement for the patient. Stimulating an "unnatural" inflammation is not the same as a spontaneously generated healing inflammation, and in the absence of increasing the oxidative metabolism and facilitating toxic elimination, the burden still lies within the body and the patient can, at most, only hope for a short remission. You have to remember that Dr. Gerson, with his therapy, was talking about cure, not control.

Dr. Gerson stated that malignancy is cell adaptation to local conditions; an adjustment to the preceding pathologies (p105). He surmised, quite accurately, that if you changed the internal environment so that the malignancy could not survive, if the body was brought to a vitality where it could generate a healing inflammation (digestion of the tumour), if the body was then able to eliminate tumour products along with other toxicity within the body, then you would indeed see cure. The following quote encapsulates his work. "After I recognised the healing of cancer to be a parenteral digestion, the entire therapeutic endeavour was subordinated to this purpose." (p217)

# The sodium/potassium balance

Throughout history healing diets have depended upon a high intake of fruit and vegetables; or a diet high in potassium while low in sodium. One of the fundamental principles which comes to light initially through Dr. Gerson's work and later through studies using NMRI technology, was that the cell, in its diseased state, will lose intracellular potassium and sodium will enter the cell. This shift in the major minerals causes inhibition of the oxidative function, leading to fermentation (sodium is an enzyme inhibitor). Otto Warburg's research into oxidative metabolism and his conclusions on the anaerobic metabolism of malignant cells (fermentation) was already current at that time and Dr. Gerson was familiar with this research. In an oxygen-deprived environment cells have to derive their energy through anaerobic glycolysis and in the process produce high volumes of lactic acid which need to be metabolised back to pyruvic acid by the liver. (*See diagram 4, p29.*) The cancer metabolism, as such, places a huge burden on the liver. Dr. Gerson argued that this type of environment supported the growth and replication of cells which have no requirement for oxygen (and indeed the lack of a cytochrome system in malignant cells lent support to this hypothesis). Cancer cells obviously cannot revert to normal metabolism, therefore the parenteral digestion and removal of malignant cells becomes crucial for the recovering patient (p125). Restoring oxidative metabolism is now a cornerstone of many alternative cancer treatments, and the conclusions reached by Dr. Gerson on the cellular sodium/potassium balance through his observation of patients placed on a high potassium diet of vegetables/juices are now well-supported scientifically and form the basis of many nutritional approaches to chronic degenerative diseases and cancer.

When one reads the scientific data that Dr. Gerson was confronted with at that time, one can appreciate how vast his task was to prove his observations in the light of opposing scientific opinion. For example, the available facts on sodium and potassium at that time were not clear (p94). Some authors stated that sodium was the most stimulating neoplastic growth agent, while others stated that the diet for a cancer patient should be rich in salt and spices. The literature on potassium stated that it promoted tumour development, tests revealed that there was an undiminished potassium content in cancer tissues (in reality there is a lack of ionised intracellular K) and that the concentration of potassium in serum was an adequate indicator of potassium levels. So all the current literature opposed the notion of the loss of intracellular potassium and the entry of sodium into the cell. Dr. Gerson, fortunately, was not one to reject his own observations on the basis of the current literature, and when he became convinced of the validity of his deductions, he gained the confidence to progress his therapy in order to treat the cancer patient effectively. Although some of his patients were responding on a very modified approach to the final therapy, many were not responding at all. It was Dr. Gerson's work in this field that confirmed that the more chronic the disease, the greater the potassium deficiencies, and that stronger measures were required to initiate healing.

**Dr. Gerson's observations:**

- X-ray studies revealed an area of oedematous swelling around damaged tissue and malignancies. On the high potassium diet/no salt therapy the oedemas reduced, tumours started shrinking and the patient started to heal. Dr. Gerson observed that once the oedema or sodium ring around tumours was drained, then the tumour would lose its protection or defence. It is a similar principle today where we are encouraged to reduce swelling around a visible injury through ice packs to restore the circulation and hence the healing to the area. The longer that inflammatory exudate remains around the injury, the slower the healing. Reduction of internal oedemas requires a high potassium/low salt therapy. It is a first stage requirement to healing.

- Dr. Gerson observed losses of up to 8g per day of sodium in the urine (day 10-14) and then at periodic intervals during flare-ups (pp97, 132, 165-166).

- Supplementing with a specific potassium compound speeded up this process. Over a six year period Dr. Gerson undertook 300 experiments to determine the exact combination of potassium salts (33% of each potassium acetate, gluconate and mono-phosphate) which would be most congenial to the body and facilitate intracellular potassium uptake (p409). With the application of these larger doses of potassium to the already high potassium diet, Dr. Gerson started seeing the results he was looking for. He ascertained that it took between one to two years to restore potassium to the vital organs. Nowadays this can be much longer.

- Dr. Gerson observed that the saltless diet and detoxification caused the reduction of Na, Cl and water in the whole system, the removal of cell oedema and the reduction of negative potential. Malignant tumours are characterized by considerable negativity associated with the accumulation of the extra-cellular group of minerals (mainly sodium) (p107). Studies in the last 30 years have verified this negative potential at tumour sites and have further shown that the insertion of an anode into the tumour site reverses this polarity, causing the tumour to shrink.

- Dr. Gerson observed that serum potassium is never high in patients during restoration time and he deduced correctly that this indicated uptake by the tissues and healing (p208).

To summarize:

- In sickness tissues lose the power to retain the intracellular minerals (namely potassium). The cellular metabolism breaks down and the cells drop into a fermentative state, a precursor for malignant change.

- On a saltless diet Dr. Gerson saw the elimination of Na, Cl and water, toxins and poisons. He asserted that all poisons were stimulants for sick tissues (pp164-165).

- The therapy paved the way for activated recharged potassium and iodine components; this increased the defences, but cancer cells could not adapt to the new intensive changes, ensuring their breakdown and death (p164).

- Serum potassium is only a passage channel; low serum potassium invariably indicated uptake by healing tissues (shows best healing) while high serum potassium indicated tissue breakdown/destruction/advancement of disease.

- As potassium is a key activator in many enzyme systems and critically in the oxidative cycle (governs the entry of acetyl groups into the Citric Acid (Krebs) cycle), it "sets the scene"(diagram 3, p.28). The oxidative cycle cannot occur in a high sodium environment. Sodium is an enzyme inhibitor and furthermore the acidity thus produced during fermentation destroys enzyme function (unravels the enzymes). For example, preservation with vinegars/lactic acid/whey acts by destroying the enzymes so that the food cannot react with oxygen. The lactic acid produced by tumours as a consequence of anaerobic glycolysis acts as a growth stimulant to the tumours themselves (diagram 4, p.29).

- Protein in the diet was seen to reduce urine secretion and sodium elimination (p80). Dr. Gerson observed that protein retarded detoxification and delayed the disappearance of harmful allergic reactions. He found that by eliminating dietary protein the sodium elimination was increased ("sodium outpouring"), which was precisely what he wanted to achieve. But he knew that he couldn't do it for too long or it would compromise immunity. He saw that sodium was trapped with protein, and the removal of protein for 6-8 weeks was sufficient time to allow for the resorption of oedemas and the initiation of the healing process.

We now understand that protein metabolism increases the acidity of the body and the excess acidity ($H^+$) is eliminated in exchange for sodium ions by the kidneys. Therefore it is extremely difficult to reduce body sodium on a high protein diet where the elimination and/or buffering of acidity takes priority over sodium elimination.

- ◆ Potassium in this special composition was seen to stimulate the autonomic nervous system (digestion).

It is important to remember in detoxification that a dietary elimination of salt is not sufficient by itself to produce cure or reversal of a degenerative disease, but is an important supporting factor of a nutritional healing program. Of greater importance is the inclusion of the high potassium content (diet and supplemental) which forces the existing sodium from the cells, drains the oedemas and stimulates cellular metabolism.

## Scientific corroboration of Dr. Gerson's work on the Na/K balance

**Clarence Cone** - a physiologist who generated substantial experimental data concerning changes in potassium and sodium levels in cancer cells. He found that elevated sodium forces cancer cells to continually divide and produce tumours.[2] Sodium is shown to have a mitotic regulating effect. He is now involved in extensive human trials.

**Christine Waterhouse and Alba Craig** (National Cancer Institute) 1957, measured water retention in cancer patients. On this study the normal calories were doubled (high fat diet), but the gain in weight was not due to forced fat feeding but an increase in intracellular fluids. This confirms that the metabolism of the body is altered; the excess calories are not converted to body tissue but the gain in weight is due to the stimulation of malignant cells to take up sodium along with water. A sick body will take up sodium which exacerbates the condition (sick cell syndrome). In my own experience, I have seen this to be the case with a terminally ill patient who was on a detoxification therapy and then admitted to hospital. He was given a high protein diet and he gained 2kg overnight. The only possible cause of this weight gain in such a short period of time is sodium and fluid retention.

Often terminally ill patients suffer cachexia (weight loss, fever, anaemia) and may be given greater quantities to eat to meet the increased energy/nutrient requirements. This treatment has no positive outcome but can be a factor in precipitating a disease crisis.

You will find that textbooks will confirm that blood sodium levels start to fall in the end-stages of terminal disease. The cause is unknown, but current medical literature indicates the possibility that the body resets its osmostat. Of course, another possibility, from the work of Christine Waterhouse and Alba Craig, is that the significant amounts of tumour tissue are taking up sodium, as this is a requirement for the cancer metabolism.

**Freeman Cope's table** of damaged muscle cell to illustrate changes in tissue content of potassium, sodium and water (referred to by Cope as the *tissue damage syndrome*):

|  | Normal tissue | Poisoned Tissue |
| --- | --- | --- |
| potassium (mM) | 105 | 6 |
| sodium (mM) | 20 | 120 |
| % of water normal content | 100% | 121% |

# Scientists involved in NMRI - Ling, Damadian and Cope

It was through the technological advancement of NMRI (Nuclear Magnetic Resonance Imaging) which linked the world of biochemistry with biophysics, that we have the most conclusive validation of Dr. Gerson's methods. NMRI reads tissue chemistry electronically; the large magnet picks up spin energy released by hydrogen nuclei, which is reproduced as an image. Therefore we are able to record and interpret the electrical fields within the body. Dr. Gerson was aware of the dynamic energies behind the chemical substances. He was aware of a force, which energized and thus gave life to tissues, minerals and chemical substances. His work makes many references which indicate this perspective.

*"We now know that what we have inherited is not a set of chemical substances but a pattern of dynamic energies" (p90).*

and when he talks about mineral supplements, which he found to be stimulating rather than replenishing

*"The system needs animating energies besides the pure substances" (p99).*

We now know that the potassium measurements taken in cancer cells may not be a measurement of the ionized potassium, which is low in malignancy. Dr. Gerson would have been one of the first physicians to truly embrace the new wave of biophysics as an instrument to measure the vital metabolism of tissues and thus healing capacity. Rather than as a purely diagnostic tool he would have employed the technology to pursue his goal of perfecting a therapy which so clearly is centred on the healing metabolism.

**Ling** (biophysicist - won the Boxer award in Biology 1940 and invented the intracellular micro-electrode, head of Molecular Biology Laboratory of Pennsylvania Hospital in Philadelphia) in 1962 approached the cell as an electrical model and had great difficulties with the sodium pump theory which was said to maintain the concentration/electrical gradient of the cell. This pump maintained 97% of body potassium intra-cellularly and 93% of body sodium extra-cellularly. He calculated by the laws of physics that the pump, operating under the given conditions, would require between 15-30 times the amount of energy that was available. He said that this was impossible.

Ling constructed a cell model based on the electrical field generated around the intracellular latticework of macromolecules: the cytoskeleton (microfilaments) and intracellular membranes. He stated that potassium gathers at negatively charged association sites along the macromolecules where, once in place, a force of attraction is generated which causes the structuring of water. Under this field, molecules of water polarise and line up, forming layers which become less structured the further they are from the electrical field. Ling hypothesized that salt water (from the ECF) passes through the cell at the rate of nearly 100 times the volume of the cell each second and that a rapid exchange of ions would occur, but the association sites preferentially choose potassium over sodium. He maintained that it was the electrical field of the cytoskeleton that governed the ionic environment (not the Na/K pump) and that no energy was required other than the attractive forces at the association sites. Additionally, structured water will not readily accept any other ions or toxins. This can be likened to the freezing of water to ice, it becomes purified of foreign substances and cannot accept more water. Ling called this theory the *Association-Induction Theory.* [3]

Ling went further to confirm this theory by paralysing the energy system of the cell so that no ATP (adenosine triphosphate or energy currency of the cell) could be formed. He found that the cell maintained a high level of potassium for many hours, indicating that it was not the energy derived from ATP (and hence driving the energy-dependent Na/K pump) that was keeping the potassium within the cell.

**Freeman Cope** - trained in medicine and physics (Chief of Biochemistry of the Naval Air Development Centre, Pennsylvania, USA) reviewed the Gerson therapy for the Journal of Physiological Chemistry and Physics in 1978 [4]. In this article he used the word "cure" with regard to the Gerson Therapy. His interest in the link between biochemistry and biophysics led him to Ling's work where he found himself to be in agreement with its logic. He tested the model with **Damadian** (received Presidential medal of honour for science and the discovery of NMR) using magnetic resonance techniques. They verified Ling's model and the type of water structuring Ling had described. Cope further predicted that large amounts of potassium could be added to a low sodium diet to reduce what he labelled the tissue damage syndrome.

# Tissue damage syndrome - Cope

*The cells in health:*

ATP
Protein configuration      }      structured water
K⁺ association sites

- ATP joins with the cell protein macromolecule which is then correctly configured. ATP is used to keep cell protein in its normal configuration.
- 20 association sites for K are formed.
- Once the potassium ions are in place, a force of attraction causes water molecules to polarize (oxygen atoms facing one direction and hydrogen atoms the other) around the latticework. This produces layers of structured water. When water is structured, it will not readily accept ions of foreign materials. Sodium cannot dissolve in structured water. So the cytoskeleton controls the ion concentration by choosing K⁺ over Na⁺ and structuring the water.

*The tissue damage syndrome:*
Electrostatic forces hold the potassium in place. However, in tissue trauma (any tissue injury mechanical, chemical) cells respond in the following way:

- Lose potassium
- Accept sodium
- Swell with too much water.

A vicious cycle is set up with any damage to the cell; it loses its cation association and structuring of water, which in turn adversely affects the production of ATP. ATP is required to keep the cell macromolecules in their correct configuration. In the damaged configurational state the cell proteins lose their preference for association with K and the water content of the cell increases. This intensifies the disturbances which further impairs ATP production, and so on. When the cell swells with water, cellular burning of sugars is impaired and so is production of ATP. Without ATP the cell dies.

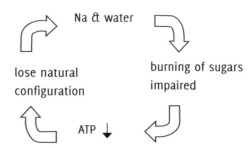

Na & water

lose natural
configuration

burning of sugars
impaired

ATP ↓

Extreme damage to the cell is irreversible. However, if the cell is not too damaged, it can be encouraged to regain its configurational state. This can be likened to the domino effect where the binding of potassium at one site triggers the binding of potassium at other sites. Cope was able to show that potassium competes with sodium for binding sites and that if the cell was bombarded with potassium, then the desired effects could be achieved. This was the success of Gerson - putting additional potassium into the diet (on an hourly basis during the day) helps potassium to compete for association sites, which removes the sodium. Once the cellular potassium is re-instated, ATP production, oxidation and cellular metabolism are restored. Cope was convinced that if you were able to control the type of salts and the water content, then you affect the way that cell functions and to this he attributed Dr. Gerson's success and rate of cure.

# Increasing oxidation and free energy (ATP)

Cancer cells derive their energy anaerobically and thrive in an oxygen-starved environment. Increasing oxidation to healthy tissue, particularly the tissue surrounding tumours, is a key factor in the healing equation. Tissue adjacent to the tumour site is particularly vulnerable, as the puffy oedematous area around the tumour is very toxic, containing cancer metabolites and lactic acid, which will poison healthy surrounding tissue (p123).

In order to both inhibit cells from falling into fermentation (anaerobic glycolysis) and from becoming poisoned by the tumours, it becomes a necessary part of any healing therapy to increase the capacity for cellular oxidation which involves:

- reinstatement of potassium in the cells
- increasing replication of cellular mitochondria (energy factories of the cell where oxygen is "burned" and ATP is formed). The energy metabolism of the body is influenced by the thyroid hormones. Many cancer patients have a low basal metabolic rate and therefore an under-active thyroid. Dr. Gerson used both thyroid and Lugol's solution (iodine) as medications. Thyroid signals cellular mitochondria to replicate and thus stimulates the cells to make more energy by burning sugars fast to generate ATP (increased energy production). Dr. Gerson found iodine to be the decisive factor in the normal differentiation of cells and used it to counteract the decrease in cell differentiation (p32). He also found that iodine invades cancer tissue when inflamed, not otherwise (p205). Smaller iodine doses appeared to make cancer cells grow more rapidly but the larger dose given at the beginning was seen to inhibit excessive growth (p206). The combination of iodine, thyroid and niacin helped check cancerous growth and aided surrounding tissues to regain their electrical potentials. Dr. Gerson states that the thyroid and Lugol's medication speeded up Na, Cl and water elimination and paved the way for the re-filling of the cell with potassium. Healing was also found to be accelerated when the thyroid and Lugol's was increased (pp126, 206).

- Niacin is a key vitamin in oxidative metabolism. It is one of the vitamins responsible for the shuttling of hydrogen and its electrons down the electron transport chain (diagram 2, p.27; diagram 3, p.28, diagram 4, p.29). Without niacin (B3) the electron transport chain would come to a standstill and no oxidation or formation of ATP would take place. Dr. Gerson saw improved results with the inclusion of this vitamin into the therapy. Niacin also causes dilatation of the blood capillaries, through stimulating the release of histamine, which accounts for the flushing often experienced by patients (pp32, 99, 100, 209). Patients who have allergic profiles may suffer increased reactions to this vitamin.

- CoQ10 has been subsequently introduced as its activity in the cytochrome system (part of the electron transport chain) which is reduced in malignancy (diagram 3, p.28). Raw calves' liver is rich in CoQ10, but as it is no longer safe to take this in its raw form (increased risk of camphylobacter from cross-contamination in the abattoir) CoQ10 may be used in supplemental form. The studies to date with breast cancer have been most encouraging. [5]

- Flaxseed oil. The use of flaxseed oil followed the successful work of Dr. Johanna Budwig who used flaxseed oil and milk protein together in her work with cancer sufferers. Dietary fat has been found to stimulate tumour growth and therefore fat should be omitted on any detoxification diet for cancer sufferers. However, the flaxseed oil has proved to be beneficial. It transports fat soluble vitamins (vitamin A) and I would also suspect that it has a part to play in the detoxification of fat soluble toxins. More importantly Johanna Budwig entertained a conviction that the flaxseed oil, when incorporated as part of the cell membrane structure, increased the cell's affinity for oxygen, drawing it to the cell like a magnet. [6] Due to the molecular structure of the omega 3 series fatty acid found in flaxseed oil, it carries a partial negative charge at its double bonds. This increases the cell membrane's electrical field, which then attracts the oxygen. Hence the entry of oxygen is facilitated into the cell and cellular respiration is improved.

- Fresh juices taken every hour are replete with living enzymes which is of added value to the body. The more "live" the food is, the greater its antioxidant capacity and the easier they are to digest. Foods that have a shelf-life only do so because all the enzymes have been destroyed in the preserving process (whether it be pasteurization or the addition of preservatives). The electrons or the electrical fields of these foods have been stripped away so that they cannot oxidize (go bad). It is important to make and drink the juices fresh, as up to 60% of the oxidizing enzymes are lost within an hour. They become technically "dead", as they have no electron fields. Furthermore, through the work of Patrick Flanagan, MD, we have found that organic vegetables/fruits are rich in hydride ions which form an energy re-fuelling system and regenerator of anti-oxidant systems of the plant. Food grown commercially with chemicals does not have hydride ions, and Flanagan suspects that they are used up by the plant as part of its defence against chemical insult.

# The healing inflammation

*"Where the inflammation metabolism begins, the cancer metabolism stops."*
*Dr. Gerson  quoting Professor G. von Bergmann (p43)*

The poisoned body cannot produce an inflammation, the detoxified body can.

*Cancer metabolism starts where the body is no longer able to produce a healing inflammation.*
*Dr. Gerson  quoting Professor G. von Bergmann (p42)*

The role of the immune system in cancer was a growing science, and Dr. Gerson had already studied inflammatory effects of the immune system and their effect on tumours. He knew that the parenteral digestion of tumour tissue was accomplished by cells of the immune system, and that in order to secure a cure, the metabolism of the patient must generate a natural and spontaneous healing inflammation described as a *flare-up*. These flare-ups were inflammatory healing reactions involving fever and often pain, redness and swelling at the site of the tumour (p130). Invariably, old injuries or tissue that had been previously damaged through infectious or chemical assault, were re-visited with similar symptoms to the original injury which resolved after a relatively short period of time. These flare-ups would repeat at longer intervals with less intensity as the healing progressed. During these periods Dr. Gerson would also notice increased elimination of sodium and toxins. Old poisons/drugs would enter the circulation, and the symptoms, as they were leaving the system, would mimic the original effects that they had in the first instance.

It was a practice at that time, in the treatment of cancer, to deliberately and repeatedly invoke fevers. It had been observed during the 18th and 19th centuries that cancer patients often went into remission following a serious infectious illness such as tuberculosis, malaria and syphilis.  So the logic behind such an approach was valid; some physicians tried to induce a disease, but by the end of the 19th century  a search was on for a serum which would, without adverse side-effects, put the patient in a state of fever. It was William Coley who came up with the famous Coley's toxins (p128). Dr. Coley used the non-infectious by-products (toxins) of live germs (namely those originating from the Streptococcus Pyogenes and Serratia Marcescens). Coley's initial success was good; however, as time went on, the treatment proved less effective. [7] Others partially succeeded in producing a sufficient defence reaction through inoculating cancerous tissue or extracts from cancer tissues but no cure was obtained, only temporary improvement (pp 43, 127). Dr. Gerson was open to this line of development and he states, "It may be advisable to stimulate, in addition to my treatment, the liberated visceral nervous system and reticulo-endothelial apparatus with a measured bacterial reagens" (p129).

However, where Dr. Gerson differed in his approach was, as always, through his concept of totality. He saw the cause of cancer to be the accumulation of numerous damaging factors and that, therefore, no single therapeutic approach would effect cure, but a combined approach could. Today, as back in the mid 1900s, the same difficulties beset researchers trying to prove the therapeutic effect of a single treatment. This is no more so than in the field of immunology and the situation has not changed over the last seventy years. While researchers focussed on single factors or treatments to stimulate an inflammatory reaction, Dr. Gerson, understood, through his own observations that the determining factor of any therapy would depend upon the "energy-capacity of the healing apparatus" for any given patient. It was already widely established that cancer patients were "anergic" (unable to produce an inflammatory reaction) to a greater or lesser degree. Dr. Gerson believed, from his observations, that the "anergia" increased, the more advanced the disease became. In advanced cases, the differential count for lymphocytes often fell below 10% (p124-125), which, as Dr. Gerson points out, indicated that the body was no longer capable of producing the necessary amount of lymphocytes for defence and healing. We now know that when the ratio reaches this level, that it reflects rapid tumoural progression with no hope of cure. However, Dr. Gerson observed that when patients were detoxified the inflammatory response was restored, or in other words, the energy-capacity of the healing apparatus was increased. "It therefore appears that the body's capacity to produce an allergic inflammation (healing power) depends on a most complete detoxication and an equilibrium in the metabolism to near normal" (pp128-129, 197). He attributed the failure in experimental research to solve the cancer problem to the fragmented scientific approach, which made the development of any systematic therapeutic treatment impossible. He further states, "In my opinion, primarily because comprehension of the detoxication has always been overlooked in clinics, we are not sufficiently trained in that direction" (p124), and later, "We do know that a healing apparatus is present and functions in a healthy body - and we learned, in addition, by means of this treatment that it can be reactivated if the body can be sufficiently detoxified (in degenerative diseases and cancer)." (p131).

Dr. Gerson maintained it was essential that the body was brought to a natural healing inflammation; that the vitality of the body had to be raised (through detoxification, remineralisation and increasing oxidative capacity) to a spontaneous inflammation. He states, "It is not enough to introduce a temporary inflammation into the body. The body itself must be able to do it and do it continuously, because many cancer cells remain hidden in some areas where even the bloodstream cannot reach them. In order to maintain this healing process, it is, of course, necessary to apply the treatment for long enough to restore all vital organs to normal function to reproduce the same reactive processes as used by the body itself, for healing purposes" (p125). Dr. Gerson knew that the prognosis was better if the patient had a healing inflammation (healing crisis/flare-up) which is a nonspecific healing inducing inflammation, a structural response to an immune process which would not only devour the tumour but also rebuild the tissues. To his mind this enabled cure and to merely induce an artificial fever while neglecting the fundamental cause of the disease was of no long-term benefit.

Currently, immunotherapy, as part of a treatment for cancer, is gaining ground in many scientific circles. The work of Thomas Tallberg, MD (Helsinki University Central Hospital) using metabolic, hormonal and immunological therapy has had some good results in improving the disease-free interval in some patients. [8] Part of the treatment involves autologous vaccination of the patient every 4-6 weeks (an autologous vaccine is prepared from the patient's own tumour tissue using polymerised tumour marker antigens admixed with tuberculin PPD - a harmless adjuvant) and/ or repeated vaccinations against influenza A and B strains. However, it is necessary to keep giving vaccinations in order to control the cancer and this method is not seen as a cure.

The role of inflammation is critical to the treatment and cure of cancer. Cells in an inflammatory exudate have aerobic glycolysis greater than normal blood leucocytes. Malignant tissue is killed fast as the inflammatory exudate inhibits glycolysis in the cancer cell (pp43, 120, 121, 127, 129). The inflammatory process also produces TNF (tumour necrosis factor), which acts to inhibit capillaries' growth into the tumour. The fever that accompanies the immune response not only amplifies the lymphocyte response and mobilisation of white blood cells, but also is thought to have a damaging effect on cancer cells.

However, there is no evidence to support the idea that hyperthermia, on its own, can control cancer. Less than 1 in 100 human cancers are destroyed by temperatures above 41.8C (the maximum tolerance temperature of the human liver). The cytoplasm of certain tumour cells is only "poached" by hyperthermia (at 39°C) and dies at 46°-47°C. It has been found that many cancer cells are actually stimulated and grow faster with hyperthermia as a sole treatment.

As a side note on infectious illness in the immune deficient patient - the condition of these patients, if they have an infection, will worsen, as tumoural growth will be accelerated as the cancer metabolism can hijack inflammatory chemicals for its own growth. Dr. Gerson was particularly vigilant in the adequate control of infection in the cancer patient during the first nine months of the therapy, as he found that the cancer patient had little or no resistance to infection at the beginning of treatment (p122). It took at least nine months, on the therapy, to build a stronger immunity. Therefore it is imperative to deal with any infectious illness appropriately, using antibiotics if necessary. As with a newborn baby, the cancer patient is advised not to have anyone visiting who has a cold or is harbouring an infection. The disease inflammation (either from infectious illness or from tumoural activity) is not the same as the healing inflammation and will impede the healing inflammation, so an infectious illness needs to be dealt with immediately and appropriately.

# Protein and the immune profile

In the 1930's Dr. Gerson observed through laboratory findings that his tuberculosis (TB) patients following a restricted protein diet would have an increased white T-cell count; in other words the branch of the immune system that fights tumours, viruses and TB was showing increased activity. So restricted protein became an integral part of the therapy. Since then the work of several scientists have validated Dr. Gerson's clinical observations:

- protein and calorie restriction affects the T-cell branch of the immune system positively
- serum blocking antibody is reduced (humoral immunity), which enables more efficient destruction of the tumour by the T cells.

**Dr. Robert Good** discovered that malnourished children had a disturbed immune profile.[9] He went on to experiment to find which dietary deficiency produced this. In animals he noted that the T-lymphocyte activity increased and remained aggressive for a long time; he noted that mice predisposed to genetically determined diseases (mouse NZB - SLE), on a protein and calorie reduced diet that was implemented at weaning, did not manifest the disease; if the disease was allowed to develop it could be caused to regress by initiating protein and calorie restriction. He reproduced his findings with mice predisposed to mammary tumours, and those on a protein and calorie restricted diet did not go on to develop tumours. Similarly tumour regression was caused by initiating these dietary restrictions. This has very important ramifications for any dietary-based healing therapy. It has been found that this type of nutritional program is particularly successful in the treatment of autoimmune disease. Very often patients suffering from an autoimmune disorder are found to be immune-compromised, although current medical treatments are aimed at suppressing an "over-active" immune system with corticosteroid therapy.

Current research has shown that on protein restriction T-cell immunity is raised, serum immunity is stable, but serum-blocking antibody is depressed (humoral immunity). In cancer, tumour-specific antibody is produced by B-cells which attaches to the antigenic sites on the tumour cells, in effect covering the antigenic sites. This prevents the T-cell from having access to the tumour and destroying it. However, when serum blocking anti-body production is depressed, the tumour is then exposed to T-cell activity and destruction.[10]

It is advisable to restrict protein during the first 6 - 12 weeks of a detoxification therapy. However, if protein restriction is continued for too long, then T-cell activity becomes compromised also. The introduction of sufficient amounts of cultured non-fat milk protein into the diet will keep the immune system intact. Studies undertaken in 1973 (Cancer Research program) showed that animals fed limited amounts of milk protein (casein) kept them with an intact T-cell activity while at the same time depressing humoral antibody activity. This was sufficient to keep the immune system intact.

## Further comments on protein and fat restriction

### Protein restriction

The work of Thomas Tallberg[8] also pinpointed specific amino acids as growth factors for tumours. He has identified methionine in leukaemia; alanine in prostate cancer; arginine in colon and ovarian cancer. He also maintains that deficiencies of other specific amino acids complexed to trace element salts in biologically active ionic form is one of the nutritional causes of cancer. Tallberg recommends that a protein restricted diet should be followed during the initial phase of his therapy where the tumours are deprived of certain simple dietary growth factors, until the biological deficiencies are made good. He also recommends, as a way forward, the genetic modification of foods by non-pathogenic bacteria to induce them to consume these deleterious growth factors.

Cancer cells forage and compete for nutrients and they are greedy for protein: protein feeds tumours, and as they grow they produce greater toxic waste from the protein which seeps into the surrounding environment, causing local trauma (toxicity) to the surrounding healthy tissue. The oedema increases around the tumour "protecting" it from the immune system. By restricting protein, the tumour loses its defence and can be attacked by the immune system. Dr. Gerson found that patients with higher protein intake could not be saved and in some cases protein led to quicker cancer growth or metastases (p146). The combined protein restriction, high potassium/low sodium regime removed the sodium ring (oedema) from the tumour, improving circulation and immune activity at the site.

### Fat restriction

Dr. Gerson found that tumours came back when fat was introduced into the diet, even a low fat yoghurt. However, flaxseed oil had only beneficial effects. In addition to those discussed, as the cells regenerate the essential fatty acids derived from flaxseed oil will replace saturated fats and cholesterol in the cell wall which will lead to a reduction in cholesterol deposits. Cholesterol readings may rise in the initial phases of detoxification, but this is likely associated with the increase in triglycerides which can occur on a high vegetable juice intake.

# Pancreatic enzymes

Our understanding of the role of pancreatic enzymes in modulating, regulating and increasing the efficacy of the immune system has grown since the 1950s. Dr. Gerson was ambivalent towards the use of pancreatic enzymes in cancer, largely due to the disappointing results obtained by Beard et al (pp 211-212) and he indicated that they were largely ineffective in digestive disorders, but did appear to have some value in alleviating gas spasms and appeared to help with improving weight and stamina. Dr. Gerson applied pancreatin *after* the detoxification part of the program, to be taken with meals. However, new studies over the last forty years have shed light on the potential role of a combination of plant and animal enzymes in chronic inflammatory disease and cancer, and more recently through the work of Dr. Nicholas Gonzalez who developed his cancer program based on the work of Beard and then later Dr. William Donald Kelley.[11]

## A brief history

### Early 1900s

### John Beard: The trophoblast theory

In 1902, Professor Beard (Professor of Embryology at the University of Scotland) explored the therapeutic value of pancreatic enzymes in cancer. He put forward his trophoblast thesis of cancer where he stated that the cancer cell shared histological and behavioural characteristics with the pregnancy trophoblast, and that cancer was, in short, trophoblastic. The trophoblast is one of the most primitive embryonic cells, which gives rise to the placenta. It is capable of rapid mitosis, and has invasive, erosive and metastasizing properties which mediate the parasitization of the uterus with a new life form. Beard confirmed that the pancreatic enzymes, amylase, trypsin and chymotrypsin are especially important in trophoblast destruction. Around the 8th week of pregnancy the foetal trophoblast cells stop dividing and are destroyed. It is around the same time that the foetal pancreas starts functioning. He maintained, through conclusive studies, that the enzymes released from the foetal pancreas (namely trypsin and chymotrypsin) digest the outer coat of the trophoblast, which exposes it to parenteral digestion by the cells of the immune system. Maternal pancreatic amylase (the foetal pancreas does not produce amylase) was also found to be a factor in the destruction of the trophoblast. Dr. Beard logically concluded that these enzymes would act against cancer as well.

Shortly after Dr. Beard advanced his theory, scientists started experimenting with pancreatic enzymes in the treatment of cancer, with favourable results. It was found that the best results obtained were those which included the administration of both chymotrypsin and amylase. It was also recognized that both the trophoblast and cancer cell were able to protect themselves against the pancreatic enzymes, through their production of specific antitryptic substances (or those that oppose trypsin). Successful treatment required quantities of the enzymes in sufficient amounts to overcome the inhibitory effects of the antitryptic substances. Various researchers have supported this. "In 1949 West and Hilliard, in the study of sera of over 3,000 cancer patients, reported the specific antithesis of the malignant cell to chymotrypsin by showing that 15 grams of crystalline chymotrypsin would be necessary, in a single dose, to neutralize all of the *average excess of* chymotrypsin inhibitor in the serum of the advanced cancer patient." [12]

There have been many eminent supporters for Beard's theory over the last century. Dr Krebs Sr. (of the Kreb's or Citric Acid cycle), in 1952 upheld the theory as being "the only explanation which finds total congruence with all established facts on cancer." Both he and his son, Dr. Krebs Jr., confirmed hundreds of products and functions shared exclusively by the trophoblast and cancer, including hormone expression, enzymes and other products of gene activity, none of which are expressed by the somatic cells.

The evidence for a shared fundamental genetic identity between cancers of all types and trophoblasts was growing. In the 1940s, Howard Beard (no relation to John Beard) developed techniques focusing on hCG (human chorionic gonadotrophin), which was found in all cancer sera. hCG is produced by both the trophoblast and cancer cell, and is found as a perfusing and membrane bound expression in cancer.[13]

As recently as 1995, the report of a study undertaken at Allegheny Medical College in Pittsburgh by Drs Acevedo, Tong and Hartsock, involving the genetic characteristics of human chorionic gonadotrophin hormone, provided the first quantitative genetic analysis that confirmed that all cancers, regardless of type or origin, expressed hCG. [14] Furthermore, there is shown to be a correlation between the degree of malignancy and the amount of hCG detected. The less differentiated the cell (greatest malignancy), the more hCG produced. This is why hCG can be used as an indicator of tumour progression in many cancers.

We now know that hCG is the potent enzyme inhibitor, or the antitryptic substance. In the embryo hCG protects against the digestion of the uterine tissues which would normally occur around menstruation, but in cancer this hormone inhibits enzymatic digestion of the cancer cells. Cancer cells can resist immunological detection through the dual activity of hCG: hCG can act as a screen to hide the antigenic sites from immune recognition and it can also inhibit trypsin activity.

hCG is a glycoprotein; the protein moiety is embedded in the cell membrane, while specific sugar side chains (sialic acid) provide an outer, negatively charged coating, which bends over and masks the membrane bound proteins. [14] This renders the cancer cell immunologically invisible as the protein part, which allows immunological detection, is hidden. Enzymatic digestion of these sugars by amylase would expose the antigenic sites (proteins) for digestion by trypsin, but the high quantity of hCG found in cancer sera inhibits trypsin activity. However, in the presence of sufficient amylase, or with factors that reactivate and accelerate the activity of the inhibited enzymes (laetrile is one such factor) the sugar coating is digested and, once unmasked, the plasma proteases may attack the membrane bound proteins to which they are specific. Once the proteases attack, then the contact immune cells, the killer T-cells and helper cells, along with other components, are activated. This constitutes parenteral digestion.

Parenteral digestion of cancer is therefore dependent upon a sequence of events:
- The unmasking of its antigenic sites through the enzymatic digestion of fibrin and mucin and hCG by the carbohydrate digesting enzymes (amylase) and the proteinases (trypsin and chymotrypsin). The activity of enzymes within the circulation are fundamental to this initial phase.
- Once the antigenic protein sites are unmasked, they undergo further enzymatic digestion (trypsin and chymotrypsin).
- Normal cellular immune components (contact immune cells such as the T-cells, killer cells and helper cells) are potentiated by this prior attack, and enzymatic destruction of the cancer cells occurs.

### 1930 - 1960s
### Ernst Freund and Gisa Kaminer: Blocking factor theory
In 1932 Freund and Kaminer (Vienna) "found that tumour cells kept *in vitro* broke down when the serum of healthy blood donors was added to a culture medium of the cancer cells. In contrast, the serum of cancer patients proved to be oncocytologically inactive. Freund assumed that this lack of reaction was due to an inhibitory agent present in the blood of individuals suffering from cancer. Other researches, the Hellstrom siblings, suspected that immunosuppressive immune complexes were responsible for the action of these "blocking factors". [15]

### Max Wolf and Helene Benitez: Birth of the WoBe enzymes
Following the research undertaken by Freund and Kaminer and later Adolf Gaschler's published results (1955) of the effects of enzyme therapy (trypsin) in cancer and inflammatory disease, Max Wolf and Helene Benitez carried out thousands of tests and isolated the enzymes with therapeutic activity, namely papain, trypsin and chymotrypsin. They discovered through *in vitro* experiments that these blocking factors could be eliminated through the administration of small amounts of chymotrypsin or plasmin. These findings compelled him to test such enzymes under *in vivo* conditions for the treatment of malignant tumours. They developed two enzyme combinations for the treatment of inflammation and degenerative disease which were called "Wolf-Benitez-Enzyme combinations" later shortened to *Wobenzym*.

### Registration of WoBe
In 1959 the WoBe enzymes were registered as pharmaceutical product in Spain (1959) and in Germany (1960). Later, in 1963, Karl Ransberger, CEO of the Munich enterprise Mucos, won approval for another WoBe–enzyme combination, later called Wobe Mucos E, for the treatment of cancer and metastasis prophylaxis. The studies that Wolf and Ransberger conducted demonstrated that a combination of vegetable and animal enzymes is substantially more effective than the use of individual enzymes.

Numerous studies in cancer patients have been conducted in Germany and Eastern Europe from the 1960s with favourable results using enzyme therapy (WobeMugos) in combination with conventional treatment and other complementary treatments. Studies demonstrated that many of the side effects of the primary therapy (chemotherapy and radiotherapy) were reduced, including limiting the degree of early damage induced by radiation and hindering the later damage, such as fibrosis and scar formation. There was also an increased regeneration of healthy tissue and a greater resistance against metastasis, and in chemotherapy there was a reduction in adverse effects, reduction in pain, faster recovery and weight gain. Generally the studies confirmed improvements in patients' general state of health and a reduction in the amount of medications and length of hospitalizations normally required to manage adverse events related to conventional treatment or the disease itself.

However, In 2005 WOBE-MUCOS E was taken off the market due to legal formalities and not for reasons of quality or effectiveness. Since then we have to source enzyme combinations within the proven therapeutic range, of which there are a few brands that contain both the plant enzyme papain, and the animal enzymes trypsin and chymotrypsin. The application of these enzymes are used in complementary cancer treatments around the world, not only for their role in reducing inflammation and oedemas, speeding the healing process and reducing metastatic potential, but also as an adjunct to chemotherapy as studies have also shown that enzymes increase the concentration of chemotherapy agents within the tumoural tissue, which increases the effectiveness of treatment.

## Immune suppression and blocking factors explained

Inflammatory chemicals, also known as cytokines, including tumour necrosis factor (TNF), interleukins (IL-6, IL-2, IL-1ß), interferons (INF), have the express task of stimulating and amplifying the immune response; they activate immune cells, such as macrophages, monocytes and natural killer cells to migrate to the area of insult, and to communicate with each other and establish an attack on either pathogens or diseased and damaged tissue. It is a complex set of events which causes a host of side effects, such as tissue oedema, the formation of fibrin and a shift of the metabolism towards thrombosis (blood clotting). When the immune system becomes dysregulated, through chronic and persistent inflammation, as seen in cancer and autoimmune diseases, it can start to work against the host, and in malignancy immune cells can be recruited by the cancer (tumour-associated macrophages or TAMs) and start to work on behalf of the cancer increasing its own cytokine production, fibrin formation, angiogenesis, and its metastatic potential.

Inflammatory cytokines cause changes at the surface of immune cells, the endothelium of blood vessels and cancer cells. These changes include the expression of adhesion molecules at the surface of these cells, and depending on the family of molecules expressed, they will exhibit different functions. As the name suggests, they cause a binding of one cell to another.

There are four main groups of adhesion molecules: the integrins, the selectins, the immunoglobulins and the cartilage link proteins and they can work both for and against the host. In metastasis, for example, the selectins enable the cancer cell to start rolling along the blood vessel wall, the integrins and immunoglobulins allow it to adhere to the blood vessel wall, and the integrins and cartilage link proteins allow it to migrate through the wall into the tissues and set up home. In mounting an immune attack both the immunoglobulins and the integrins support antigen presentation, activation of T lymphocytes and facilitation of communication between the T-cells and B-cells. In addition the immunoglobulins are responsible for antigen/antibody binding (formation of immune complexes) and the integrins stimulate phagocytosis.

Many people believe that the immune system is deficient in cancer, but it is probably more true to say that it becomes paralyzed. Cancer cells foil the immune system by shedding their antigens (also known as tumour markers, such as carbohydrate antigens CA 19-9 or CA 15-3) and shedding their receptors. The antigens are picked up by the immune system and form immune complexes, and the receptors (such as TNF receptors) are picked up by the cytokines (such as TNF) to form cytokine polymers. The shedding of antigens and receptors creates a problem for the immune system, for in order for the cancer cell to be recognized as such and destroyed, the antigens and receptors must be attached to the cancer cell itself. Therefore with this shedding the cancer cell can avoid detection and destruction.

The situation can progressively worsen as an increase in immune complexes and cytokine polymers (blocking factors) in the circulation will suppress macrophage, NK cell and cytotoxic T cell activity. The larger the tumoural mass, the higher the inflammatory activity and the shedding of receptors and antigens, and the more compromised the immune system becomes.

One can appreciate that if you could either reduce the inflammation or down-regulate the cytokines that stimulate the over-expression of adhesion molecules you could make an impact on the growth and metastasis of the cancer, and if you could increase the clearance of immune complexes and cytokine polymers you could reactivate the immune system.

This is where enzyme therapy come in. Through the years of research scientists have been able to determine the activities of these enzymes. In cancer, the application of both animal and plant enzymes are required for their diverse actions. Of the animal enzymes, chymotrypsin is the most valuable as it down-regulates the integrins (MAC and vitronectin) and selectins (MEL) and significantly reduces the potential for metastasis; while  trypsin is important in down-regulating immunoglobulins (ICAM) which reduces immune complex formation and the potential for metastases. The plant enzymes, bromelain and papain down-regulate the cartilage link proteins, CD44, which reduce the potential for metastases into the tissues. Papain works with trypsin in down-regulating immune complex formation.

Trypsin:
- stimulates the clearance of inflammatory chemicals which, in turn, will down-regulate the expression of adhesion molecules;
- down-regulates immunoglobulin expression and hence immune complex formation and reduces the potential for metastasis;
- stimulates complement activation and macrophage phagocytosis of immune complexes;
- has anti-clotting/fibrinolytic activity; and
- increases tumour cell apoptosis

Chymoptrypsin:
- down-regulates expression of selectins and so reduces the potential for metastases;
- down-regulates expression of integrins which reduces the potential for metastasis;
- reduces the capacity for immune complex formation
- stimulates complement activation and macrophage phagocytosis of immune complexes;
- has anti-clotting/fibrinolytic activity; and
- increases tumour cell apoptosis

Papain
- down-regulates the cartilage link proteins which reduces the potential for metastasis;
- reduces the immune complex load by inhibiting antigen/antibody binding, digesting antibodies and stimulating phagocytosis of immune complexes
- has anti-clotting/fibrinolytic activity; and
- increases tumour cell apoptosis

Bromelain:

- down-regulates cartilage link proteins;
- has anti-inflammatory activity
- has anti-clotting/fibrinolytic activity; and
- increases tumour cell apoptosis

# Detoxification & the role of the liver

## The coffee enema

The capacity of the liver to detoxify is paramount to the success of any detoxification therapy. When the release of toxins into the blood circulation is stimulated, the liver must be able to take these up and detoxify them for elimination. A detoxification therapy, without facilitating the removal of toxins by the liver will accelerate the disease process, because the toxicity will not be removed and the liver will become more damaged. It is vital to keep the metabolism free of poison and to help the patient eliminate the poisonous substances, not least those from the tumour masses themselves. Dr. Gerson found that with some patients the therapy (without enemas) was accelerating the disease process and subsequently he lost a few patients in what he described as "hepatic coma" (pp123, 197, 198).

In cancer the liver is not only damaged but also toxic. It is also an organ that is fully restorable. Dr. Gerson maintained that when the liver is fully restorable, then the patient survives. Dr. Gerson was quick to recognise that patients with cancer carry a greater toxic burden than other patients and that the liver was more compromised, as tumour tissue perpetually creates toxins, and the larger the tumoural mass the more toxins produced. He stated that in chronic disease the liver was damaged, but in malignancy it was toxic. Therefore he had to find a way to manage this situation without compromising the speed of toxic removal from the tissues.

In the 1930s Dr. Gerson was aware of experiments at the Göettingen University, undertaken by Heubner and Meyer, on the rectal administration of caffeine in animals, which indicated dilatation of the bile ducts and increased flow of bile for elimination. Excretion of toxicity from the liver is governed by bile production and flow. Toxins are conjugated in the liver with bile, which enables its safe elimination. Dr. Gerson proceeded to add the coffee enema to the regime, to support toxic elimination by the liver, and as a consequence he found that his patients could then tolerate the vigorous cleansing. The coffee enema was applied more frequently at times of flare-up and when the body was resorbing malignancies (necrotic tissue in the blood stream). The literature at that time also advocated the role of coffee enemas for pain reduction and it has been found that they do relieve pain in up to 90% of patients, as well as depression, confusion and nervous tension. Pain is often caused by circulating toxins irritating the nervous system. These toxins can also set up an inflammatory response, but through their detoxification and removal from the blood stream this inflammatory cycle is curbed.

In the 1970s to 1990s further research by Wattenberg and later Lechner [16] identified in experiments that the palmitates extracted from coffee increased the glutathione S transferase system - an enzyme system responsible for detoxifying carcinogens and free radicals in the liver and small intestine. Its activity was increased 600% in the liver and 700% in the small intestine. This is critical for the removal of serum toxins and to facilitate the removal of toxic cancer breakdown products (ammonia, toxin bound nitrogen, both protein derivatives).

1. Caffeine, theobromine and theophylline dilate bile ducts and works as a choleretic to cause increased bile flow (also counteract inflammation in the gut).

2.  Palmitates increase glutathione-S-transferase. This increases the conjugation of toxic elements with bile for elimination. Bile is normally reabsorbed 9-10 times before making its way out via the colon. However, the enzyme enhancing ability of the coffee in the liver and small intestine reduces the reabsorption of the toxic bile. Most choleretic agents do not ensure removal of toxins, they only increase the bile flow.
3.  The litre of fluid dilutes the portal blood and the bile, stimulating a flushing. It also encourages peristalsis, which ensures the transit of toxic bile from the duodenum to the outside.
4.  The retention of the coffee enema for 15 minutes ensures the cleansing of the blood five times. The entire blood circulation passes through the liver every three minutes.

The studies undertaken by Lechner reported the observed effects on cancer patients following traditional treatment (chemotherapy, radiotherapy etc.) in conjunction with a dietary regime which involved lacto-vegetarian foods, the strictest reduction of salt, juices and *the addition of coffee enemas* showed that this group were in a better general condition with less risk of complications and also tolerated radiation and chemotherapy better than those who did not do the program. It was found that the coffee enema played a key role in exerting a liver protective effect against the chemotherapy, due to its activation of enzymes (glutathione-S-transferase) within the liver and the rapid clearance of free radicals. It was further recommended that "The continuations of these investigations is beyond our scope and should be reserved for the pharmaceutical industry, together with a possible clinical test. As long as the substances under discussion, which, in our view could make a highly effective drug for protecting the liver, are not produced industrially and no relevant studies are planned, we have to continue administering them in the awkward form of enemas." [16]

Dr. Gerson added the raw liver, juiced, for the explicit reason of restoring the liver in patients where he felt that the liver was too compromised. We now understand that although the coffee enemas can facilitate one of the detoxification pathways, it will have little impact on the other five pathways which are involved in the detoxification of an entire range of toxins.[17] So although the coffee enema can play a vital role in damage limitation or risk mitigation (as in chemotherapy), it will not rebuild the liver; for this, Dr. Gerson determined that we needed an increased quota of nutrients that could be supplied by the raw liver.

Dr. Gerson was very astute in recognising the capacity of the liver in individual patients. Whether this was intuition or based upon observation of symptoms/past case history I cannot say, other than that his expertise often led to accurate prognoses. In many cases you will observe that the initial response of patients to the therapy is good, but it is often after 2-3 months that clinical symptoms will indicate to you whether the liver and/or other vital organs are too damaged to be sufficiently reactivated to maintain the healing process (p33). The killing of tumour mass, its dissolution and absorption is a very heavy burden on the eliminative organs. It is essential that you keep the metabolism free of poison. Sadly it is the poisoning of the liver from tumour tissue which becomes the underlying cause of liver disease in later stages, and I have witnessed this a few times. (p69)

Since Dr. Gerson's time many more patients are coming to the therapy with metastases after the original cancer was treated with chemotherapy. These patients are carrying an additional toxic load, their immune systems are more compromised and their liver is very damaged. It is not possible to put these patients on a the very intensive program, unlike patients who have not received chemotherapy, as the risk of an onslaught on the liver of too great a quantity of powerful toxins will compromise the patients and their condition will worsen. Additionally, in severe liver damage (liver disease, chemotherapy) you cannot afford to stimulate the liver too much with the enemas and must use a reduced juice/medication protocol so as not to place a heavy burden on the liver and weaken it further.

# The castor oil treatment

In spite of an average of five coffee enemas daily, it was found by Dr. Gerson that the cancer patient needed additional help for the liver during the initial stages. The body was so toxic and, certainly within the first month with the high doses of potassium, Lugol's and thyroid, the pressure on the system to release toxicity was great. Dr. Gerson found that by introducing the castor oil treatment he was able to fulfil the requirements for adequate elimination.

Castor oil is not metabolised/absorbed in the gut, but when taken orally will create a huge stimulus to the liver to release large quantities of bile (in the case of the cancer patient, toxic bile). Castor oil by mouth effectively exploits the role of the bile in fat digestion and it has a far greater stimulatory effect on the bile system than the coffee enema. Once the toxic bile is released, it binds with the castor oil. As the oil is not digested and absorbed, it traps the toxins inhibiting the re-circulation of both the toxins and bile acids back to the liver. Consequently toxins are removed from the body more effectively with the castor oil treatment. We must not forget that we are not just getting rid of toxins from the liver, we have to remove them from the body. Under normal circumstances a proportion of the toxic bile is reabsorbed in the small intestine, but the binding capacity of the castor oil inhibits this. The strength of the castor oil treatment in removing toxicity has been well documented, as it is on the castor oil days that you are more likely to smell toxic fumes that are released with the enemas. In patients who have had a lot of chemical exposure, the castor oil treatment becomes essential, providing that the liver is strong enough to cope with this treatment.

The castor oil treatment is an extremely aggressive treatment affecting the liver and is contra-indicated for the patient who has a weakened liver (chemotherapy, hepatitis, liver disease) or ulcers anywhere along the digestive tract.

# Liver juice, crude liver extract injections & ox bile powder

## Liver juice

The liver juice was added to the therapy in 1949 when Dr. Gerson noticed a drop in his success rate. He investigated the mineral content of the main groups of vegetables he was using (tomatoes, potatoes, carrots) and found a deteriorating nutritional value. He also felt that the increase in toxic chemicals, namely DDT, was responsible for the poorer healing capacity experienced by his patients. (p220)

The liver juice was obtained from fresh (not frozen) calves liver, from animals no older than 48 - 60 hours and the liver no greater than 4 lbs in weight. It was used in 3 juices a day (carrot and liver juice) and approximately 250g of raw liver would be used for each juice. The living enzymes and nutrients were used to replenish the sick liver which could not build and activate these substances for itself.  It was found that the therapy was more successful with the inclusion of the liver juice.  However, nowadays there is substantial risk of cross contamination in the abattoir of the camphylobacter (found not in the liver but in the digestive tract of the cow), and it can prove fatal for patients with a compromised immune system.  The livers can be sterilized by dipping in hot water (80°C) for 10 seconds and then packed in ice and couriered to the patient. This has to be done at the abattoir and there appears to be a logistic problem on two counts: the first is setting up the facility to do this, and secondly, most of the calves that come into the abattoir are not divided into organic/non-organic. If these difficulties could be surmounted then it would be possible to re-introduce the raw liver into the regime.

We are now living in an age of severe exposure to environmental toxins. Dr. Gerson blamed toxic chemicals as a major factor in the poisoning of the liver, compromising detoxification and making the liver more difficult to restore. He knew that the success of his therapy lay in the restoration of the liver. We are now in a position to confirm Dr. Gerson's intuitive insight.

Modern research in molecular toxicology has made the startling discovery that the determining factor leading to health problems associated with low-dose chemical exposure is dependent on the genetics and biochemistry of the exposed individual. "In particular, it depends on the *capacity of their [liver] detoxification pathways* and antioxidant protective systems, among others, to prevent such harm. Inadequate nutrition, stress, infection and genetic susceptibility are now implicated as secondary factors in increased health risks from toxic agents." Dr. Mark Donohoe. Emphasis mine). See also Dr. Mark Donohoe's article on The Human Liver. [18]

Additional studies have linked certain defects in the liver's detoxification capacity with diseases of the brain, namely Parkinson's and Alzheimer's diseases. Exposure to occupational toxins is a known co-factor in those suffering from Parkinson's disease, but a recent study carried out at the University of Birmingham Medical School in 1991, has indicated that individuals with compromised liver detoxification ability are more prone to developing these diseases. [19, 20] This research by Williams, Steventon and colleagues identified significant variation in detoxification metabolism amongst patients with Parkinson's disease, Alzheimer's disease and motor neurone disease. They commented, "The possibility exists that the ability to cope safely with endogenous and exogenous substances which have neurotoxic properties is important in the pathogenesis of these diseases. Potentially such individuals could be identified pre-clinically and these diseases postponed by reduction in the load of toxin or modification of the relevant enzymatic activity."[20] It is proposed that deficiencies in the liver's detoxification capacity are the result of genetic variance.

Recent studies have also indicated a relationship between cow's milk protein and schizophrenia, autism, insulin dependent diabetes and heart disease. The milk protein in question is A1 beta casein, found in milk specifically from Friesian cows. This milk protein is resistant to complete digestion and leaves a peptide called beta-casomorphine which is absorbed into the system. This peptide has been found to have immunomodulatory properties, and it is suggested that early exposure to cow's milk in youngsters genetically predisposed to insulin dependent diabetes can be one environmental factor which triggers the autoimmune response. This same peptide is taken up by areas of the brain known to be involved in autism and schizophrenia. The preliminary findings of a study by University of Florida physiologist, Dr. Robert Cade,[21] showed that 95% of 81 autistic children had 100 times the normal levels of the milk protein in their blood and urine. When these children went on a milk-free diet, 80% no longer showed symptoms of autism or schizophrenia. He suggests that an intestinal flaw, such as a malfunctioning enzyme, is the cause. However, many potential allergens enter the systemic circulation on a daily basis. These are normally detoxified by a healthy liver. If there is any deficiency in the liver's detoxification system, then a build-up of certain toxins or allergens is bound to occur.

It would appear that there is a strong role for the raw liver juice in the Gerson treatment as it reactivates detoxification pathways. However, serious caution should be applied when using the raw liver juice as the risk of camphylobacter contamination for the cancer patient can be life-threatening.

The role of the liver is central to the nutritional healing and detoxification. As the body becomes more toxic, so the liver becomes more damaged, adversely affecting the genetic inheritance with a rising incidence of chronic degenerative disease in ever younger age groups. We are also witnessing an increase in mental disease throughout the generations, with dementia now the fourth leading cause of death in the western world. In simple terms, if the liver cannot detoxify endogenous or exogenous toxins, whether they are from the food we eat or exposure to environmental chemicals, then a toxic residue accumulates in the system which gives rise to a spectrum of diseases determined by the individual's genetic predisposition. The weaker the genetic line, the more chronic the disease.

**GM foods**

Since the mid 1990s, with the introduction of GM foods, the incidence of chronic inflammatory disease of the gastrointestinal tract, including cancers of the stomach, pancreas and intestines, and a rise in multiple allergy syndromes, autoimmune conditions (including coeliac disease) and autism, is reaching epidemic proportions. These foods, and their derivatives (particularly soy, corn and sugar) are now endemic in the food chain, and in livestock raised on this food, particularly corn and soy.

GM crops are genetically modified to produce toxins that confer greater plant resistance to both insects and to survive the deadly doses of the herbicide, RoundUp. However, there is now sufficient scientific evidence that the residual toxins from RoundUp and the toxins produced by the GM plants (such as Bt-toxin, or specific lectins) are not inert in humans, and they induce the equivalent damage to human cells as they do in insects, by disrupting their membranes. From studies on animals fed on GM foods we can see what can best be described as a corrosive effect on the gut wall along with severe dysbiosis, defects in the liver and pancreas with a profound reduction in digestive enzyme production. Additional health risks that were identified are infertility and an increase in birth defects.

Glyphosate is a broad spectrum biocide, or a powerful antibiotic, that wipes out beneficial bacteria in favour of the more pathogenic strains that are now being blamed for the increase in botulism in cattle. In addition, Bt-toxin has been found in the circulation of those who eat GM foods and also in the foetus. That Bt-toxin persists, and its destructive effects are not limited to insects, is extremely worrying as we now know that the genes from a genetically modified food can be transferred into the DNA of our gut bacteria giving rise to a living pesticide factory within us, producing the toxin on a continual basis. It is not known by how much these ill-effects are due to the synergistic activity of both these groups of toxins (glyphosate and GM toxins), but what is understood is that the knock on effect of chronic inflammation in the gut leads to a permanent loading on the immune system and also a persistent suppressive effect on digestive enzyme responses (both from the pancreas and the liver) leading to malabsorption syndromes.

The primary cause of food-reactive symptoms or disease-states related to the toxic fractions of either proteins which enter the systemic circulation, or the toxins from GM foods or from our indigenous bowel flora, lies in the toxic food source itself. Whilst one could quibble over which diet is best, which food groups one should avoid, which bowel flora products or what range of digestive enzymes work the best, the truth is that if one continues to eat the contaminated food that is causing the problem, then one simply perpetuates the problem.

In the healthy system, the visceral or autonomic nervous system of the gut works in tandem; as one part of the digestive system activates, messages pass to start the activation of the next part of the process. Finally, the digestive enzymes liberated by the small intestinal mucosa complete the end-stage of digestion where foods are finally broken down into their single components. If the pancreatic function is suppressed or the small intestinal mucosa is inflamed or damaged then we will see incomplete digestion and the entry of food products into the portal circulation. If these cannot be cleared by the liver, then they will enter the systemic circulation and cause immune responses, which may include allergic and autoimmune reactions.

Chronic weakening of the entire body, including the digestive system, comes about through years of nutritional deficiency and accumulating toxicity. This weakness in the constitution is passed down through the generations, with each generation becoming successively weaker. When the digestive system fails to respond adequately, the body is unable to nourish itself, and toxic fractions of foods enter the system. The combination of systemic food antigens, which exacerbate an immunological response, in the presence of degenerate tissue, leads to the exacerbation of a pre-existing or inherited condition. While the removal of such potential antigens (proteins) from the diet, will result in regression, this as a treatment alone would be ineffective. The only recourse for restoring health is a diet capable of reversing the tissue damage syndrome; an organic diet, low in sodium, fat and protein, but high in nutrients that are easily assimilable. It is then that regeneration will start to occur.

### Crude Liver Extract Injections
These injections return some nutrients and enzymes, also minute quantities of hormones, to the body. They have been found to be essential in the healing process. (p211)

### Ox bile powder
This is used in the castor oil enema for the emulsification of the castor oil. Dr. Gerson also felt that it was of value if the bile system was damaged by adhesions or scarring. (p211) Lubile (defatted bile powder from young calves) was also used extensively by Dr. Gerson in cases where the liver was damaged and the bile system impaired. He stopped the use of Lubile shortly after he introduced the raw liver juice.

# The organic diet

*"Using organically grown foods brings both the discovered and undiscovered ones (nutrients) together in the proper quantity, mixture and composition" (Dr. Gerson).*

The case for organic produce is manifold:
- No toxic chemicals (insecticides and pesticides accumulate in the body, their oestrogenic activity not only affects fertility but also potentiates many of the hormone dependent cancers)
- Organically fertilized soil ensures that the uptake of minerals by the crop is optimally balanced. Synthetic fertilizers, such as NPK, forces plant growth, disturbs its metabolism and balance of nutrients leading to a high crop yield of a poor nutritional quality prone to disease. NPK also disturbs the Na/K balance in favour of Na)
- Replete with anti-oxidants and hydride ions (usually used up by the plant's self-defence on commercially grown crops). Hydride ions refuel enzyme systems.

The patient must be aware that organic produce does not necessarily mean good nutrient status. Farmers nowadays traditionally prefer monoculture (single crop) farming. It has been found that a monoculture system is not diverse enough to ensure good ecological balance and balanced nutrient delivery by the soil to that crop. Diversity ensures that the different plants access different minerals at the various levels that their roots reach into the soil. They will pull these nutrients to the surface, and when the land is mulched with the excess of the crop, then these nutrients become available to the vegetables whose roots scavenge the upper layers of soil strata. Hydroponic is not organic. It relies on force-feeding the plant through artificial means and deprives the plant of its selective mechanisms for absorbing specific nutrients. The nutrient content is unbalanced and leads to a poor quality food.

# Supplements

*"The system needs animating energies besides the pure substances"* *(p99)*

In detoxification we are looking to replenish the body through food. Nutrients are not well-absorbed when out of their colloidal state. The nutrients as found in natural foods have specific energetic blueprints or patterns, which enable absorption both at gut level and into the cell. They are able therefore to replenish the body. Supplements seem to have stimulant value only. Many patients may appear to improve on supplementation, only to deteriorate a few months later often with a progression of the disease. Dr. Gerson states, "Several times I observed that vitamins in good combinations, with or without minerals, produced a *regrowth* of cancer or new spreadings in a few days. The patient felt better for a shorter or longer period through what may be regarded as the stimulation of the entire metabolism. However, the cancer re-grew, caused by what some other authors explained as the greater attraction power of the cancerous tissue"(p210). It seems that it is only through replenishment that the body can heal. It is interesting to note that Dr. Gerson found that even with the wrong potassium combination he failed to get the expected results (p220).

The emphasis on the raw foods (live juices) is not only for the quantity of enzymes they contain but also for their mineral activity and their high antioxidant value. Dr. Gerson observed that patients had difficulty in healing if they consumed juices that were not taken freshly made, or prepared using a centrifugal machine. Obviously one loses the antioxidant potential which is of significant value in fighting cancer and neutralising the free radicals, but minerals are also incorporated into oxidizing enzyme systems and when these enzymes are destroyed, then mineral activity may alter. It may be debated that on a nutritional program for cancer we are looking to feed the healthy tissue, while starving the tumour tissue. We are looking at two separate metabolisms, the cancer metabolism and the healthy cell metabolism. Both are quite different. The cancer cell derives its energy through fermentation, the healthy cell, through oxidation. The cancer cell is greedy for nutrients, but whether it can readily accept nutrients that are delivered as part of actively oxidizing systems could be a topic of scientific interest. If this were the case, then taking nutrients in their living state could have the impact of feeding healthy tissues while starving tumour tissue.

Although the diet contains food that is cooked, in fact the bulk of the meals are cooked, and although cooking destroys enzyme systems, [18] the greater volume of the diet is raw but in juiced form. It is essential, from the digestive aspect of the cancer patient, that the diet is cooked as a totally raw diet will exacerbate digestive difficulties where the patient would fail to adequately nourish and heal. Cooked food is predigested in that cooking starts the breaking down of carbohydrate to glucose, and also breaks down the tough cell membranes increasing both the nutritional and energy value of the food. This is vital for the healing patient where maximum nutrition for minimum digestive output makes a significant impact on improving the capacity to heal.

Dr. Gerson was also concerned with the hereditary effects of nutritional deficiencies. It is interesting to note that certain inherited mineral deficiencies in animals could not be corrected in the next generation. For example, it took five to six generations to redress iron deficiencies. Iodine deficiency, however, was easily corrected in the offspring of the new generation (p181).

## Diagram 1

# Entry of fuels into the citric acid (Krebs) cycle

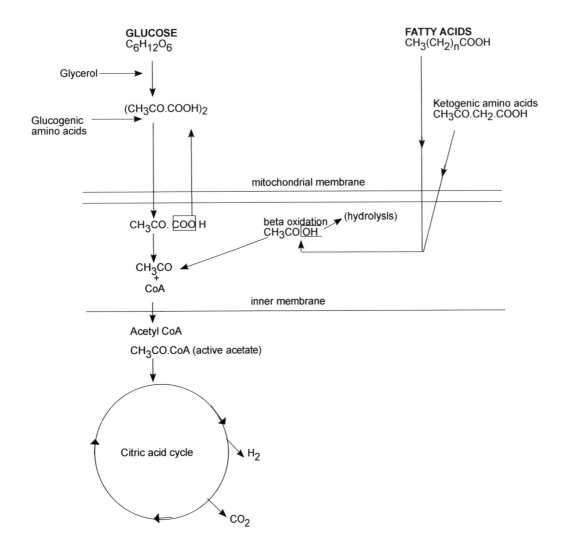

Glucose, fatty acids and amino acids do not pass into the citric acid cycle until they have been broken down into 2 carbon acetyl units. Then they pass across the inner mitochondrial membrane where they combine with acetyl CoA and enter the energy cycle.

**Diagram 2**

# The citric acid cycle (Krebs) and the formation of ATP

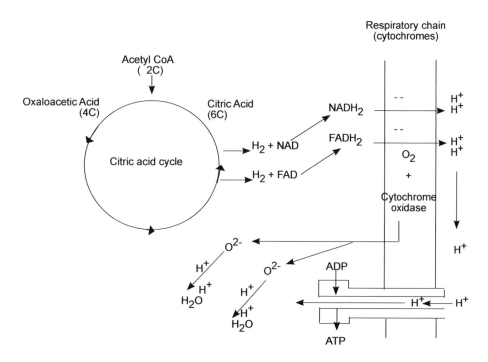

Hydrogen atoms are stripped off the carbon skeleton in the citric acid cycle. They are transported by NAD (B3 dependent) and FAD (B2 dependent) to the electron transport chain located on the inner mitochondrial membrane. Here H atoms off-load their electrons and the H ion (H$^+$) passes across the inner membrane to the space between the inner and outer mitochondrial membrane. The electrons are transported via a number of enzymes systems until they reach the enzyme cytochrome oxidase at the end of the chain. Cytochrome oxidase donates the electrons to oxygen (always hungry for electrons). Meanwhile H ions diffuse down their concentration gradient and back through the mitochondrial membrane, and in the process the energy generated is used to form ATP from ADP. The positively charged hydrogen ions then unite with the negatively charged oxygen ions to form water.

**Diagram 3**

# Metabolism of fuel substrates in the energy cycle

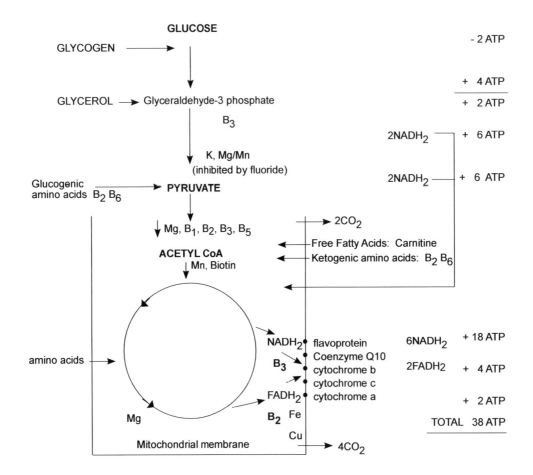

NADH$_2$ generated in the initial stages of glycolysis transports its hydrogen atoms to the electron transport chain in the inner mitochondrial membrane. This diagram indicates the essential nutrients involved in the production of energy. Fluoride is an inhibitor of the conversion of glucose to pyruvate prior to its entry into the citric acid cycle (Krebs cycle).

**Diagram 4**

## Anaerobic Glycolysis

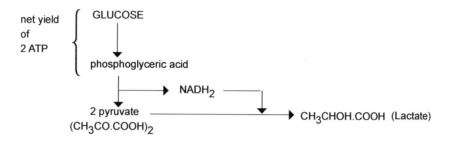

In the absence of oxygen the electron transport chain comes to a standstill. The hydrogen atoms are unable to be transported by NAD. Instead they are dumped onto pyruvic acid converting it to lactic acid where it is taken up by the liver and converted back to glucose through the Cori cycle.

## Aerobic Glycolysis

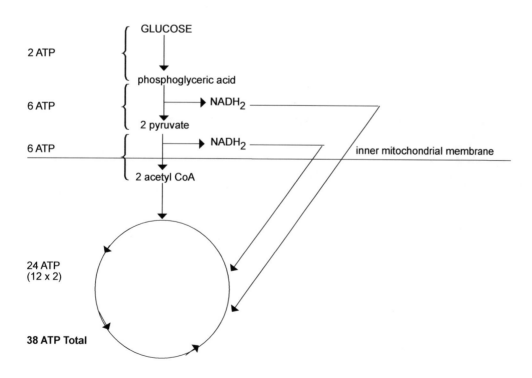

# References

1.  Dr. Patricia Spain Ward: *A History of the Gerson Therapy,*
    http://www.gerson-research.org/docs/WardPS-1988-1/index.html

2.  Cone, Clarence D. Jr.: *Unified theory on the Basic Mechanism of Normal Mitotic Control and Oncogenesis.* Journal of Theoretical Biology 30: 151-181, 1971

3.  Ling, Gilbert: *A Revolution in the Physiology of the Living Cell,* 1992. www.gilbertling.org/

4.  Cope, Freeman W., *A Medical Application of the Ling Association-Induction Hypothesis: The High Potassium, Low Sodium diet of the Gerson Cancer Therapy,* Physiological Chemistry and Physics 10: 456-467, 1978
    http://www.gerson-research.org/docs/CopeFW-1978-1/index.html

5.  Lockwood, K., et al: *Partial and complete regression of breast cancer in patients in relation to dosage of co-enzyme Q10.* Biochemical and Biophysical Research Communications, Vol. 199, 1994, pp. 1504-08

6.  Budwig, Johanna: *Flax Oil as a True Aid Against Arthritis, Heart Infarction, Cancer and Other Diseases,* 1992

7.  Hoption Cann, S. A., van Netten, J. P., van Netten, C; *Dr William Coley and tumour regression: a place in history or in the future;* Postgrad Med J 2003;79:672-680 http://pmj.bmj.com/content/79/938/672.full

8.  Tallberg, Thomas: *Cancer treatment, based on active nutritional biomodulation, hormonal therapy and specific autologous immunotherapy,* Journal of Australasian College of Nutrition & Environmental Medicine, Vol. 15 No 1, April 1996, pp 5-23.

9.  Good, Robert A., Fernandes, Gabriel, and Day, Noorbibi D., *The Influence of Nutrition on Development of Cancer Immunity and Resistance to Mesenchymal Diseases,* 1982, New York Raven Press, Molecular Interrelations of Nutrition and Cancer.

10. Evelyne Kirkwood and Catriona Lewis: *Understanding Medical Immunology;* 1989, pp 84-85: John Wiley and Sons

11. Gonzalez, N, M.D. *Enzyme Therapy and Cancer;* http://www.dr-gonzalez.com/history_of_treatment.htm

12. Krebs, Ernst T. Jr., Krebs, Ernst T. Sr., Howard H. Beard: *The Unitarian or Trophoblastic Thesis of Cancer,*
    http://users.navi.net/~rsc/unitari1.htm

13. Cathey, Robert: *On the Cause of Birth and Its Relation to Cancer Regression;*
    http://users.navi.net/~rsc/thesis.htm

14. Cathey, Robert; *Amylase attacks hCG; and the importance of amylase as precursive enzyme activity before proteinase;* http://users.navi.net/~rsc/sialo.htm

15. Klaschka, F.; *Oral Enzymes - New Approach to Cancer Treatment;* Forum Medizin; ISBN3 910075 22 3

16. Lechner, P. et al; *Experiences in the use of dietary therapy in Surgical Oncology;* Oncological Outpatient department, Graz, Austria, Topical Nutritional Medicine, 1990

17. Alexander, K; *Dietary Healing, the complete detox program,* ISBN 9780980376289

18. Donohoe, Mark J; *The Detoxification System, Part I: The Human Liver;*
    http://www.toxipedia.org/download/ attachments/17044484/Report%20%239%20-%20Human%20Liver.pdf?version=1&modificationDate=1388194068000&api=v2

19. Kimber, Helen B.Sc., *Liver Detoxification and Optimal Liver Function, A Nutritional Approach:* 2001, Denor Press: Parkinson's Disease, The Way Forward: Dr. Geoffrey Leader, Lucille Leader, Ch 9.6 pp 144-152

20. Williams, A.C., Steventon, G.B., et al., *Hereditary variation of liver enzymes involved with detoxification and neurodegenerative diseases.* Journal of Inherited Metabolic Disorders 1991, Vol. 14: pp 431-435

21. Cade, Robert et al.; *Autism and Schizophrenia: Intestinal Disorders;* 1999 Department of Medicine, Physiology, Psychology and Psychiatry, University of Florida, Gainesville, FL, USA;
    http://www.fooddetective.pl/download/No%2038.%20Cade%20Autism%20and%20Schizophrenia%20Paper.pdf

# *Chapter 2*

# TAKING ON THE PATIENT

Before taking on a cancer patient, you will need to be clear about your role and your responsibilities. Having this clarity will enable you to operate more efficiently as many patients are making hard decisions regarding treatment, and may wish to follow an integrative path, but would like your input or comment on this, or wish you to monitor a range of treatments in addition to the program you are recommending. At the end of the day patients need to make their own choice on treatment, and it is unwise to unduly influence this, particularly when you cannot promise cure. Improving the outcome is where you can make a difference, and many patients, particularly if they do not come too late to the therapy, will achieve results far beyond their expectations or their attending physicians. Many cancer patients need a great deal of support both from their family, friends and practitioner, and the patient may expect more support from you than you can give, or indeed that would be truly beneficial to the patient. Being there for your patient is essential and by determining your own framework you will be able to work through the responsibilities, reach an understanding of your role and help the patient to make informed decisions.[1] A detoxification therapy is about getting the job done. It is a practical application of a methodical therapy; it is a means to an end, but not the end itself, where its correct application will instigate the healing process. Try not to become sidelined in this goal and always tread with caution when other therapies are being applied in relation to their impact, negative or positive, on the healing process as you will need to make a determination whether the benefits outweigh the risks for the patient which will largely depend on their healing potential and the relative resistance of the disease. The patient will need emotional support and you may or may not be able to give this over and above the treatment. It is important that you can refer the patient to support groups or therapists that you feel can offer appropriate guidance while not undermining their therapy. You do not want to find yourself in the position of picking up the pieces after a well-meaning therapist, who understands nothing of the therapy, has made some adverse comments or recommendations to your patient.

New patients will probably approach you via the telephone. They may have already investigated the Gerson treatment and have a firm understanding, or they may be looking for an hour of your time in which to explain detoxification and convince them that yes, they should definitely do this type of therapy. Your conversation will flow more smoothly and you can be of more help to the client if you are able to establish at the outset the following:

**Establish:**

**1. Their overall condition** including their current diagnosis, the stage and grade of the disease.

- The name of the cancer/s, the stage which will determine the degree of metastatic spread, and the grade which will determine how quickly it is likely to spread. It is important to establish the number of primary cancers, and which organs may be involved, particularly when this involves brain metastases. The latter information will indicate whether there are likely to be acute medical events which could necessitate urgent treatment;
- The date of diagnosis, and if it is a recurrence, when did the cancer relapse;
- The treatment they have received, whether they are currently on any treatment, and are they thinking of doing the therapy in conjunction with allopathic treatment (chemotherapy, radiotherapy, hormone treatment etc.);
- Do they have any other diseases, such as heart disease, thyroid disorders, diabetes, and if so, what medication/s are they taking;

- What major surgeries have they had (cancer and other, including implants etc.); and
- Why are they choosing this program (have all other treatments failed?)

**2. Their knowledge of the program:** establish whether their knowledge is scant, or whether they have studied the treatment thoroughly, before deciding on this course of action.

**3. Establish how much support/opposition they have at home,** both practically and emotionally.

Having confirmed all of the above, you are now in a position to tell the patient whether the treatment is suitable for them. They will often ask for your prognosis and here it is important that you are completely honest. I would recommend that at the beginning of your journey in treating cancer patients you take on the best cases, those that have had no prior treatment with chemotherapy, those who do not have concomitant disease (heart disease, diabetes etc.) or have undertaken multiple surgeries. However, non-cancer patients with chronic disease can be treated effectively with this program providing you factor in the potential risk of acute events and monitor this appropriately. This is easier said than done when you are faced with a desperate situation, and at the end of the day you have to use your own judgement. However, some people do come when it is a last ditch attempt and they may expect miracles, and others just want to use the treatment for more effective palliative management of their deteriorating condition. Patients who opt for this treatment on the basis of better care usually do so because both they, themselves, and their close relatives need to be involved and not impotent in the face of the disease, the doctor, oncologist and hospital. These patients often die at home peacefully, surrounded by those they love.

The prospective client must be completely committed to the therapy. It is a very difficult and disciplined therapy, and without total commitment the patient may not achieve the expected results. They will be continually looking to you to bolster their flagging convictions, which you may never fulfil, and these patients are always tempted to give up the therapy even at the smallest hiccough.

Once you have established if you can take the patient on, please request them to familiarize themselves with the therapy prior to the initial appointment as you will not have time in your initial consultation to go through all the finer details of the therapy, only to answer questions about areas that need more clarification for the patient.

## Before they come for their consultation patients need to:

1. Read all the material available and recommend that they view any recordings of food preparation and set-up;
2. Resource a vegetable supplier and any equipment they need;
3. Fill out a health questionnaire (it is easier if you receive this prior to the appointment);
4. Send all the medical reports relating to scans (PET, MRI, CAT, CT, X-ray), histology and other relevant pathology reports;
5. Send a recent blood test which must include a complete blood count, blood chemistry panel, thyroid function test (TSH, fT4 and fT3 if possible) and any tumour markers if applicable. You cannot "guess" the blood work and will not be able to prescribe potassium, thyroid or Lugol's without the recent blood test results; and
6. Arrange to bring their companion/carer to the first appointment.

It is advisable to send out a package to the patient detailing suppliers etc., and specific requests prior to consultation, together with a case questionnaire. It is better that they wait a couple of weeks for their first consultation to get everything in place. You may find that some patients are evasive in their answers, often down-playing the extent of their illness, so it is imperative that you obtain all the reports.

# Practitioner health warning

This is a nutritional program where the client must take self-responsibility and learn to self-manage. Make sure that none of your patients are doing the therapy because you think it works: they must have confidence that it works, or every symptom that these patients have may be interpreted as negative, and it can turn into a no win situation. The patient needs to develop a real understanding of the healing process and detoxification, so that they are able to interpret their reactions correctly. Patients need to accept that the program works slowly and that we need to give it time, especially if there are bone metastases or if they have had their condition for many years. They also have to understand that we are using different techniques to control pain and inflammation (enemas, packs, not Tylenol or anti-inflammatories). They must also understand the importance and reasoning behind the diet and medications, and have a sensible attitude to rest and a positive outlook. Of course there will be ups and downs, but the stronger the commitment, the stronger the conviction and the more positive the attitude, the more likelihood of success.

## The practitioner's role

This is going to vary from practitioner to practitioner, but the bottom line is that you must be prepared to be available to the patient both as practitioner and teacher. You will need to explain thoroughly at every stage, what is going on and why. Sometimes you will be their mentor and you may have to liaise with other health professionals on their team. You will also have to be vigilant about ensuring correct practice of the therapy. Never assume that the patient is doing every aspect correctly; mistakes do happen even when people have been on the therapy a long while.

It is better if you have a good working relationship with the patient's doctor. Your patient will be attending the surgery at least once a month in the initial stages for a blood test, and if you take on a very sick patient, then they will need their doctor to monitor them and if they worsen they could require acute care. The level of care of your patient is paramount and ideally this should not be compromised by a poor relationship with the doctor. Some patients may feel the need to change their doctor to one who is more open to the treatment.

You may need to communicate with the patient's oncologist. Specialists are bound by ethical standards and medical procedures which tend to influence their recommendations for treatment. For example, an oncologist will not give a less toxic chemotherapy to a patient if it has been proven to be an inadequate treatment in clinical trials, regardless of the fact that the patient is on an intensive nutritional program where it may, under these circumstances, prove to be an appropriate alternative. This is a very difficult situation for both patient, practitioner and oncologist, and constructive communication needs to occur to find a solution that is acceptable to all.

# Taking the case

For your ease, I have included in this handbook a number of forms to help you organise your case taking, so that it is not only complete but makes reference easy when assessing the progress of the case on a month by month basis.

## Practitioner's case study form

The first page of this form is for patient details, diagnosis and chronological treatment to date. More fields can be added as treatment progresses to include the results of further scans/treatments etc. If the patient has filled out and sent you a complete case consultation form before they arrive (Patient Case Study Form), then you will have already completed your form as far as possible, and be ready to fill in the gaps, seeking further clarification on the case history. Your first consultation will be more productive, less time-consuming for both yourself and the patient if you can have all the details prior to the consultation.

- The front page must indicate the name of the disease, recurrence, metastases and treatment to date so that you can see at a glance precisely the prior history. You will also need to know how long they were they feeling ill, or when the symptoms first started (and what they were) before the diagnosis. You will also need to establish whether they had any recommended treatment, whether it was taken within the time frame recommended and, if not, how long they waited.
- You also need to know at a glance the location and size of the tumour/s and their proximity to any organs/arteries. This will be evident from the scan reports. This is vitally important if main structures/organs are involved, as many of the symptoms can relate to obstruction/compression by the tumour and can indicate the likelihood of an acute event that would require medical intervention.
- Treatment received, such as chemotherapy/radiotherapy/surgery/other drugs/hormones. Establish specific medication (chemotherapy, targeted treatment) and treatment (radiotherapy, surgery); the doses and dates given. This will indicate whether to recommend the full or modified therapy and to what extent the immune system is compromised and how toxic the body/liver is.
- Any other current disease/disorder and medication taken. Establish if there is any concomitant disease, when it was diagnosed, which medical drugs were taken and for how long.
- Alternative treatments. It is useful to list all alternative treatments/medications that the patient has tried or is currently taking.

# The clinical history

You will need to take a full clinical history with details of inheritance, birth, illnesses, surgeries and medications from childhood on. Details surrounding the female reproductive cycle/pregnancy/menopause along with any hormonal treatment taken are also important. Details of past and current diet along with any habits/addictions will be useful in terms of building the case and understanding the patient's constitution, or how resilient they are. It represents the fabric that you will be working with, so to speak, which is relevant for assessing the patient's starting point in relation to the program. It will indicate the amount of restoration and detoxification required and the time frames for monitoring the patient's progress.

## Inheritance factors

We normally inherit predominantly from one side of the family or the other, and the patient will usually be aware of where their weaknesses may lie. You will be able to ascertain weaknesses and may be able to link current symptoms with predisposing factors in the inheritance picture. For example, the patient may take after the maternal line where there appears a high incidence of gallstones and they may be unaware that they too have accumulated gallstones. So symptoms, which may manifest in the liver/gall area during a healing flare-up, may relate to this underlying condition. When the inheritance picture indicates a great deal of chronic degenerative illness in the preceding generations, this is often an indication of the strength of the inherited constitution of your patient. In these patients their constitutional vitality may be low and there may be many inherited nutritional deficiencies present. The incidence of cancer often runs in families. Although cancer is not inherited, the predisposition, triggered by epigenetic factors, is. By attending to known risk factors one may successfully reduce one's suspectibility to cancer and this becomes an important focus in treatment.

## Progression of disease

You will be looking for health patterns, seeing the movement of disease in that patient from birth to the current time. Chronic degenerative illness does not appear out of the blue. In most circumstances the health picture will be seen to have worsened over a long period of time before cancer eventually manifests. Stress cannot be underestimated in its effect on health. Periods of ongoing stress will often appear in the case history. Many people feel that particular types of stress feature as causative factors in the type of cancer suffered. In general, the greater, the deeper or more chronic the illness, the greater the toxicity and the longer the time frame to healing.

Symptoms arise as an indication that things are not well, the body is struggling, and unless the imbalance is corrected, or healing takes place, then the situation will continue to deteriorate until a new symptom, which seems to be unrelated to the original complaint, arises. This symptom will be more chronic and more difficult to resolve. Unfortunately we usually only bother to take action and address the symptoms when they have become a permanent or disabling feature of our lives. Below I have given a couple of examples of two common health patterns:

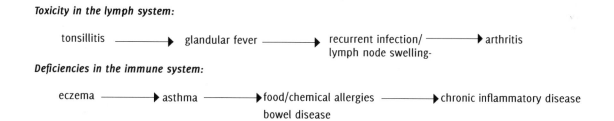

*Toxicity in the lymph system:*

tonsillitis ⟶ glandular fever ⟶ recurrent infection/ ⟶ arthritis
lymph node swelling-

*Deficiencies in the immune system:*

eczema ⟶ asthma ⟶ food/chemical allergies ⟶ chronic inflammatory disease
bowel disease

## Assessment of liver capacity

It is very useful to be able to assess the health of the liver as cure is dependent upon the liver's capacity to eliminate toxicity and regenerate, therefore the starting point of the liver will be a useful indicator of the patient's capacity to both undertake the program and the speed at which the program can progress. There are many indicators in the health picture which can indicate a toxic, deficient liver. Recognising these patterns is the skill of the practitioner. The most obvious indications are a past history of hepatic insult, such as infectious illness (including hepatitis, glandular fever, malaria, dengue fever), and alcohol abuse. Some chemicals and medical drugs are also known to specifically damage the liver. So you need to take all these elements into account when taking the case.

Other useful indicators of liver capacity:
- ◆ Constipation
- ◆ Poor blood sugar control
- ◆ Difficulties in digesting fats
- ◆ Gallstones

- Stomach/duodenal ulcers
- Food allergies/intolerances
- Ulcerative disease of the gastrointestinal tract
- Disorders/imbalances in the reproductive cycle from puberty to menopause governing menstruation, pregnancy and health of the reproductive organs (fibroids, cysts, endometriosis, oestrogen dominance, infertility, premenstrual syndrome)
- Headaches
- Hepatitis, jaundice (including that of the new-born)
- Alcohol abuse
- Chemicals/drugs - most are liver-toxic

Having identified these areas, we must remember that as the disease becomes more chronic, so liver toxicity increases. The liver, or its functional capacity, as far as detoxification is concerned, is always going to be implicated in the aetiology of disease; the more chronic the disease or level of degeneracy, the less the capacity of the liver.

## Toxicity

It is useful to ascertain specific toxicity and the type of toxins involved. You are going to question your patient on any chemicals used over a period of time, any exposure to chemicals (agricultural/industrial), when/for how long, and any habits that the patient may have had that are known to increase toxicity and deplete the body. Below is a list of the more common areas to investigate:

- Chemicals: workplace, industrial or agricultural chemicals
- Electro-magnetic radiation exposure
- Alcohol/smoking
- Social drugs (these patients appear to do well during the first 6 months but may deteriorate thereafter)
- Current and previous medication for all conditions, including hormone therapy (contraception, HRT)

## Surgeries

Which bits are missing! Which bits are new! It is important to investigate thoroughly any foreign material in the body such as implants, pacemakers, metal rods/pins, as the body will attempt to reject these on the full therapy.

## Dental history

It is important to ask your patient about the health of their mouth, specifically whether they have any root canal and amalgam fillings. While we may not be particularly concerned with amalgam fillings (the patient may have these removed once their immune system is strengthened as mercury vapours are released during their removal), we are concerned with root canals as it is the experience of health professionals that patients often fail to respond adequately to the therapy if they have root canals. In essence, when the nerve is removed from the tooth then the tooth is dead, no longer has a circulation or is supplied with nutrients. This dead tooth can become a focus of infection and the root canal, when the packing shrinks, also becomes a seat of infection. A chronic, low-grade infection sets in which is often without symptoms. However, in the immune compromised patient, this can be enough to continuously deplete the vital immune resources, create a low-grade chronic inflammatory situation where the inflammatory chemicals can feed and drive the cancer metabolism. Infections in the mouth can easily spread and become systemic, and the burden upon the immune system deepens. Infection in the tonsils can also impair the immune response to a significant degree and inhibit healing, so it is worth while considering these facts when taking patient case notes.

# Dietary history

**Current Diet** - ask about the current dietary habits of your patient. Remember that, even for the patient with the most health conscious diet, the Gerson treatment is still a major transition. You will be able to assess how difficult that transition is going to be for that patient. Assessing past and current diet will also indicate the nutritional value of the diet, the amount of salt, fat and protein consumed and over what period of time. If the childhood diet has been inadequate, this will contribute to the constitutional status/strength in adulthood.

**Allergies** - foods and drugs. Be careful not to confuse food allergies with food intolerances. Food intolerances refer to digestive difficulties with certain foods which cause bloating and flatulence. Many patients may have allergies to gluten (rye and oats), dairy (non-fat yoghurt, pot cheese) oranges or the nightshade family (potatoes, tomatoes, capsicum [peppers] and eggplant). Any food allergens must be removed but the practitioner may need to substitute with an alternate grain or protein source to ensure that deficiencies do not occur. Allergic reactions to foods may abate once the program is underway and one can then often add these foods into the regime.

# Check list

- **Digestion** - can they eat or drink, or do enemas? Is there a history of reflux/ ulceration/ bleeding? As the patient will be required to take a lot of food and juices, we need to ascertain the digestive capacity. When there are obvious digestive difficulties, we are going to use our common sense over amounts of foods and in certain cases may have to limit the foods given to very easily digested items, such as mashed potato, oatmeal, Hippocrates soup and stewed apple. You need to take into account if there is any gastrointestinal obstruction. If there is a history of ulceration in the colon, then enemas may be introduced cautiously, first as the chamomile tea enema, and later add small amounts of coffee to the mixture until the patient is able to take the full-strength coffee enema. Stress is a major factor in digestive capacity; if a patient is stressed then this impairs the circulation to the organs of digestion and reduces any digestive capacity.
- **Respiratory system** - can they breathe comfortably? If a patient is having difficulty in breathing, you need to determine whether the cause is anaemia, infection/consolidation, metastases to the lungs or pleural effusion.
- **Cardiovascular system** - you need to enquire whether your patient has had any heart conditions. Pain in the chest area and/or breathing difficulties can indicate pericardial effusion, cardiac insufficiency, heart disease. If a patient is on heart medication, do not take them off the medication until the patient is seen to be responding to the therapy. Always let the patient reduce their medication under the guidance of their doctor who can adequately monitor them. The therapy with its high fluid volume and the additional, K, Lugols and thyroid is taxing on the heart and lungs. You must check the blood serum potassium and, if necessary, adjust the fluids.
- **Renal function** - is the patient voiding without difficulty? You will need to check the blood urea, creatinine and serum potassium.
- **Brain and nervous system** - does the patient suffer any disturbance of vision, balance, black-outs, nausea or vomiting or any other symptoms relating to nerve function? If there are metastases to the brain, then the overall prognosis changes. The therapy must progress more slowly as the patient cannot afford healing inflammations which affect the brain. The patient could react with seizures.
- **Does the patient have any pain?** Ascertain the location, and if there are any difficulties in movement. You will need to be aware that pain or difficulty in movement can inhibit the physical aspect of the therapy, especially the preparation of the diet and juicing and even the administration of enemas.

Once you have determined your patient's case history and taken all the above points into consideration, you will be able to prescribe the diet and the medications. You will probably request follow-up scans every six months to determine disease progression/regression. Occasionally, the blood test results may indicate progression of the disease and you may request additional scans. In general, MRI scans are a superior imaging technique for the brain and spine, while CAT or CT scans are better for the internal organs. PET scans are useful for determining how active the cancer is. Ultrasound imaging gives a less accurate interpretation. Many patients do not wish to take the radioactive contrast media with the CT scan, but the imaging is that much clearer leading to a more accurate interpretation, so it is generally preferred. Patients are recommended to do additional coffee enemas after these scans to help with the detoxification.

# Contra-indications to the intensive program

There will be many patients whose illness would not be treatable by the full Gerson treatment. The therapy is a diet therapy, so if clients simply can't eat or drink, then they would not be able to do the therapy. If the patient has a disease where the tissue is dead and will never repair (as in certain brain and nervous disorders) then these clients will not respond. However, these patients may be able to derive benefit from some of the principles and guidelines, and your understanding of its capacity to reduce the toxic burden on the system and make good nutritional deficiencies will allow you to confidently prescribe some of the medications, enemas, juices and diet protocol. Below is a list of conditions that may contra-indicate the full therapy.

- If the patient can't eat of drink. This may be due to a gastrointestinal obstruction/tumour growth or gastrostomy. If they can eat something, then you can start slowly with the soup, oatmeal, mashed potato and a few juices, but you have to be mindful that the patients may become nutritionally compromised if you are unable to meet their requirements.
- Patients with colostomies can follow the therapy, using special irrigation equipment. Many patients, upon healing, are able to reverse temporary colostomies (see p118).
- Enlarged liver: it is difficult for these patients to do the therapy and recover as the liver is pushed too hard. Their condition may be aggravated on such a treatment.
- Ascites: either from liver failure or inflammatory activity from cancers, such as ovarian cancer or metastases to the peritoneum. These patients have to reduce their fluid intake and the high volume of fluid on the therapy, both in the juicing and the coffee enemas, is counter-productive and will exacerbate the condition. These patients are often terminal and need specialist care.
- Brain metastases: any inflammatory healing reactions in the brain can be very serious. They are normally on corticosteroid and anti-convulsant treatment to suppress inflammation and seizures, respectively.
- Bleeding in the gastrointestinal tract, ulcers/gastritis, colitis/diverticulitis: the bleeding must be resolved through modifications to the program. Remove salads and use cooked food only, that is fibre free (potato, soup, oatmeal, apple sauce, Hippocrates soup) and do not introduce the coffee enemas, potassium, niacin, Lugol's, or thyroid until the condition is resolved. You may then start adding the medication slowly.
- Acute leukaemias: recommend orthodox medicine, as the Gerson protocol may speed the progress of the disease.
- Low breathing capacity, including pleural effusions. Under these circumstances you cannot give the high volume fluids or the enemas, as these would increase total body fluids and cause the heart to work harder and the effusions present would increase in volume. You cannot do the coffee enemas (caffeine), potassium, Lugol's or thyroid. If 75% of the lung function is gone, then you cannot help the patient with the Gerson treatment.
- Cardio-respiratory failure: as above. You cannot afford to place an additional burden on the heart.

- Foreign bodies: implants (including breast), valves, pacemaker, metal plates, screen mesh (prolapse/hernia). You need to be aware that inflammatory reactions on the full therapy will occur and the body will try to reject these foreign objects. We have not found problems with patients who have hip replacements.
- Dialysis, renal failure.
- Patients on Warfarin should not do the coffee enemas as the enema clears the drug too quickly.
- Parkinson's; when parts of the brain are destroyed, then this cannot be regenerated. The patient with Parkinson's needs to continue with their medication in order to be able to function.
- The white cell differential indicating a lymphocyte count under 10% of the white cell differential. This means that the neutrophil count is 90% or higher which occurs when there is aggressive tumoural progression and the patient will be in a terminal phase of their cancer and the prognosis is very poor.
- Radiation therapy in the pelvic area. Most of the immune cells are made in the bone marrow of this area, and once the tissue is burned it will not restore quickly enough to allow the body to respond. However, the restorative capacity is much greater in children than adults.
- Patients who have been receiving corticosteroid therapy for longer than two years may not respond to detoxification adequately. By this stage too much of the functional reserve of the liver may have been eroded and there may be deleterious effects on the immune system. You will never produce a healing inflammation in a patient who is currently taking corticosteroid treatment.
- Patients currently on morphine (except those heavily pretreated with chemotherapy or with severe bone pain) respond very quickly to coffee enemas and the high potassium for detoxification. Usually pain is controlled within 1½ to 3 days, so morphine can be discontinued and the therapy becomes effective. If the patient is unable to reduce this medication, then the practitioner must be aware that morphine suppresses autonomic nerve activity in the gastrointestinal tract, nervous stimulus to the liver, digestive tract and the colon. Without an intact digestive and eliminative system, the effects of the program will be limited.

# Follow-up consultations

Once the patient understands how vitally important the monitoring of their case is, they will be happy to comply with the monthly follow-up appointments. Once again, during the first six months of treatment you will be requesting blood tests on a monthly basis. It is quite a good idea to ask the patient to fill in a follow-up consultation form and send it prior to their appointment, along with their blood results. A sample follow-up form is included in this manual for your guidance. This ensures that the patient cannot arrive for an appointment without their follow-up or blood work!

You need to ascertain a great deal of information at each follow-up to enable you to make an accurate assessment of the progress of your patient. It is easy to forget to ask specifics, particularly if the patient wishes to talk about their problems/concerns. If you have already read through the patient's update and latest blood results, you will have a good idea of the patient's progress and be sufficiently prepared to address the main issues arising each month and offer appropriate advice and modifications.

The questions on the follow-up consultation form have been carefully selected to obtain the maximum information that you require to make a full assessment. When you start to use the form you will be surprised at how many mistakes are made by the patient with regard to their treatment and how many "alternatives" or even medical drugs the patient may resort to during their treatment. For example, at the first flare-up or discomfort the patient may reach for the Paracetamol, completely forgetting that we do not use this medication for pain/fever etc. So the consultation follow-up is a fail-safe mechanism to ensure patient compliance and correct interpretation by the practitioner, of the patient's progress.

Below is a list of the types of mistakes/symptoms to watch out for:

- Medication/enema mistakes: sometimes the patient can misinterpret their chart and take the wrong amounts of medication, skipping the last enema, not doing enough castor oil enemas or administering them wrongly.
- Dietary mistakes: very common. You may discover that the patient is only eating raw food and none cooked because they read somewhere that the raw food diet is best; the Hippocrates soup only once a day (or not at all because they don't like it or can't find all the ingredients); potatoes only once daily; cooking with yoghurt; skipping the porridge and taking raw oats; or simply not eating enough!
- Juice mistakes: taking two juices at once to reduce time spent juicing and cleaning the juicing machine.
- Weight loss: this is expected, but if it continues then you would need to check the amount of food consumed and the amount of exercise undertaken, and the amount of thyroid medication.
- Other medications/treatments/medical procedures they have incorporated without telling you.
- Detoxification symptoms which the patient may not think of as being important (for example difficulty in holding the first enema of the day), nausea, diarrhoea.
- Flare-ups and their symptoms (the list of symptoms on the form will help the patient to "jog their memory").
- Pulse and temperature: asking the patient to record these ensures that the patient takes both regularly
- Energy levels: when these are low check the amount of rest and quality of sleep, and if they are eating enough.
- Major concerns: answering and advising the patient's concerns is vitally important to the success of the therapy and the patient/practitioner relationship.

Most practitioners monitor the disease process, exclusively. Practitioners using a naturopathic philosophy of cure, such as the Gerson treatment, monitor the healing process where any reduction in the disease is a side-effect of that process. Unless the practitioner asks and interprets the relevant questions and their answers in relation to the progress of the case, then there can be no clear idea on that progress or whether the patient is heading in the right direction, and how far. It is the repair of the whole body that will ultimately secure cure.

*"Therefore one has to separate two basic components in cancer: a general one and a local one. The general component is mostly a very slow, progressing, imperceptible symptom caused by poisoning of the liver and simultaneously an impairment of the whole intestinal tract, later producing appearances of vitally important consequences all over the body." (pp35-36)*

# References

1.   Alexander, K; *Managing the Patient's Journey*; an online practitioner training course using the Smart Patient® case management framework for case-taking, follow-up, interpretation, monitoring and fostering the practitioner/patient partnership.
http://www.kathrynalexander.com.au/store/p38/Managing_the_Patient%27s_Journey_%28online_course%29.html

# Recommended Reading

Bates, Barbara: *A Guide to Physical Examination and History Taking*, 1991, 5th edition, J.B. Lippincott, pp 5-33, 37-65

Alexander, K; *Smart Patient Journey Road Map, increasing your odds for success*; ISBN 9780980376296

# Chapter 3

# BLOOD PATHOLOGY

I t is essential that the client has regular blood tests. These are invaluable to the practitioner, as the results will indicate how the patient is progressing and if you need to make any modifications to the diet or medications. In the initial phase you would be advised not to prescribe potassium, Lugol's or thyroid without recent blood results. The tests requested include:

- Blood chemistry (includes liver function tests; kidney function tests, glucose)
- Complete Blood Count
- Thyroid function test (TSH, fT4, fT3)
- Tumour markers (if applicable)
- Urinalysis

Follow-up monthly tests are essential during the first six months. Thereafter the patient should send their blood results prior to each appointment.

Generally the tests will indicate a trend and must be read in the context of previous test results and current symptoms. Tests can be unreliable if the patient is experiencing a healing flare-up. Under these circumstances the liver enzymes and alkaline phosphatase may be elevated. A single test result of elevated levels is not diagnostic. Reference ranges and units of measurement will vary from laboratory to laboratory.

The tests will indicate:

- Liver function - active/chronic disease, biliary obstruction, (LFT, bilirubin, albumin)
- Renal function - (potassium, urea and creatinine)
- Thyroid function - (TSH, fT4, fT3)
- Bone metastases - (ALP)
- Dehydration/electrolyte imbalance - (Na, K, urea)
- Immune response - infection, flare-ups, tumoural activity (neutrophils/lymphocytes).
- Anaemia - (red blood cell count, haemoglobin, B12, iron)
- Tumour markers - disease progression/regression
- Paraneoplastic disorders - secretion of hormones or hormone-related peptides by the tumour

Blood pathology will be divided into the following sections:

**Complete Blood Count**
    Red cell count/haemoglobin
    Iron Status
    White cell count
    Platelets
**Liver Function Tests**
    Bilirubin
    Plasma enzymes/proteins
**Thyroid Function**
    TSH, fT4, fT3

**The Electrolytes and Kidney Function Tests**

**Urinalysis**

**Inflammatory Markers**

**Tumour Markers**

**Metabolic Complications**
    Paraneoplastic syndromes
    Carcinoid syndrome
    Cachexia

# Complete blood count

## Glossary of terms with reference ranges

| | Reference Range | Description | |
|---|---|---|---|
| Haemoglobin | 11.5-16.5 g/dL | Amount of Hb g/dL of plasma | |
| Red Cell Count (RCC) | 3.8-5.5 x10$^{12}$/L | Number of red cells / litre of plasma | |
| PCV (haemocrit) | 0.35-0.47 | % of RBCs in plasma  (0.45 = 45%) | |
| MCV (mean cell volume) | 80-99 fL | average cell volume (PCV/RCC) | |
| MCH (mean cell Hb) | 27-32 pg/cell | average Hb/cell (Hb/RCC) | |
| MCHC (mean cell  Hb conc) | 300-360 g/L | Hb in red cell mass (Hb g/L /PCV) | |
| White Cell Count (WCC) | 4-11 x10$^9$/L | total number of white cells/litre | |
| Neutrophils | 2.0-8.0 x10$^9$/L | Differential | 40% - 75% |
| Lymphocytes | 1.0-4.0 x10$^9$/L | Differential | 20% - 45% |
| Monocytes | <1.1 x10$^9$/L | Differential | 2% - 10% |
| Eosinophils | <0.6 x10$^9$/L | Differential | 1% - 6% |
| Basophils | <0.2 x10$^9$/L | Differential | 0% - 1% |
| Platelets | 150-450 x10$^9$/L | | |

### Iron Studies

| | |
|---|---|
| Ferritin | 10-250µg/L |
| Iron | 10 - 30µmols/L |
| Iron binding capacity (TIBC) | 40-75 µmols/L |
| % TFN (transferrin) saturation | 20-55% |

## Calculating the White cell Differential

The white cell differential is the ratio of the white cell type (neutrophils or lymphocytes) over the total WCC expressed as a percentage. For example:

| | |
|---|---|
| **White cell count** (4-11 x10$^9$/L) | 5.8 |
| Neutrophils (2.0-8.0 x10$^9$/L) | 3.5 |
| Lymphocytes (1.0-4.0 x10$^9$/L) | 1.8 |

The neutrophils expressed as a % of the total WCC:

$$\frac{3.5 \times 100}{5.8} = 60\%$$

The lymphocytes expressed as a % of the total WCC:

$$\frac{1.8 \times 100}{5.8} = 31\%$$

## Calculating the MCH, MCV and MCHC

If you have the haemoglobin, red cell count and haemocrit (PCV) values then you can deduce the values for the MCH, MCV and MCHC.

| | | | |
|---|---|---|---|
| MCH | Hb g/L | / RCC | 129/4.7 = 27.44 |
| MCV | PCV mls/L | / RCC | 380 mls/4.7 = 80.85 |
| MCHC | Hb g/L | / PCV% | 129/0.38 = 339 g/L (34%) |

| | |
|---|---|
| Haemoglobin (11.5-16.5 g/dL) | 12.9 |
| RBC (3.8-5.5 x10$^{12}$/L) | 4.7 |
| PCV (0.35-0.47) | 0.38 |
| MCV (80-99 fL) | 80.85 |
| MCH (27-32 pg/cell) | 27.4 |
| MCHC (300-360 g/L) | 339 |

# Red cell count and haemoglobin

The number of red cells (erythrocytes) in circulation is governed by the rate of erythropoiesis in the bone marrow. Erythropoiesis is stimulated in response to anoxia where the kidneys secrete the hormone erythropoietin which stimulates the bone marrow to produce more red blood cells.

Haemoglobin is the respiratory pigment of erythrocytes. The haem component consists of four iron-protoporphyrin molecules and its synthesis is dependent upon nutritional availability of iron, B12 and folic acid. Deficiencies in any of these nutrients, due to inadequate dietary intake or absorption, results in anaemia leading to deficient oxygenation of the tissues for metabolism. There are many different causes of anaemia and it is important to qualify the cause so that appropriate advice and treatment can be offered. Invariably a range of tests needs to be ordered and assessed against the patient's current diagnosis and condition before a full evaluation can be made.

**Indications for anaemia**

- Nutritional deficiencies (iron, B12, folate, vitamin C):
  - Iron deficiency anaemia
  - Megaloblastic anaemia (B12 and/or folate deficiency)
- Hypochlorhydria/achlorhydria (gastritis)
- Inflammatory disease (infection, autoimmune, arthritis, malignancy; hepcidin inhibits dietary iron uptake)
- Liver disease (failure to produce transferrin)
- Haemorrhage/occult bleeding/haemolysis (loss of red cells)
- Hypothyroidism
- Marrow failure (due to cytotoxic drugs [chemotherapy] or myeloproliferative disorders/leukaemia)
- Renal disease (failure to produce erythropoietin)

Clinical features

- Symptoms of inadequate oxygenation:
  - Breathlessness, rapid or irregular heart beat
  - Low energy/constant fatigue
- Pallor - general pallor, nails and eyes
- Koilonychia (brittle, spoon-shaped nails)
- Glossitis (smooth tongue)
- Angular cheilosis
- Atrophy of mucosal surfaces (tongue and vagina - B12 deficiency)
- Tingling in hands and feet
- Poor healing/recurrent infection

# Haemoglobin

**Reference range** 11.5-16.5 g/dL (115-165 g/L)

**Metabolism**

Erythropoiesis is stimulated by anoxia. The supply of oxygen to the cells is decreased by deficient haemoglobin synthesis and a deficient number of red cells. The kidneys secrete erythropoietin which stimulates red blood cell production. In high doses it also stimulates platelet production. Chemotherapy induced anaemia is often treated by recombinant erythropoietin administration.

The formation and maturation of red blood cells is dependent upon adequate supplies of B12 and folic acid. These nutrients govern DNA synthesis for cell replication and the effects of deficiency will be found in tissues with a rapid turnover, such as haemopoietic tissue which is particularly susceptible and changes in the counts for red cells, platelets and granulocytes will reflect B12 deficiency. Deficiencies of both folic acid and B12 lead to slower cell synthesis, replication and maturation giving rise to the megaloblastic anaemias. B12 deficiency specifically gives rise to pernicious anaemia, but the cause may not be a dietary deficiency of this vitamin but lack of intrinsic factor which is essential for its absorption. Pernicious anaemia is an auto-immune disease and B12 will need to be administered as an injection in such cases.

The megaloblastic anaemias are characterised by larger immature red cells being released into the circulation, but the overall numbers of red blood cells are decreased, with each cell carrying a greater concentration of haemoglobin. Tests can be made for both B12 and folate status. However, it is important to remember that the conversion of folate to its active coenzyme (tetrahydrofolate - THF) is B12 dependent and therefore B12 deficiencies will give rise to apparent folate deficiencies. There is no shortage of folate on the program (green vegetables - *foliage*) although folate is destroyed by cooking. Patients homozygous for the MTHFR gene variants will obtain sufficient folate in its active form from the green juices.

Iron deficiency also leads to low haemoglobin levels and anaemia as the formation of haem is dependent upon adequate iron status. This type of anaemia gives rise to erythrocytes that are smaller than normal (microcytic) with a low concentration of haemoglobin (hypochromic). A primary iron deficiency may account for the anaemia, where increased intake will resolve the problem, but in the chronically sick patient the cause is rarely as simple as this. In chronic inflammatory disease, including cancer, there is suppression of the uptake of dietary iron, and in liver disease the production of transferrin, an iron binding globulin, may be compromised leading to poor dietary iron uptake. The anaemia of blood loss will show erythrocytes of a normal size and haemoglobin concentration, but the numbers are low due to blood losses resulting in an overall low haemoglobin status.

## Interpreting blood results for anaemia

| Iron deficiency anaemia | Megaloblastic anaemia | Anaemia due to blood loss |
|---|---|---|
| *Microcytic and hypochromic red blood cells.* | *Macrocytic, normochromic* | |
| ↑ RCC to normal | ↓ RCC | ↓ RCC |
| ↓ Hb | ↓ Hb | ↓ Hb |
| ↓ PCV to normal | ↓ PCV | ↓ PCV |
| ↓ MCV | ↑ MCV | MCV normal |
| ↓ MCH | ↑ MCH | MCH normal |
| ↓ MCHC | ↑ MCHC to normal | ↓ MCHC to normal (due to both Hb and PCV being lower) |
| | ↓ Neutrophils | |
| ↑ Platelets to normal | ↓ Platelets | ↑ Platelets to normal |
| ↓ Serum iron | Serum iron normal | ↓ Serum iron |
| ↑ Iron Binding Capacity (Transferrin) | Iron Binding Capacity normal | ↑ Iron Binding Capacity |
| ↓ TFN saturation | TFN saturation normal | ↑ TFN saturation |
| ↓ Ferritin (with prolonged anaemia) | Ferritin normal | ↓ Ferritin (with prolonged haemorrhage) |

## Megaloblastic anaemia due to B12 deficiency

| | |
|---|---|
| Haemoglobin (11.5-16.5 g/dL) | **10.5** |
| RBC (3.8-5.5 x10$^{12}$/L) | 3.17 |
| PCV (0.35-0.47) | 0.32 |
| MCV (80-99 fL) | 99.5 |
| MCH (27-32 pg/cell) | 33.2 |
| Neutrophils (2.0-8.0 x10$^9$/L) | **1.5** |
| **Platelets** (150-450 x10$^9$/L) | **106.0** |
| Iron (9-27µmols/L) | 13.0 |
| Transferrin (1.8-3.7 g/L) | 2.8 |
| TFN saturation (20-55%) | 18.0 |
| Ferritin (20-300 µg/L) | 68.0 |
| Serum vitamin B12 (150-600 pmol/L) | **123.0** |
| Serum Folate (5.9-45.0 nmol/L) | **37.4** |

## Anaemia due to iron deficiency

| | |
|---|---|
| Haemoglobin (11.5-16.5g/dL) | **11.2** |
| RBC (3.8-5.5 x10$^{12}$/L) | **4.1** |
| PCV (0.35-0.47) | **0.35** |
| MCV (80-99 fL) | 85 |
| MCH (27-32 pg/cell) | 27 |
| Platelets (150-450 x10$^9$/L) | 340 |
| Iron (9-27 µmols/L) | **8.0** |
| Transferrin (45-72 g/L) | 75 |
| Fe saturation (20-55%) | **11** |
| Ferritin (20-300 µg/L) | 6 |
| Serum vitamin B12 (150-600 pmol/L) | 420.0 |

## Anaemia due to chronic inflammatory disease

*Elevated WCC, CRP and ESR indicate inflammation. The anaemia is not due to a dietary iron deficiency or blood loss, but due to chronic inflammatory disease which inhibits the absorption of dietary iron.*

| | | | |
|---|---|---|---|
| Haemoglobin (11.5-16.5g/dL) | **10.8** | Iron (9-27 µmols/L) | **6** |
| MCV (80-99 fL) | 86.0 | Transferrin (20-45 µmol/L) | 25 |
| MCHC (320-360 g/L) | **334** | TFN saturation (20-55%) | **12** |
| WCC (4-11 x10$^9$/L) | **8.0** | Ferritin (20-300 µg/L) | 58 |
| **Platelets** (150-450 x10$^9$/L) | **372** | CRP (<4.0) | **21** |
| Serum vitamin B12 (150-600 pmol/L) | 428 | ESR (<15) | **51** |

## Anaemia due to the thalassaemias

Thalassaemia is an inherited impairment of haemoglobin formation where there is a failure to synthesise either the alpha or beta chains of the globin chain. A high frequency of beta-thalassaemia is found among Mediterraneans and alpha-thalassaemia in the SE Asian population. Individuals heterozygous for this gene are mildly affected and a variable degree of anaemia is often present with hypochromic and microcytic erythrocytes.

## Blood results of a patient with thalassaemia

*Red cell count is normal but both the average size of the cell and its haemoglobin concentration are low leading to hypochromic, microcytic anaemia.*

| Haematology | |
|---|---|
| Haemoglobin (11.5-16.5 g/dL) | 10.5 |
| RBC (3.8-5.5 x10$^{12}$/L) | 5.1 |
| PCV (0.35-0.47) | 33 |
| MCV (80-99 fL) | 65 |
| MCH (27-32 pg/cell) | 20.6 |
| **Platelets** (150-450 x10$^9$/L) | 341 |

*Same patient in end-stage of disease. The rise in platelets is a morbid sign and may be caused by erythropoietin stimulation in response to anoxia (low Hb and RBC). High platelet counts are invariably seen in patients with terminal disease.*

| Haematology | |
|---|---|
| Haemoglobin (11.5-16.5 g/dL) | 5.2 |
| RBC (3.8-5.5 x10$^{12}$/L) | 2.92 |
| PCV (0.35-0.47) | 16.9% |
| MCV (80-99 fL) | 58 |
| MCH (27-32 pg/cell) | 17.8 |
| **Platelets** (150-450 x10$^9$/L) | 677 |

# Iron status

The most common cause of microcytic, hypochromic anaemia is iron deficiency. Dietary deficiencies are rare amongst meat eaters and vegetarians who consume adequate amounts of green, leafy vegetables. Other good sources are the dried fruits (prunes, raisins, apricots, dates). However, absorption is dependent upon gastric acid secretion in the stomach which liberates iron from food and promotes conversion from $Fe^{3+}$ to $Fe^{2+}$. So anaemia may present in patients with achlorhydria or hypochlorhydria and those suffering from gastritis. Vitamin C (reducing agent) facilitates the absorption of iron derived from vegetable sources; however, the iron bound in haem, found in red meat, is absorbed intact. Iron absorption is increased in erythropoiesis and depletion of stores.

Haemorrhage will cause anaemia through the loss of red blood cells and hence the overall haemoglobin status. This is why it is important to determine the cause of the anaemia, particularly if dietary iron is adequate and occult bleeding is suspected.

Iron can either be transported directly into the circulation or, when body stores are full, will combine with apoferritin in the mucous membrane cells and is shed with the lining. Once in the circulation, iron is bound to transferrin as free iron is very toxic. In tissues it is bound to ferritin and haemosiderin. Iron injections will lead to rapid oxidative damage throughout the system.

There are several measurements for iron: serum iron, ferritin, iron-binding capacity and saturation (transferrin [TFN] saturation).

### Reference range

| | |
|---|---|
| Ferritin | 10-250 µg/L |
| Iron | 10-30 µmols/L |
| Iron binding capacity (TIBC) | 40-75 µmols/L |
| % TFN saturation | 20-55% |

**Ferritin** (10-250 µg/L) - this is the best assessment for iron stores. A low plasma ferritin indicates low stores. Levels less than 12µg/L indicate complete absence of stored iron. High ferritin levels may be used as a tumour marker for disease progression. Low serum iron with high ferritin is a marker for inflammatory disease and active cancer, where dietary iron uptake is suppressed through the action of the iron-regulatory hormone, hepcidin, but serum iron is rapidly used in the inflammatory process but accumulates increasing serum ferritin.[1,2] A persistently elevated ferritin may herald recurrent disease. Serum ferritin seems to increase with increased oestrogen levels and is elevated in many suffering from prostate or breast cancer. High ferritin levels may also occur with inherited haemochromatosis and therefore you may need to request a genetic test if you suspect this to be the case.

### Female - Breast cancer with bone metastases, aged 53 years
*Ferritin is used as a marker for disease progression.*

| Haematology | 8/4/98 | 24/6/98 | 13/8/98 | 02/11/98 | 25/02/99 |
|---|---|---|---|---|---|
| Haemoglobin (11.5-16.5 g/dL) | 15.1 | 14.6 | 14.6 | 15.0 | 14.5 |
| RBC (3.8-5.5 x10$^{12}$/L) | 4.66 | 4.55 | 4.53 | 4.79 | 4.77 |
| PCV (0.35-0.47) | 0.42 | 0.42 | 0.41 | 0.44 | 0.43 |
| MCV (80-99 fL) | 90 | 92 | 91 | 91 | 90 |
| MCH (27-32 pg/cell) | 32 | 32 | 32 | 31 | 30 |
| **Tumour markers** | | | | | |
| Ferritin (15-185 µg/L) | 497 | 530 | 398 | 400 | 646 |
| CA15.3 (<34) | 39 | 74 | 81 | 158 | 403 |

**Serum or plasma iron** (10 - 30 μmols/L) - indicates the amount of iron in the plasma. This is often reduced in chronic inflammatory disease and neoplastic disease. These patients may also have microcytic, hypochromic anaemia and yet show a normal ferritin reading. Iron mobilisation from ferritin stores is often inhibited for haemoglobin synthesis in chronic disease. Plasma iron can fluctuate considerably and is invariably low during infection.

**Total Iron-binding capacity** (40-75 μmols/L) - is a measurement of transferrin concentration, an iron-binding globulin produced by the liver in response to iron requirements which will be increased in anaemia. It is also increased during pregnancy.

**% TFN saturation** (20%-55%) - this measurement indicates how much transferrin is saturated with iron and is represented by the equation below. Normal saturation is around 33%.

$$\frac{\text{Plasma iron x 100}}{\text{Transferrin}}$$

### Female - Cervical cancer with heavy bleeding, aged 47 years

*Comment: Cause of anaemia is haemorrhage. Normal MCV and MCH indicates normal synthesis of red cells but the low Hb, RCC and PCV indicate blood loss. Iron studies indicate that iron stores are depleted. Iron-binding capacity is low/normal. Following a further haemorrhage the iron status fell again.*

| | 18/2/99 | 10/3/99 | 12/4/99 | 15/5/99 | 12/6/99 | 19/6/99 | 18/7/99 | 21/8/99 | 12/10/99 |
|---|---|---|---|---|---|---|---|---|---|
| **Haematology** | | | | | | | | | |
| Haemoglobin (11.5-16.5 g/dL) | 10.9 | 9.5 | 10.5 | 10.1 | 10.4 | 11.0 | 12.5 | 13.1 | 10.8 |
| RBC (3.8-5.5 x10¹²/L) | | 3.06 | | | | | 4.01 | 4.12 | 3.5 |
| PCV (0.35-0.47) | 0.32 | 0.28 | 0.33 | 0.31 | 0.34 | 0.33 | 0.36 | 37 | 0.34 |
| MCV (80-99 fL) | 96 | 93 | 86 | 83 | 85 | 85 | 90 | 90 | 96 |
| MCH (27-32 pg/cell) | 33 | 31.1 | 27 | 27 | 26 | 28 | 31 | 32 | 31 |
| Ferritin (10-250 μg/L) | 14 | | | | | | | | |
| Iron (10 - 30 μmols/L) | 4.4 | | 4.0 | 5.7 | 4.6 | 6.6 | 12.4 | 9.8 | 6.5 |
| TIBC (40-75 μmol/L) | 45 | | 50 | 51 | 51 | 46 | 61 | 59 | 60 |
| % iron saturation (20-55%) | 10 | 5 | 8 | 11 | 9 | 14 | 20 | 17 | 11 |

### Female - Primary colon carcinoma with liver metastases, aged 67 years

*Comment: Anaemia with low ferritin and serum iron. Hb levels are improving with the diet. No values for iron binding capacity although both serum iron and TIBC would be expected to fall in response to inflammation due to the inhibitory action of hepcidin on dietary iron uptake.*

| | 25/04/00 | 23/05/00 | 1/8/00 | 19/9/00 | 17/10/00 |
|---|---|---|---|---|---|
| **Haematology** | | | | | |
| Haemoglobin (11.5-16.5 g/dL) | 8.0 | 7.7 | 7.2 | 9.3 | 10.2 |
| RBC (3.8-5.5 x10¹²/L) | 4.5 | 4.27 | 3.89 | 3.22 | 3.62 |
| PCV (0.35-0.47) | 0.38 | 0.38 | 0.35 | 0.30 | 0.32 |
| MCV (80-99 fL) | 86 | 90 | 92 | 92 | 89 |
| MCH (27-32 pg/cell) | 27.7 | 28.1 | 28.9 | 28.9 | 28.2 |
| Serum Fe (10-30 μmols/L) | | | 6 | 7 | 5 |
| Ferritin (10-250 μg/L) | | | 19 | | |

**Male - Colo-rectal carcinoma with metastases to liver and lungs, aged 55 years**

*These results indicate chronic tumoural inflammation resulting in low serum Fe and TFN saturation. The patient was able to eat only 30% of his normal intake and could not tolerate the green juices. He was advised to take iron by his GP which has increased the ferritin value, but made no difference to his haemoglobin levels. The cause of the anaemia is both dietary iron deficiency but, more importantly, chronic inflammation. Under these circumstances prescribing iron will only aggravate the ferritin levels and have little impact on haemoglobin or red cell synthesis. In order to resolve the anaemia of chronic disease one has to treat the cause of the inflammation.*

| | 9/1/01 | 23/02/01 |
|---|---|---|
| **Haematology** | | |
| Haemoglobin (11.5-16.5 g/dL) | 10.4 | 9.9 |
| RBC (3.8-5.5 x10$^{12}$/L) | 3.52 | 3.7 |
| PCV (0.35-0.47) | 30.6 | 30 |
| MCV (80-99 fL) | 87 | 81 |
| MCH (27-32 pg/cell) | 29.5 | 26.8 |
| **white cell count** (4-11 x10$^9$/L) | 7.9 | 9.3 |
| Neutrophils (2.0-8.0 x10$^9$/L) | 5.8 | 6.6 |
| Lymphocytes (1.0-4.0 x10$^9$/L) | 1.0 | 1.7 |
| **Platelets** (150-450 x10$^9$/L) | 606 | 967 |
| Serum Fe (10-30 µmol/L) | 3 | 2 |
| TNF Saturation (13-47%) | 5% | 4% |
| TIBC (44-74 µmol/L) | 58 | 51 |
| Ferritin (20-300 µg/L) | 17 | 27 |

# White cell count

All the white blood cells, granulocytes (neutrophils, oesinophils and basophils), monocytes and lymphocytes are produced by the bone marrow. Lymphocytes also proliferate outside the bone marrow in lymphoid organs (thymus, lymph nodes and spleen) and lymphoid tissue/follicles. Granulocytes and monocytes derive from myeloblasts and monoblasts respectively, whereas the lymphocytes derive from lymphoblasts.

**Reference ranges for white cells**

| | | | | |
|---|---|---|---|---|
| White Cell Count | 4-11 $\times 10^9$/L | total number of white cells/litre | | |
| Neutrophils | 2.0-8.0 $\times 10^9$/L | Differential | 40% - 75% | |
| Lymphocytes | 1.0-4.0 $\times 10^9$/L | Differential | 20% - 45% | |
| Monocytes | <1.1 $\times 10^9$/L | Differential | 2% - 10% | |
| Eosinophils | <0.6 $\times 10^9$/L | Differential | 1% - 6% | |
| Basophils | <0.2 $\times 10^9$/L | Differential | 0% - 1% | |

# White cells from the myeloid line

The white cells form an important part of the body's defence system. **Neutrophils** and monocytes form the first-line defence against invasion from micro-organisms in a non-specific manner and engulf cell debris and particulate matter. Granulopoiesis is stimulated by bacterial and tissue extracts. The neutrophil count will increase during infection and necrosis (granulocytosis). In the absence of infection it is a useful indicator of tumoral activity/ progression/flare-up. The bone marrow pool of granulocytes contains 15 times the amount in the peripheral circulation, thus the bone marrow is able to respond to acute inflammation by the release of both mature and immature granulocytes. Neutrophils are the most common leucocyte in circulating blood and make up to between 40 - 75% of the differential.

**Eosinophils** may be raised in response to parasitic infestations but more likely in the allergic individual to specific dietary or environmental factors. Patients with known allergies should be monitored for any adverse reactions and/or a raised eosinophil count, when cultured milk products are introduced into the diet. Eosinophils deactivate vasoactive substances such as histamine produced during the allergic inflammatory response. Eosinophilia is associated with malignant disease, particularly Hodgkin's disease.

**Basophils** are the least common leucocyte and bear close resemblance to mast cells, and similar stimuli induce de-granulation of these cells and the release of histamine. This type of reaction occurs in hypersensitive states to external allergens.

**Monocytes** circulate in the blood for only 1 or 2 days before they migrate to the tissues where they remain as tissue macrophages. They have a long life span.

*Indications for neutropenia:*
- Severe infection
- Bone marrow infiltration
- Hypersplenism
- Radiation
- Cytotoxic drugs/during detoxification of cytotoxic drugs
- Corticosteroids
- Nutritional deficiencies (B12, folate)

*Indications for granulocytosis:*

- ◆  Bacterial infection
- ◆  Tumoral activity/progression
- ◆  Neoplastic proliferation in bone marrow (myeloid leukaemia or leukaemic phase of metastatic cancer)

# White cells from the lymphoid line

**Lymphocytes** play a key role in all immune responses, but in contrast to the non-specific response of the neutrophils, their action is always directed against specific antigens. Lymphocytes are divided into two main populations: the T-cells and the B cells. The T cells (cellular immunity) are important in tumour destruction/viral infection/fungal infection, whereas the B cells (humoral immunity) produce antibodies in response to bacterial invasion. The lymphocyte count is a measure of the total T and B populations. Around 75% of circulating lymphocytes are T-cells. Lymphocytes are the second most common leucocyte in circulating blood and make up to between 20 - 45% of the differential.

*Indications for lymphopenia* $(<1.5 \times 10^9/L)$

- ◆  Radiation
- ◆  Cytotoxic drugs
- ◆  Corticosteroids
- ◆  Nutritional deficiencies (B12, folate)
- ◆  During detoxification of cytotoxic drugs

The effects of radiation on the bone marrow, particularly in the pelvic area, are most damaging to the lymphocyte population. If the differential either drops below 10% or remains below the lymphocyte lower level of normal, then the prognosis is poor.

*Indications for lymphocytosis* $(>4.0 \times 10^9/L)$

- ◆  Viral infection
- ◆  Neoplastic proliferation of lymphocytes (such as lymphocytic leukaemia)

### *Female - Primary colon carcinoma with liver metastases, aged 67 years*
*The white cell count (specifically the neutrophils) is raised due to tumour progression. The lymphocyte differential is continuing to fall.*

| | | | |
|---|---|---|---|
| **White cell count** (4-11 x10⁹/L) | 7.2 | 6.5 | 9.1 |
| Neutrophils (2.0-8.0 x10⁹/L) | 5.1 (71.4%) | 4.69 (72%) | 6.93 (76%) |
| Lymphocytes (1.0-4.0 x10⁹/L) | 1.5 (20.9%) | 1.31(20%) | 1.34 (15%) |
| Monocytes (<1.1 x10⁹/L) | 0.34 | 0.31 | 0.67 |
| Eosinophils (<0.6 x10⁹/L) | 0.12 | 0.16 | 0.13 |
| Basophils (<0.2 x10⁹/L) | 0.04 | 0.03 | 0.04 |
| **Platelets** (150-450 x10⁹/L) | 472 | 570 | 556 |

### *Male - Malignant squamous cell carcinoma, aged 65 years*
*The neutrophil count is elevated due to tumour progression. The lymphocyte differential is continuing to fall.*

| | | | | | |
|---|---|---|---|---|---|
| **White cell count** (4-11 x10⁹/L) | 10.2 | 16.4 | 13.8 | 29.4 | 47.7 |
| Neutrophils (2.0-8.0 x10⁹/L) | 7.5 (74%) | 12.6 77% | 10.3 (75%) | 20.6 (70%) | 45.7 (95%) |
| Lymphocytes (1.0-4.0 x10⁹/L) | 1.9 (19%) | 2.6 (16%) | 2.3 (17%) | 3.2 (11%) | 1.7 (3.5%) |
| **Platelets** (150-450 x10⁹/L) | 341 | 462 | 477 | 716 | 676 |

# The leukaemias

A group of malignant disorders of the white blood cells. The myeloid leukaemias refer to neoplastic proliferation of cells of the granulocytic series, and the lymphocytic leukaemias refer to cells of the lymphoid series. Classification of the leukaemias is made through histochemical staining techniques, morphological appearance and the identification of specific cell markers. The complications of anaemia and thrombocytopenia result from bone marrow infiltration of the neoplasm. Hypo-gammaglobulinaemia is also common.

## Male - diagnosed CLL 1996, aged 58 years

*The lymphocyte count is greatly elevated. Anaemia is found to be caused by a B12 deficiency as the iron study is normal. The patient started a modified Gerson Therapy in early 2000 and we saw an improvement in the WCC.*

|  | 17/06/96 | 27/02/97 | 18/01/99 | 20/3/00 | 10/01/01 | 08/02/01 |
|---|---|---|---|---|---|---|
| Haemoglobin (11.5-16.5 g/dL) | 15.5 | 14.5 | 12.9 | 11.8 | 10.5 | |
| RBC (3.8-5.5 x10$^{12}$/L) | 4.86 | 4.62 | 4.15 | | 3.17 | |
| PCV (0.35-0.47) | 0.45 | 0.45 | 0.42 | 0.35 | 0.32 | |
| MCV (80-99 fL) | 93 | 97 | 100 | 102.2 | 99.5 | |
| MCH (27-32 pg/cell) | 31.9 | 31.4 | 31.1 | | 33.2 | |
| **White cell count** (4-11 x10$^9$/L) | **66.9** | **96.5** | **207** | **142** | **148** | |
| Neutrophils (2.0-8.0 x10$^9$/L) | 3.7 | 4.2 | 16.8 | 1.4 | 1.5 | |
| Lymphocytes (1.0-4.0x 10$^9$/L) | **59.4** | **87.5** | **178.4** | **137.7** | **142.1** | |
| Monocytes (<1.1 x10$^9$/L) | 3.7 | 4.4 | 11.8 | 2.8 | 4.4 | |
| **Platelets** (150-450 x10$^9$/L) | 150 | 132 | | | 106 | |
| Iron (9-27 µmols/L) | | | | | | 13 |
| Transferrin (1.8-3.7 g/L) | | | | | | 2.8 |
| TIBC (10-55%) | | | | | | 18 |
| Ferritin (20-300 µg/L) | | | | | | 68 |
| Serum B12 (150-600 pmol/L) | | | | | | 123 |
| Serum Folate (5.9-45.0 nmol/L) | | | | | | 37.4 |

# Platelets

## Reference range  150-450x109/L

Platelets are derived from the megakaryocyte precursor in the bone marrow. Platelets are shed from the megakaryocyte, as areas of cytoplasm become demarcated by membranes. Thrombopoietin is a glycoprotein hormone produced by the liver and kidney which regulates the production of platelets. Thrombopoiesis is stimulated after haemorrhage, surgery, infection, tumoural activity and myeloid metaplasia. Tissue extracts from necrotic tumoural masses stimulate granulopoiesis (increased neutrophil count) and may stimulate thrombopoiesis. Sustained high levels of platelets are often a morbid sign in the terminally ill patient. There is a poor correlation between low platelet count and a bleeding tendency. Chronic liver disease, such as hepatitis C, predispose to thrombocytopenia.

## Indications for thrombocytopenia

- Cytotoxic drugs/during detoxification of chemotherapy
- Nutritional deficiencies (folic acid and B12)
- Bone marrow disease

- Viral infections
- Drugs (heparin, alcohol)
- Autoimmune disease (SLE, idiopathic thrombocytopenia purpura  (ITP), pernicious anaemia)
- Liver disease (hepatitis)
- Hypertension

### Female  - diagnosed chronic Hepatitis C, aged 65 years

The platelet count is greatly reduced due to liver damage by the Hepatitis C virus. As both the red and white cell counts were low, she was tested for B12 which was found to be sufficient.

|  | 23/11/09 | 01/05/10 | 05/07/10 |
|---|---|---|---|
| Alk. Phos (30-120 U/L) | 132 | 172 | 173 |
| Bilirubin (<25 µmol/L) | 18 | 31 | 28 |
| GGPT (<50 U/L) | 54 | 94 | 63 |
| AST (<41 U/L) | 182 | 374 | 259 |
| ALT (0-50 U/L) | 147 | 338 | 227 |
| RCC (3.8-5.5 x10$^{12}$/L) | 4.0 | 3.79 | 3.94 |
| WCC (4-11 x10$^9$/L) | 4.4 | 3.3 | 3.7 |
| Platelets (150-450 x10$^9$/L) | 56 | 49 | 50 |
| Ferritin (15-165 µg/L) |  |  | 312 |
| B12 (190-900 ng/mL) |  | 1159 |  |
| ESR (0-15 mm/hr) |  |  | 25 |
| CRP (<6 mg/L) |  |  | 6 |
| Comment | Thrombocytopenia is due to liver damage | B12 levels are normal | Chronic inflammation increases ferritin |

# Liver function tests

There are several blood indicators which are used to assess liver function: bilirubin, the liver enzymes (ALP, AST, ALT, GGTP, LDH) and the plasma proteins (albumin and globulin). The most sensitive indicators of liver disease are the hepatic enzymes. Elevated bilirubin levels indicate disorders of the bile metabolism/excretion, while abnormal levels of the plasma proteins can reflect an impaired functional capacity of the liver (decreased albumin) and chronic liver disease, acute or chronic infection, auto-immune disease, myeloma (increase in globulins). Abnormal results are a reflection of the disease process, not its cause. We can monitor these results as an indication of disease progression, flare-up and disease regression.

## Reference Ranges

| | | |
|---|---|---|
| Total Protein | 60-82 | g/L |
| Albumin | 35-50 | g/L |
| Globulin | 20-35 | g/L |
| Alk. Phos | 30-120 | U/L |
| Bilirubin | <25 | µmols /L |
| Bilirubin conjugated | < 1 | µmols/L |
| GGTP | <50 | U/L |
| AST | <41 | U/L |
| ALT | 0-50 | U/L |
| LDH | 50-280 | U/L |

# Bilirubin

## Bilirubin metabolism

Bilirubin is formed from the degradation of haemoglobin. The haem part of the molecule contains iron and bilirubin. The iron is recycled and the bilirubin is transported, bound to albumin, to the liver. Here it is taken up by the hepatocytes and undergoes conjugation with glucuronic acid before being excreted in the bile. In the gut it is oxidised to a brown pigment, urobilin, which gives the stools their characteristic colour.

### Indications for elevated bilirubin

- cholestasis (biliary obstruction)
- liver disease
- haemolysis
- Gilbert's syndrome

### Symptoms

Jaundice, anorexia, vomiting, weight loss, pale stools, dark orange urine

### Reference range

| | | |
|---|---|---|
| Total | 3-25 | µmols/L |
| Conjugated | <1 | µmols/L |

## Interpreting Blood Results for Bilirubin

The total bilirubin refers to the conjugated and unconjugated bilirubin in plasma. Under normal conditions most of the bilirubin in plasma will be unconjugated. Unconjugated bilirubin is not water soluble and therefore cannot be excreted by the kidneys.

### Unconjugated hyperbilirubinaemia

- Liver disease - defective conjugation
- Haemolysis - exceeds the capacity of the liver to remove and conjugate the pigment
- Gilbert's syndrome - defective conjugation

### Conjugated hyperbilirubinaemia

Increased levels of conjugated bilirubin occurs in cholestasis and a leakage of conjugated bilirubin enters the circulation. Conjugated bilirubin is water soluble and therefore the urine will be deep orange. In complete obstruction no bilirubin will reach the gastrointestinal tract, no urobilin will be formed and the stools will be pale.

## Causes of cholestasis

- Gallstones
- Primary or secondary tumours in the liver pressing and occluding the bile ducts
- Tumour deposits in small bile ducts
- Advanced pancreatic carcinoma
- Carcinoma of the bile ducts (cholangiocarcinoma)
- Cirrhosis
- Hepatitis

### Indications in the blood results for the differential diagnosis of cholestasis and jaundice

#### Intrinsic hepatocellular disease

↑ unconjugated bilirubin
↑ transaminases

#### Intra- and extra-hepatic cholestasis

↑ conjugated bilirubin
↑ alkaline phosphatase (ALP)

### Female - Primary colon carcinoma with liver metastases, aged 67 years

Cholestasis due to obstruction of the biliary tree by liver metastases. ALP and GGTP are elevated due to enzyme induction and may occur before cholestasis is apparent (elevated conjugated plasma bilirubin). Elevated transaminase levels indicate hepatocellular damage and appear post cholestasis. The elevated cholesterol may reflect defective bile acid synthesis by the hepatocytes.

| | 19/9/00 | 8/10/00 | 12/11/00 |
|---|---|---|---|
| Alk. Phos (30-120 U/L) | 496 | 294 | 1700 |
| Bilirubin (<25 μmol/L) | 3 | 4 | 285 |
| Bilirubin conjugated (<1 μmol/L) | | | 210 |
| GGTP (<50U/L) | 197 | 120 | 860 |
| AST (<41 U/L) | 65 | 37 | 302 |
| ALT (<50 U/L) | 60 | 30 | 361 |
| LD (50-280 U/L) | 192 | 195 | 296 |
| Cholesterol (<5.5 mmol/L) | 4.3 | 4.2 | 17.2 |

# Plasma enzymes

There are five plasma enzymes that are routinely measured as indicators of liver function:

> aspartate transaminase (AST)
> alanine transaminase (ALT)
> alkaline phosphatase (ALP)
> gamma-glutamyl transpeptidase (GGTP)
> lactate dehydrogenase (LDH)

# Transaminases: ALT and AST

AST (aspartate transaminase) and ALT (alanine transaminase) are both widely distributed in body tissues. These enzymes are released from tissues as a consequence of tissue destruction. Therefore high levels of these enzymes indicate tissue destruction, and specific iso-enzyme studies will reveal the tissue of origination. ALT is more specific to liver disease than AST.

## *Indications*

- ◆ AST levels are increased in liver disease, hypoxaemia, myocardial infarction, skeletal muscle disease, cholestasis, pancreatitis, haemolysis, alcohol abuse.
- ◆ ALT levels are increased liver disease

## *Reference Ranges*

AST    < 41 U/L
ALT    < 50 U/L

## Interpreting blood results for AST and ALT

In liver disease where there is liver cell destruction the transaminases may be increased by 20 times ULN (upper level of normal). ALT levels are a more reliable indication of liver disease than AST. If cholestasis occurs secondary to hepatocellular damage, then both AST and ALT will be increased along with bilirubin levels prior to cholestasis.

# Alkaline Phosphatase (ALP)

## *Indications*

- ◆ Liver metastases/liver disease
- ◆ Cholestasis
- ◆ Bone metastases
- ◆ Bronchial carcinoma

## *Reference range*

ALP    30-120 U/L

## Interpreting blood results for ALP

High concentrations of the enzyme alkaline phosphatase are found in the liver, bone (osteoblasts) and the intestinal epithelium. Elevated levels, depending upon the diagnosis and total pattern of plasma enzyme activities, may indicate malignancies of the bone or liver (primary or secondary tumours). It is not uncommon for levels to be elevated in flare-ups and therefore one reading is not diagnostically reliable. Iso-enzyme studies can identify the tissue source of ALP, if there is doubt with the interpretation of blood results. ALP may also be elevated in bronchial carcinoma where there is ectopic production of ALP by the tumour.

## Bone metastases/re-modelling

ALP is most specific for bone metastases and indicates increased osteoblastic activity. Osteoblastic activity is stimulated in response to increased osteoclastic activity which occurs both in disease progression and during bone healing. It can indicate either an exacerbation of the disease, or recalcification due to bone re-modelling. Several readings need to be obtained over a period of a few months to reach a diagnosis.

### Female - Breast cancer with bone metastases, aged 53 years

*The current diagnosis of bone metastases and the absence of abnormal liver function readings indicate progression of the bone metastases. The elevated calcium readings also confirm this diagnosis.*

|  | 08/04/98 | 24/06/98 | 13/8/98 | 02/11/98 | 25/02/99 |
|---|---|---|---|---|---|
| Calcium (2.10-2.55 mmol/L) | 2.35 | 2.34 | 2.41 | 2.47 | 2.82 |
| Phosphate (0.75-1.35 mmol/L) | 1.26 | 1.39 | 1.05 | 1.12 | 1.32 |
| Alk. Phos (30-120 U/L) | 46 | 48 | 55 | 86 | 121 |
| Bilirubin (<25 µmol/L) | 16 | 12 | 14 | 6 | 10 |
| GGTP (<50 U/L) | 20 | 19 | 16 | 29 | 42 |
| AST (<41 U/L) | 27 | 26 | 26 | 19 | 37 |
| ALT (0-50 U/L) | 30 | 19 | 16 | 21 | 18 |
| LD (50-280 U/L) | 171 | 161 | 165 | 166 | 209 |
| Cholesterol (<5.5 mmol/L) | 5.0 | 4.8 | 5.1 | 5.0 | 5.5 |

## Liver disease

Elevated levels of ALP occur as a consequence of cholestasis where ALP may be increased 10 times ULN (upper level of normal). Elevated levels are not due to cell damage but to enzyme induction caused by the disease process. Other indicators of liver disease, such as elevated bilirubin levels and/or AST/ALT, will preclude other causes such as bone cancer.

### Male - Colo-rectal carcinoma with metastases to liver and lungs, aged 55 years

*Abnormal liver function tests reveal hepatocellular damage and cholestasis. A stent was placed in the blocked bile duct alleviating the condition.*

|  | 22/05/00 | 30/06/00 | 14/07/00 | 08/08/00 | 06/009/00 | 18/09/00 |
|---|---|---|---|---|---|---|
| Alk. Phos (30-120 U/L) | 87 | 896 | 870 | 260 | 2584 | 736 |
| Bilirubin (<25 µmol/L) | 11 | 11 | 139 | 61 | 194 | 30 |
| GGTP (<50 U/L) | 41 | 1123 | 1283 | 120 | 1696 | 494 |
| AST (<41 U/L) | 25 | 308 | | | 287 | 58 |
| ALT (0-50 U/L) | 33 | 369 | | | 476 | 67 |
| LD (50-280 U/L) (370-680) | 441 | 1048 | | | | 403 |

# Gamma-glutamyl transpeptidase (GGTP)

GGTP is found in the liver, kidney and pancreas. Elevated levels, due to enzyme induction, indicate hepatobiliary disease, and this is of no value in distinguishing between hepatocellular disease or cholestasis.

## Indications
- Cholestasis
- Hepatocellular damage (liver disease, alcohol, cytotoxic drugs, cirrhosis, autoimmune hepatitis)

## Reference range
GGTP < 50 U/L

## Interpreting blood results for GGTP
Elevated levels of GGTP are not due to cell damage but to enzyme induction caused by the disease process. In cases of obstruction GGTP may rise before ALP.

# Lactate dehydrogenase (LDH)

High concentrations of this enzyme are found in the liver, skeletal muscle and kidneys, heart muscle, red blood cells, white blood cells. High levels reflect rapid cell turnover and/or damage to these tissues, and iso-enzyme studies will reveal the tissue of origin. High levels in lymphoma indicate a poor prognosis as there is a correlation between enzyme activity and tumour bulk.

## Indications
- liver disease
- megaloblastic and haemolytic anaemias
- lymphoma
- myocardial infarction
- haemolytic crises
- pulmonary disease

## Reference range
LDH      50 - 280 U/L

### Female - Non-Hodgkin's Lymphoma, aged 24 years

|  | 8/11/99 | 8/12/99 | 10/01/00 | 11/02/00 | 24/02/00 | 16/03/00 |
|---|---|---|---|---|---|---|
| General chemistry |  |  |  |  |  |  |
| Alk. Phos (30-120 U/L) | 95 | 77 | 86 | 83 | 84 | 89 |
| Bilirubin (<25 µmol/L) | 13 | 4 | 5 | 4 | 5 | 8 |
| GGTP (<50U/L) | 7 | 9 | 9 | 7 | 5 | 6 |
| AST (<41 U/L) | 23 | 16 | 23 |  | 19 | 21 |
| ALT (0-50 U/L) | 17 | 15 | 20 | 18 | 17 | 20 |
| LD (50-280 U/L) |  | 199 |  |  | 334 | 316 |

# Plasma proteins

There are over 100 different types of plasma proteins in serum which are divided into two groups: albumin and the globulins. The globulins include transport proteins, such as hormone binding globulins, metal transport globulins (transferrin and caeruloplasmin), enzymes, low density lipoproteins and the immunoglobulins. Electrophoresis can separate the globulins into discrete bands (alpha, beta, and gamma globulins) if a specific diagnosis is required (say auto-immune disease with increased circulation of auto-antibodies, inflammatory disease, multiple myeloma, B cell lymphomas, CLL) but in general the globulin concentration represents the gamma globulin group (immuno-globulins, specifically IgG, as its concentration is much higher than the other immunoglobulins in this group). Any significant changes in the total protein concentration will usually only reflect changes in the albumin and gamma globulin concentrations, as these two plasma proteins are the more abundant.

# Albumin

The albumin concentration is a useful assessment of liver function, as the liver synthesizes this protein. In known liver disease a decrease in albumin indicates liver failure. Albumin is a carrier protein and has the greatest influence on the plasma oncotic pressure (80%). Low albumin levels lead to leakage of plasma into the ECF leading to oedema, and if chronic, ascites, a late feature of liver failure. As albumin has a half-life of 20 days, the true clinical picture may not become apparent for 3 weeks or so.

Hypo-albuminaemia can also occur as a consequence of the nephrotic syndrome where albumin is lost via the urine or in chronic inflammation due to malignancy, such as in cancers with peritoneal/omental involvement, where albumin moves into the extracellular space along with the inflammatory fluid leading to ascites. This occurs in the terminal phase, such as in ovarian cancer or cancers that have metastased to the peritoneum.

### Female - Rheumatoid arthritis and NIDDM aged 49 years
*In the absence of known liver disease then abnormal albumin results initiated further tests which indicated NIDDM with related nephropathy causing urinary albumin losses.*

| | 17/07/14 | 16/09/14 | 29/10/14 | 17/03/15 |
|---|---|---|---|---|
| Glucose (3.0-6.0 mmol/L) | | | 7.3 | 6.2 |
| HbA1c (<7%) | | 5.6 | 5.8 | |
| Albumin (35-50 g/L) | 29 | 30 | 29 | 32 |
| Globulin (20-35 g/L) | 45 | 45 | 51 | 45 |
| Urea (2.5-8.0 mmol/L) | | 3.6 | 3.5 | 2.2 |
| Creatinine (40-110 umol/L) | 62 | 64 | 54 | 55 |
| White cell count (4-11 x109/L) | 13.4 | 12.0 | 12.5 | 10.1 |
| Neutrophils (2.0-8.0 x109/L) | 9.1 | 8.9 | 8.3 | 6.0 |
| ESR (<15 mm/h) | 44 | 41 | 2 | 8 |
| CRP (<6 mg/L) | 83.8 | 47.6 | 42.2 | 41.8 |
| RF (<20) | 117 | 112 | 101 | |
| Urinary Albumin (<20 mg/L) | | | 37 | 13 |
| Urinary Creatinine (8-16 mmol/L) | | | 29.4 | 20.1 |

It is important to monitor the albumin levels, particularly through the early phase of the therapy. On the very restricted protein diet occasionally the albumin falls below the lower level of normal, and this may indicate insufficient dietary protein. Under these circumstances, it is wise to enquire about general quantities of foods taken, as many patients do not feel like eating because they feel full with all the juices, specifically the oatmeal and potatoes, before you introduce other forms of protein, such as the non-fat soured milk protein. If the patient is indeed taking all the foods in sufficient quantities, then you may need to increase the protein in the diet.

# Globulins

In malignancy and chronic inflammatory conditions you will see a diffuse increase in the globulins.

## Hypergammaglobulinaemia
- Acute and chronic infection
- Chronic liver disease (especially if autoimmune in origin)
- Autoimmune disease (rheumatoid arthritis, SLE)

## Hypogammaglobulinaemia
Haematological malignancies, due to the replacement of normal bone marrow by malignant cells, frequently results in anaemia and decreased synthesis of normal immunoglobulins:

- CLL
- Multiple myeloma
- Hodgkin's
- Cytotoxic drugs
- Severe protein-losing states (nephrotic syndrome)
- Increased catabolism (uncontrolled diabetes, corticosteroid therapy)

# The paraproteins

A paraprotein is an immunoglobulin produced by a single clone of B cells. They are characteristic of malignant proliferation of B cells, occurring most frequently in multiple myeloma, solitary plasmacytoma, Waldenström's macroglobulinaemia and to a lesser extent in CLL and B cell lymphomas. In Multiple Myeloma, the tumour produces light chain immunoglobulins only (Bence Jones proteins) which are rapidly cleared in the urine and will not be detected in the serum. They are a useful marker indicating disease progression/regression, as the amount of paraprotein produced in myeloma is a reflection of the tumour mass.

# Thyroid function tests

*Reference ranges*

TSH      0.4-4.0  mIU/L

fT4      10-25    pmol/L

fT3      2.5-5.3  pmol/L

The thyroid hormones, thyroxine (T4) and triiodothyronine (T3) are synthesized and secreted by the thyroid gland. They are under the control of TSH (Thyroglobulin Stimulating Hormone) which is secreted from the pituitary gland in response to low circulating levels of these hormones (positive feed-back mechanism). TSH is the most sensitive index of thyroid function and is the preferred test for thyroid function. If the TSH is outside the normal reference range, then further tests on free thyroid levels are the best means of assessing the degree of thyroid dysfunction. It is usual to find low TSH levels in patients who are taking thyroid supplementation, as the medication will naturally suppress TSH.

Both T3 (triiodothyronine) and T4 (thyroxine) are produced by the thyroid gland. 99.95 percent of both these hormones are bound to TBG (thyroid binding globulin) which is produced by the liver, while the 0.05 percent remains in its free state and biologically active. It is the measurements of the free thyroid hormones (fT3, fT4) which indicate thyroid activity.

It is the fT3 which is physiologically active and although serum levels are 2-3 times lower than fT4, fT4 converts at the liver and other tissues to fT3 through a process known as de-iodination. 80 percent of fT3 is derived from fT4. The anterior pituitary also converts fT4 to fT3 and it is believed that the pituitary measures thyroid hormone status through the change in the concentration of fT3.

Thyroxine (T4)

Triiodothyronine (T3)

Reverse Triiodothyronine (T3)

Under stress adrenal production of cortisol leads to low T4 production by the thyroid and poor conversion of T4 to T3 by the tissues, or results in increased reverse triiodothyronine (rT3) which is inactive. This is a protective measure which reduces the basal metabolic rate to help conserve our energy resources. The minerals selenium, zinc, and copper are cofactors for the enzyme that is necessary for conversion of T4 to T3. A vitamin B12 deficiency also appears to interfere with the activity of thyroid hormones throughout the body.

## Mode of action

fT3 enters the cells and binds to specific receptors in the nuclei, which stimulates the synthesis of mRNA, leading to increased protein synthesis including that of hormones and enzymes. Thyroid hormones stimulate the basal metabolic rate, but the precise mechanism is unknown. Thyroid hormone signals cellular mitochondria to replicate and hence increases cellular respiration, potentiates the action of catecholamines and increases cardiac output (tachycardia, arrhythmias, palpitation). These effects increase pulse rate, temperature and anxiety levels. They may also be accompanied by weight loss, but with an increased appetite. The liver determines the availability of fT4 through its production of thyroid binding globulins and the subsequent binding of thyroid hormone. Oestrogen increases the liver's production of TBGs which then binds with and inactivates more thyroid hormone. As a consequence we may see an increased rate of goitre or the onset of autoimmune thyroiditis in women during pregnancy or during the peri-menopausal period. Supporting the liver in its detoxification of oestrogen will reduce the burden on the thyroid gland, by default of reducing the stimulation for liver TBG production.

# Natural thyroid hormone

Natural thyroid hormone contains both T3 and T4 and therefore replaces both the inactive and active hormone and reduces conversion requirements. Thyroxine is a synthetic form of T4 and requires conversion to its active form. The body can then regulate the degree of conversions to T3 and protect itself against over-prescribing. Occasionally, patients may not be able to rapidly clear excess T3 and this may lead to a state of thyrotoxicosis, and they may need to switch from the natural thyroid to the synthetic form. On the other hand, patients who do not do well on thyroxine, will do much better on natural thyroid or compounds that include T3 as their conversion rates may be slow, or they may be under stress.

# Interpreting thyroid function tests

## Hypothyroidism

An elevated TSH indicates the earliest change in the development of hypothyroidism. fT4, on its own, is not a sufficient indicator of thyroid function, as it may be normal in the presence of a lowered fT3. Even though the reference range for TSH is <4.0, a reading above 2.0 can be regarded as a subclinical hypothyroid state, and treatment is best instigated at this juncture rather than waiting until the gland loses its capacity to produce thyroid hormone or be responsive to iodine supplementation. If there is a sub-clinical undiagnosed autoimmune hypothyroid condition then treatment with iodine (Lugol's solution) may aggravate the gland and suppress thyroid hormone output. You will then see a further increase in TSH which will resolve once the iodine is withdrawn. Oestrogen dominance, as mentioned above, has an adverse effect on thyroid function leading to a reduction in fT3 and fT4 and elevated TSH which forces the thyroid gland to work harder. If the gland is already subclinically hypothyroid it can lead to either goitre or Hashimoto's thyroiditis. Invariably, supporting the liver in its clearance of oestrogens during these phases can rectify the imbalance and restore thyroid function, unless it is compounded by a primary iodine deficiency.

**In hypothyroidism:**

- ↑ TSH
- ↓ to normal fT4
- ↓ to normal fT3

*Female, 33 yr - Myasthenia Gravis with Hashimoto's thyroiditis (before and after thyroid medication)*

|  | before medication | after medication |
|---|---|---|
| TSH (0.4-4.0 mIU/L) | 15.83 | 1.58 |
| FT4 (10-25 pmol/L) | 9.4 | 11.2 |

### Female, 22 yr - Primary Iodine deficiency

*Supplementing with Lugol's solution in a primary iodine deficiency state will lead to resolution of the subclinical hypothyroid readings.*

|  | 22/12/06 | 12/07/07 |
|---|---|---|
| TSH (0.4-4.0 mIU/L) | 2.38 | 1.56 |
| Comment | subclinical hypothyroid due to primary iodine deficiency. Recommended Lugol's 1/2 strength solution x 12 drops over a 4 month period | |

### Female, 63 yr - Hashimoto's thyroiditis, before and after supplementation with Lugol's solution

*Self-medicating with Lugol's solution as a standalone treatment in an autoimmune thyroiditis state led to an exacerbation of the clinical condition.*

|  | 16/04/07 | 07/08/07 | 19/09/07 |
|---|---|---|---|
| TSH (0.4-4.0 mIU/L) | 9.0 | 90 | 3.7 |
| FT4 (10-25 pmol/L) | 12.0 | 4.0 | |
| fT3 (3.5-6.0 pmol/L) | 4.6 | | |
| Comment | Based on these results decided to administer Lugol's 1/2 strength at 18 drops daily. | Iodine has dramatically suppressed thyroid output increasing TSH | Thyroid results 6 weeks post ceasing Lugol's |

### Female, 45 yr - Perimenopausal sub-clinical hypothyroidism, before and after resolving oestrogen dominance.

*Supporting liver detoxification of oestrogen naturally reduces the stress on the thyroid gland and the production of TSH.*

|  | 25/01/13 | 08/05/13 |
|---|---|---|
| TSH (0.4-4.0 mIU/L) | 2.26 | 1.26 |
| FT4 (10-25 pmol/L) | 15.0 | 14.4 |
| fT3 (3.5-6.0 pmol/L) | 5.0 | 4.5 |
| Comment | subclinical hypothyroidism due to oestrogen dominance | |

### Female, 48 yr - Hashimoto's thyroiditis

*This patient had to switch from natural thyroid to thyroxine as she had symptoms of thyrotoxicosis on the natural thyroid with an elevated fT3, and the natural thyroid failed to reduce the antibody count. Sometimes these readings cannot be explained, so the practitioner may have to go by symptoms and blood readings and switch medications until the patient feels well and the blood readings reflect a reduced antibody load.*

|  | 15/10/12 | 01/02/13 | 26/02/13 | 21/05/13 | 16/07/13 |
|---|---|---|---|---|---|
| TSH (0.4-4.0 mIU/L) | 0.02 |  | 0.19 | 0.038 | 0.01 |
| FT4 (10-25 pmol/L) | 13.5 | 14.0 | 10.3 | 13.7 | 20.5 |
| fT3 (3.5-6.0 pmol/L) |  | 7.3 | 3.36 | 7.2 | 4.1 |
| TPOAb (<60) |  | 177 | 255.3 | 207 | 140 |
| TGAb (<34) |  |  | 50.6 |  |  |
| Recommended | Thyroid 2.5 gr Lugol's 1/2 strength x 6 drops | Thyroid 2 gr Lugol's 1/2 strength x 4 drops | Thyroid 2.5 gr Lugol's 1/2 strength x 2 drops | Recommended thyroxine as fT3 was elevated | **Thyroxine** |
| Comment | *No fT3 reading* | *No TSH reading Hashimoto's diagnosed Reduced thyroid medication due to elevated fT3* | *Elevated antibodies fT3 and fT4 reduced; increased thyroid to former dose* | *Antibodies reducing but fT3 elevated* | *Antibodies reducing, fT3 and fT4 within normal range* |

## Hashimoto's thyroiditis

This often arises after a prolonged period of subclinical hyopthyroidism usually referenced when TSH lies between 2.0 -4.0 mIU/L.. The thyroid gland will be targeted by increased levels of TSH which will stimulate the activity of the iodine trap (Na/Iodide symporter) and enhance the rapid uptake of iodine.

TSH also stimulates TPO (thyroperoxidase) which forms hydrogen peroxide to rapidly oxidize iodide to become a more reactive iodine (atomic iodine). This leads to iodination of thyroglobulin and thyroid hormone synthesis. Each thyroglobulin molecule can take up either one or two iodine radicals, and couple to form the T3 or T4 residues.

You can appreciate when TSH is high, the gland can rapidly take up available iodine and is under increased oxidative stress. It is believed that intense stimulation by TSH causes a release of TPO, thyroglobulin (TG) and thyroid hormones which may lead to a transient hyperthyroid state. In fact this often precedes Hashimoto's thyroiditis. Release of these thyroid products into the circulation may stimulate an antibody response to TPO and TG (TPOAb and TGAb). The onset of Hashimoto's or autoimmune thyroiditis is believed to be triggered by a period of intense oxidative stress on the gland. One of the purposes of thyroid supplementation is to reduce the TSH, which then reduces the oxidative stress on the gland, which is then reflected by reduced antibody counts.

Selenium methionine at 400µg has been found to protect the thyroid from H2O2 excess and reduce TPOAb readings.

## Hyperthyroidism (thyrotoxicosis)

A suppressed TSH with normal fT4 and fT3 indicates the earliest phase of thyrotoxicosis. fT4, on its own, is not a sufficient indicator of thyroid function, as it may be normal in the presence of a raised fT3. In hyperthyroidism the fT3 is raised to a proportionally greater extent than fT4. An increased fT4 with a normal or lowered fT3 can indicate impaired conversion of fT4 to fT3. Treatment with corticosteroids can cause TSH to be undetectable, as cortisol inhibits TSH secretion.

- ↓ TSH
- ↑ to normal fT4
- ↑ fT3

### Female, 60 yr - Adenocarcinoma in lymph nodes in neck (secondary to possible breast cancer)

*This patient is hyperthyroid due to multi-nodular goitre. A thyroid scan was delayed, as this patient had been self-medicating with Lugol's over a six-month period. Invariably, with hyperthyroid states, low to moderate doses of iodine stimulates thyroid hormone output, whereas high doses (90mg/day or 30 drops, 1/2 strength) will suppress output. Lugol's was stopped towards the end of November.*

|                    | 24/08/00 | 17/11/00 | 11/01/01 |
|--------------------|----------|----------|----------|
| TSH (0.4-4.0 mIU/L)| 0.38     | 0.04     | 0.10     |
| FT4 (10-25 pmol/L) | 26.5     | 30.2     | 18.8     |

### On Replacement Therapy

- ↓ TSH
- normal fT4 (may be slightly elevated)
- normal fT3 (if raised, then replacement therapy is excessive)

## The sick euthyroid syndrome

The sick euthyroid syndrome occurs in sickness (non-thyroidal), infections, malignancy, starvation and stress. Thyroid readings indicate reduced TSH and fT3 levels. These abnormal results occur due to a reduced TSH output (stress/corticosteroids will suppress output), an increased conversion of fT4 to rT3 (reverse T3), which is biologically inactive, and to increased breakdown of thyroid hormone to release iodine. Iodine can be rapidly concentrated 300-fold by leucocytes increasing their defence power during infectious and/or inflammatory states. If iodine stores are low, then iodine will be diverted away from thyroid hormone synthesis and the de-iodination of existing thyroid hormone will be accelerated to generate sufficient inorganic iodine. The overall effect will be a reduction ingeneral metabolism, an important factor in stress where resources need to be protected against loss.

# Iodine

During the early to mid-1900s iodine was routinely prescribed by physicians for thyroid disorders. Large amounts were used to suppress the gland in hyperthyroidism (90mg/day = 30 drops, 1/2 strength solution; 15 drops, full-strength) and smaller amounts, ranging from 12.5mg - 50mg daily (4-16 drops, 1/2 strength or 2-8 drops full strength) for hypothyroid goitre due to primary iodine deficiency. Prescribing iodine fell out of favour with the advent of synthetically produced thyroid hormone.[3] However, although thyroid medication will address hypothyroidism it will not resolve iodine deficiency which has many diverse activities in the body. Furthermore, if hypothyroidism is caused by a primary iodine deficiency then taking thyroid hormone will inhibit the gland from taking up iodine reducing its capacity to re-iodinate.

Nowadays it is not unusual to see iodine deficiency in our population due to low dietary intake and exposure to fluoride and chlorine which competes with iodine at the thyroid gland. When hypothyroidism is due to a primary iodine deficiency and the gland is pathologically intact, supplemental iodine will correct the condition. However, in hypothyroid states due to a functionally reduced capacity to produce thyroid hormone by the gland, as in autoimmune thyroiditis (Hashimoto's), iodine supplementation may suppress output of thyroid hormone and cause increases in TSH and a worsening of the condition. It can be difficult to ascertain from the case or the TSH reading the underlying cause of the hypothyroid state unless the patient has a known autoimmune thyroiditis, but a blood test request to determine the presence of thyroid antibodies (TPOAb or TgAb) will indicate if the patient does indeed have an autoimmune condition.

On the Gerson Therapy, we rarely supplement iodine without the thyroid hormone, therefore there is little danger of suppressing the gland, but rather it is just a matter of balancing the two medications until you achieve the desired results. However, it must be remembered that a lowered TSH, fT4 and fT3 may indicate the sick euthyroid syndrome. Thyroid function tests should always be interpreted in the context of the overall blood results and the general condition of the patient.

In addition to its beneficial role in supporting optimum thyroid activity, Dr. Gerson found iodine to be a decisive factor in the normal differentiation of cells and used it to counteract the decrease in cell differentiation. He also found that iodine invaded cancer tissue when inflamed, not otherwise. Smaller iodine doses appeared to make cancer cells grow more rapidly, but the larger dose given at the beginning was seen to inhibit excessive growth. He found that the combination of iodine, thyroid and niacin helped check cancerous growth and aided surrounding tissues to regain their electrical potentials. Dr. Gerson states that the thyroid and Lugol's medication speeds up Na, Cl and water elimination and paves the way for the re-filling of the cell with potassium. Healing was also found to be accelerated when the thyroid and Lugol's medications were increased. Chlorine, from chlorinated water and table salt, and fluoride compete with iodine and patients are asked to check their water supply and take appropriate steps, such as distillation, to ensure that the water is clean of these contaminants. Bathing in chlorinated water is prohibited for these reasons.

When prescribing thyroid hormone and Lugol's for the non-cancer patient, it is recommended that you monitor thyroid function and manipulate the doses in the manner described to ensure that the thyroid is functioning optimally and not suppressed.

# The electrolytes

*Reference ranges*

| | | |
|---|---|---|
| Sodium | 136-146 | mmol/L |
| Potassium | 3.5-5.2 | mmol/L |
| Calcium | 2.10-2.55 | mmol/L |

# Sodium

*Reference range*

Sodium          136-146 mmol/L

Sodium is the principal cation of the ECF, governs the osmolality of the ECF and is the chief determinant of the extracellular fluid volume. The clinical features of sodium depletion (hyponatraemia) will arise primarily as a result of decreased ECF volume: e.g. peripheral circulatory failure, syncope, postural dizziness, and weakness. Mental symptoms include disorientation, apprehension, lethargy, apathy, confusion and coma.

The concentration of sodium in the ECF governs the osmolality of the extracellular fluids (including blood serum). Osmolality of the ECF is maintained in the range 282-295mmol/kg water, and any fluctuation outside this range (dilution or concentration) is detected by the osmoreceptors in the hypothalamus. A rise in the concentration of sodium (osmolality) stimulates the hypothalamic thirst centre (promoting a desire to drink) and the hypothalamic osmoreceptors which cause the release of vasopressin (ADH - anti-diuretic hormone) which renders the renal collecting ducts permeable to water where re-absorption of water takes place. Hence sodium is diluted in the serum and the concentration returns to normal.

A fall in osmolality leads to a fall in the blood volume (the ECF volume of the body is determined by sodium status, therefore a fall in ECF sodium causes a fall in total blood volume), and mechanisms in the kidney and adrenal glands kick in to raise the blood pressure and increase the reabsorption of sodium and water by the kidneys. In brief, a fall in the blood volume leads to a reduced glomerular filtration rate (GFR). The kidneys release an enzyme, renin, in response to this, which catalyses the formation of angiotensin 1 from angiotensinogen. Angiotensin 1 is metabolised to angiotensin 2, by angiotensin converting enzyme, during its passage through the lungs. Angiotensin 2 constricts the blood vessels, increasing the resistance and thus raising blood pressure. It also stimulates the release of aldosterone from the adrenal cortex. Aldosterone promotes sodium reabsorption (in return for potassium secretion) in the distal tubules of the kidney.  As sodium is reabsorbed, so too is water, and both blood volume and sodium concentration are returned to normal. However, any substantial decrease (10%) in blood  volume stimulates vasopressin release to restore blood volume and this will be at the expense of any decrease in osmolality. Osmolar controls are therefore over-ridden in severe hypovolaemia, and a dilutional hyponatraemia ensues.

Changes in ECF concentration of sodium are always a secondary phenomenon to an underlying pathology. Treatment is therefore dependent upon correction of the underlying disease.

## Causes of hypernatraemia

*Hypernatraemia is rarely a problem. The causes include pure water depletion and hypotonic fluid loss, as with diarrhoea. However, chronic diarrhoea leads to hyponatraemia. Sodium excess refers to total ECF sodium, not the osmolar concentration, and is usually caused by diseases that lead to renal reabsorption of both sodium and water.*

**Water depletion**

- Renal tubular disorders
- Diabetes insipidus
- Diabetes mellitus
- Osmotic diuretics
- Diarrhoea
- Decreased fluid intake

**Primary sodium excess**

*Increased intake*

- Excessive parenteral administration

*Decreased excretion*

- Acute/chronic renal failure

*Increased tubular reabsorption*

- Primary mineralocorticoid excess
- Ectopic secretion of ACTH by tumours
- Cushing's and Conn's syndrome
- Congestive cardiac failure
- Nephrotic syndrome
- Hepatic cirrhosis with ascites
- Renal artery stenosis

*With increased tubular reabsorption the rise in sodium concentration is compensated for by the rise in water retention. In cases where there is oedema, the blood sodium concentration may be reduced, while the total ECF sodium is increased.*

## Causes of hyponatraemia

- Vomiting
- Diarrhoea
- Diuretic therapy
- Mineralocorticoid deficiency (Addison's)
- Acute tubular necrosis
- Burns
- Excessive sweating
- Sick cell syndrome
- Dilutional

*Clinical conditions that increase the ECF volume*

- Congestive cardiac failure
- Nephrotic syndrome
- Hypoproteinaemic states
- Hepatic cirrhosis with ascites

*In these case the blood sodium concentration may be reduced, but paradoxically the total sodium in the ECF will be increased.*

- Hyperglycaemia *(glucose increases ECF osmolality, which causes a shift of water from the ICF to the ECF, which lowers the concentration of sodium)*
- SIADH (ectopic secretion from tumours of ADH)

## Sick cell syndrome

Sodium concentration can start to fall in a wide variety of illnesses and advanced malignancy. At the present time various hypotheses have been put forward. One theory is that the body resets its osmostat and another is the "sick cell syndrome". It is thought that in the sick cell syndrome there is an iso-osmotic shift of water between the ICF and the ECF, caused by a disturbance of the major cations, potassium and sodium. There are two possible mechanisms put forward. In the sick cell there is:

♦ increased permeability, which could result in the movement of sodium to the ICF. Water usually follows sodium and therefore under normal circumstances no decrease in overall ECF sodium concentration would be noted. However, it is thought that if sodium was bound by intracellular molecules, water would not follow the sodium into the cell, resulting in a decreased ECF osmolality, which would lead to hyponatraemia.

♦ decreased and/or partial metabolism leads to acidic build-up in the cell. Intracellular buffering of acidity (H+ moves into the cell for buffering) displaces K+ (H+ and K+ exchange to maintain electrical neutrality) and both the cellular potassium depletion and loss/decreased synthesis of intracellular organic molecules will lower the intracellular osmolality. Water will then move to the ECF (higher concentration) to maintain isotonicity. A dilutional hyponatraemia ensues.

## In health

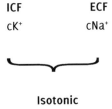

ICF       ECF
cK+       cNa+

Isotonic

## In Disease

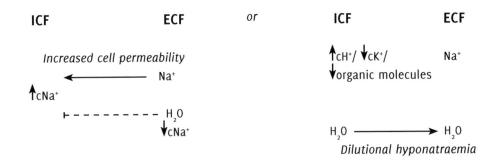

ICF       ECF     or     ICF       ECF

*Increased cell permeability*

←———— Na+

↑cNa+

⊢ – – – – – – – H₂O
↓cNa+

↑cH+/ ↓cK+/    Na+
↓organic molecules

H₂O ———→ H₂O
*Dilutional hyponatraemia*

# Dehydration

Both sodium and water losses can occur in the severely ill patient. They will experience low blood pressure, dizziness and fainting, and may need to be hospitalised to stabilize fluid volumes and blood pressure. Due to the lowered blood volume the patient will either suffer oliguria or have a very concentrated urine. There is a limit to the concentrating ability of the kidneys and therefore a typical blood reading in dehydration will give an elevated urea status. Under these circumstances vasopressin (ADH) will be secreted to maintain the fluid volume. This will be at the expense of osmolality, and the sodium concentration will decrease.

### Male, 65 yr - squamous cell carcinoma of the neck
A typical dehydration picture

|  | 29/09/99 | 30/09/99 |
|---|---|---|
| **General chemistry** | | |
| Sodium (136-146 mmol/L) | 118 | 107 |
| Potassium (3.5-5.2 mmol/L) | 6.5 | 6.1 |
| Chloride (98-109 mmol/L) | 70 | 71 |
| Bicarb. (20-33 mmol/L) | 27 | 26 |
| Albumin (35-50 g/L) | 31 | 22 |
| Globulin (20-35 g/L) | 38 | |
| Urea (2.5-8.0 mmol/L) | **6.1** | **6.4** |
| Creatinine (0.05-0.11 mmol/L) | 0.09 | **0.20** |
| **White cell count** (4-11 x10$^9$/L) | 29.4 | 47.7 |
| Neutrophils (2.0-8.0 x10$^9$/L) | 20.6(70%) | 45.7 |
| Lymphocytes (1.0-4.0 x10$^9$/L) | 3.2(11%) | 1.7 |
| Platelets (150-450 x10$^9$/L) | 716 | 676 |

Doctors will be quick to indicate to the patient on the Gerson treatment that the low salt diet is responsible for the lower sodium results and will advise the patient to increase their dietary sodium. However, this is not the cause of the hyponatraemia, and the addition of salt to the cancer patient's diet will accelerate the disease process, if dehydration is the mechanism underlying the pathology. However, the situation can become critical and the patient may have to receive an IV solution to stabilise their fluid volumes and blood pressure. This is not going to reverse the disease metabolism. Occasionally we may recommend the dietary inclusion of vegetables that can contribute to the sodium balance, such as silver beet, radish and celery and we may reduce the number of coffee enemas (these have a dialysis effect on blood sodium where they facilitate the exchange of potassium for sodium through the colon).

It is worth remembering that the daily obligatory loss for sodium is only 230mg, which is lost in the faeces, urine and through the skin. This is why you can never become sodium deficient on the Gerson treatment, unless there is concomitant disease which affects the sodium concentrations. The body is so efficient in conserving sodium that the 23g (23,000mg) secreted in the digestive tract and the 575g (575,000mg) filtered by the kidneys on a daily basis is reabsorbed and returned to the body. Additionally, the high potassium diet, although it shunts excess sodium out of the cells, will regulate the ECF sodium concentration. In response to high serum potassium, the adrenal glands secrete aldosterone to stimulate the elimination of potassium in exchange for sodium. Sodium is returned to the blood plasma to maintain normal blood concentration.

# Paraneoplastic syndromes affecting sodium/potassium balance

The practitioner must be aware that there are specific tumours that can secrete hormones. This is known as ectopic production of hormones by a non-endocrine tumour, or the paraneoplastic syndrome. The two syndromes which affect the sodium/potassium balance are SIADH (inappropriate secretion of ADH) and ectopic production of ACTH which gives rise to Cushing's syndrome (high concentration of glucocorticoids). Below is a brief indication of the types of cancer likely to be implicated in these syndromes.

- **SIADH** - small cell carcinomas of bronchus (most common), carcinoid tumours (intestinal endocrine cells), pancreatic adenocarcinomas. Also prostate, cancers of the head/neck, oesophagus, adrenal cortex, colon, lymphoma, thymoma, mesothelioma, brain metastases.

*Features:* dilutional hyponatraemia (water retention), drowsiness, confusion, fits and coma.

- **ACTH** - small cell carcinoma of bronchus, carcinoid tumours. ACTH stimulates the re-uptake of sodium by the kidneys.

*Features:* due to high levels of the glucocorticoids: glucose intolerance (high blood glucose), high sodium/low potassium, muscle weakness and wasting, truncal obesity, hypertension, bruising, thinning of skin and striae.

# Potassium

*Reference range*

Potassium        3.5-5.2 mmol/L

Serum potassium concentration does not reflect the true potassium status of the body. Only 2% of the total body potassium is readily accessible for measurement, the bulk of the remainder being in the cells. The kidneys are the main organs which control extracellular potassium. Therefore serum potassium measurements become important for determining kidney function. A high potassium concentration will imply defective control by the kidneys, a resistance of cellular uptake of potassium (diabetes or insulin resistance), or a redistribution of potassium from the ICF to the ECF (tissue catabolism). A very small shift from the ICF can cause a significant increase in ECF potassium concentration. This will occur during widespread tissue damage and catabolic states, such as uncontrolled diabetes. Unless there is severe circulatory, renal or adrenal failure, hyperkalaemia usually indicates an overall potassium depletion.

The symptoms of hyperkalaemia and hypokalaemia are indistinguishable. If the serum potassium falls outside the reference range, then serious effects occur in the nervous system. It is the large concentration gradient of potassium ions across the cell membrane which determines the electrical potential and thus the efficiency of the transmission of nervous signals which govern neuromuscular function. A lowered ECF potassium ion concentration decreases neuromuscular excitability, as potassium ions from within the cell diffuse out more rapidly down a steep concentration gradient, and the resting membrane potential becomes more negative and therefore difficult to stimulate.

A raised ECF potassium concentration will increase nerve/muscle excitability. The resting membrane potential becomes partially depolarized (increase in positive charge due to K ions diffusing less readily down its concentration gradient), so the voltage is diminished. Although the nerves and muscles are in a state of excitability, the reduction in voltage reduces the force of contraction, which can be fatal for heart contraction. The heart loses its ability to act as an effective pump and ventricular fibrillation results in cardiac arrest.

*The symptoms include:*
- weakness of muscles
- tingling in the face, hands and feet
- flaccid paralysis with loss of tendon reflexes
- neuromuscular weakness of the gastrointestinal tract, resulting in decreased intestinal motility (constipation) and paralytic ileus (paralysis of the smooth muscle of small intestine - abdominal distension)
- Inhibition of digestion (poor glandular secretion) - bloating, flatulence, fermentation and bacterial growth, diarrhoea.
- Cardiac arrhythmias, inefficient heart pumping.

## Hyperkalaemia
*Causes*

- Renal failure
- Mineralocorticoid deficiency (Addison's disease)
- Dehydration
- Transcellular movement of potassium from the ICF to ECF
  - tissue catabolism (uncontrolled diabetes)
  - corticosteroids (glucocorticoids oppose the action of insulin and cause breakdown of body tissue)
  - lack of insulin, insulin resistance (reduces uptake of potassium by the cells)
  - prolonged stress (increased glucocorticoid output)
  - trauma
  - acidosis ($H^+$ migrates inwards displacing $K^+$)

### *Male, aged 62 yr - uncontrolled diabetes before and after treatment with drugs*

|                        | 18/10/00 | 24/11/00 |
|------------------------|----------|----------|
| **General chemistry**  |          |          |
| Sodium (136-146 mmol/L) | 134      | 142      |
| Potassium (3.5-5.2 mmol/L) | 5.8  | 4.3      |
| Glucose (3.0-6.5 mmol/L) | 25     | 9.2      |

### *Female, aged 33 yr: hypothyroid, insulin resistance and oestrogen dominance*

*This patient has slightly elevated potassium due to insulin resistance (elevated fasting glucose) exacerbated by oestrogen dominance. She was treated with herbs and diet for the oestrogen dominance which, in turn, resolved the insulin resistance and the hypothyroid state. Entry of potassium into the cell is dependent upon an intact insulin/ glucose pathway and therefore correcting this metabolism is critical to healing from cell level.*

|                          | 15/05/13 | 29/08/13 | 03/12/13 | 01/02/14 |
|--------------------------|----------|----------|----------|----------|
| Potassium (3.5-5.2mmol/L) | 5.0     | 4.5      | 4.2      |          |
| Cholesterol (< 5.5 mmol/L) | 6.1    | 4.6      | 4.9      |          |
| Triglycerides (0.3-2.0 mmol/L) | 2.5 | 1.2    | 1.1      |          |
| Glucose (3.0-6.0 mmol/L) | 6.4      | 6.5      | 5.7      | 5.3      |
| HbA1c (<7%)              |          | 5.6      |          |          |
| TSH (0.4-4.0 mIU/L)      | 4.75     | 1.87     |          | 1.56     |
| 25 (OH) D (60-160 ng/mL) | 34       |          |          | 93       |
| B12 (190-900 ng/mL)     | 230      |          |          | 445      |

## Hypokalaemia

*Causes*

- ♦ Increased renal loss:
  - ▸ ectopic production of ACTH - small cell carcinoma of bronchus, carcinoid tumours.
  - ▸ Cushing's syndrome (glucocorticoid excess)
  - ▸ Conn's syndrome (mineralocorticoid excess)
  - ▸ Diuretics
  - ▸ Renal tubular acidosis

- ♦ Extra-renal loss:
  - ▸ Diarrhoea
  - ▸ Vomiting
  - ▸ Excessive sweating

It is important to note that many patients remain with a low serum potassium concentration throughout the therapy and it is not uncommon to see a lowered serum potassium concentration in recovering patients. This is not a negative sign in a normal pathology, but a sign of the body healing. Patients may misinterpret the sodium and potassium blood readings, thinking that a slight rise in sodium and fall in potassium is heading in the wrong direction. However, optimal entry of potassium into the cell occurs once the metabolism is restored, therefore the reducing potassium status is an indication of the restoration and maintenance of cellular metabolism. Dr. Gerson indicated that it would take around two years to fully restore intracellular potassium, and this may be longer by today's standards. Certainly with the increase in metabolic syndrome (insulin resistance and diabetes) it is more difficult to restore intracellular potassium, as the uptake of potassium by the cell is governed by insulin, and in insulin resistance neither glucose nor potassium can be taken up. Therefore, restoring the potassium status is compounded the more deranged the cell's metabolism becomes and can be difficult to achieve a good intracellular potassium status under these conditions. Generally, monitoring the glucose along with the potassium is a good guide as you will find as the glucose falls then so too does the potassium indicating that both are entering the cell and the metabolism is restoring.

## Supplementation of the potassium compound solution

Supplemental potassium will push the body to work harder. If there is any disturbance/impairment in kidney or heart function, or if the serum potassium concentration is high, then discretion needs to be applied with regard to this medication. It is not unusual, on the Gerson treatment, for potassium levels to reach an equilibrium, where medication with the potassium solution can proceed.

# Calcium

## Reference range
Calcium          2.10-2.55 mmol/L

Calcium metabolism is regulated by the kidneys and the parathyroid glands. In response to a low circulating concentration of calcium, the parathyroids secrete parathyroid hormone (PTH). PTH stimulates the kidneys to convert cholecalciferol to vitamin D3, which increases calcium uptake in the gut and stimulates the release of calcium from the bone. In addition, renal reabsorption of calcium is increased. Under normal conditions the kidneys will recycle 234mmols of calcium daily, only 6mmols being excreted in the urine. Losses may be incurred in renal failure and diarrhoea. Hypocalcaemia usually only occurs with low vitamin D status or with renal failure.

## Hypercalcaemia
*Features: confusion, impaired concentration, fatigue, anorexia, nausea, polyuria, polydipsia, constipation and muscle weakness and dehydration.*

### Causes
- Ectopic secretion of PTHrP by tumours (parathyroid-related peptide)
- Secretion of humoral factors by the tumour (cytokines and growth factors)
- Hyperparathyroidism
- Bone metastases

There are several factors secreted by tumours which can elevate serum calcium concentration. In 20 percent of cancers, where there is no indication of metastases to the bone, specific tumours may secrete humoral substances, such as PTHrP (ectopic production by a non-endocrine tumour), osteolytic cytokines and growth factors. Below is a list of some of the more common tumours associated with hypercalcaemia.

- Multiple myeloma - secretion of osteolytic cytokines by malignant cells, which stimulate osteoclast precursors to destroy surrounding bone and also inhibit osteoblasts, which allows the tumour to grow into the space destroyed by osteoclasts.

- Squamous cell carcinoma of head, neck, lung and oesophagus - ectopic production of PTHrP, increased bone alkaline phosphatase

- Lymphoma - certain types - ectopic production of several osteotrophic factors - e.g. osteoclast activating factor, CSF (colony stimulating factor), gamma interferon, active D metabolite.

- Bone metastases  (dissolution from bone by secondary tumour) with breast or prostate primary. In general there is poor correlation between extent of metastatic bone involvement and calcium levels. High serum calcium is not generally caused by bone metastases (unless there is also renal dysfunction), although malignant cells in bone produce growth factors. However, if the alkaline phosphatase and serum calcium are both increased in bone metastases, then this will indicate disease progression.

- Hormonal treatment with oestrogen and anti-oestrogens - stimulate breast cancer cells to produce osteolytic prostaglandins which increase bone resorption.

## Male, 65 yr - squamous cell carcinoma of the neck

The tumour is secreting PTHrP, leading to an elevated serum calcium which was treated with biphosphonates. There is also increased bone alkaline phosphatase. He is also suffering from dehydration.

| General chemistry | 10/10/99 | 12/10/99 | 18/10/99 | 25/10/99 |
|---|---|---|---|---|
| Sodium (136-146 mmol/L) | 107 | 122 | 134 | 124 |
| Potassium (3.5-5.2 mmol/L) | 5.9 | 5.9 | 4.8 | 6.6 |
| Calcium (2.10-2.55 mmol/L) | 3.57 | 3.43 | 1.96 | 1.49 |
| Phosphate (0.75-1.35 mmol/L) | 0.97 | 0.89 | | 0.8 |
| Urea (2.5-8.0 mmol/L) | 9.7 | 3.9 | 2.5 | 5.9 |
| Creatinine (0.05-0.11 mmol/L) | 0.21 | 0.08 | 0.62 | 0.07 |
| Alk. Phos (30-120 U/L) | 144 | | | 84 |
| White cell count (4-11 x$10^9$/L) | 52.3 | 28.8 | | 13.8 |
| Neutrophils (2.0-8.0 x$10^9$/L) | 49.8 | 23.4 | | 10.5 (76%) |
| Lymphocytes (1.0-4.0 x$10^9$/L) | 2.1 | 3.17 | | 2.3 (17%) |
| Platelets (150-450 x$10^9$/L) | 770 | 805 | | 677 |

# Kidney function tests

**Reference ranges**

| | | |
|---|---|---|
| Urea | 2.5-8.0 | mmol/L |
| Creatinine | 0.05-0.11 | mmol/L |
| Urate | 0.15-0.45 | mmol/L |

Three specific readings from the blood results will indicate impaired kidney function: creatinine, urea and potassium. The kidneys eliminate potassium and the waste products creatinine and urea. You will need to determine from these results the degree of renal impairment and, from the case history, the underlying pathology. An increase in serum potassium and/or urea concentrations may not necessarily indicate renal impairment, unless the plasma creatinine is also raised.

# Creatinine

**Reference range**

| | |
|---|---|
| Creatinine | 0.05-0.11 mmol/L |

Serum creatinine is the most definitive test of kidney function. Creatinine is a waste product from the turnover of creatine phosphate in muscle. Ingestion of meat and strenuous exercise may cause a slight increase in the plasma creatinine levels. Creatinine is actively secreted by the renal tubules, and elevated serum levels indicate impaired renal function with a lowered GFR (glomerular filtration rate).

### Female, 52 yr -  advanced cervical carcinoma
*Radical hysterectomy followed by 7 weeks radiotherapy, leaving patient with bowel and bladder incontinence. Three years later invasive tumour from the bladder pressing on L ureter causing obstructive nephropathy. Both kidneys enlarged and ureters dilated. Treated with bilateral nephrostomies and self-catheterisation.*

| | 9/3/99 | 15/6/99 | 6/7/99 | 20/7/99 |
|---|---|---|---|---|
| **General chemistry** | | | | |
| Sodium (136-146 mmol/L) | 144 | 139 | 141 | 141 |
| Potassium (3.5-5.2 mmol/L) | 4.5 | 4.5 | 4.3 | 4.7 |
| Urea (2.5-8.0 mmol/L) | 8.1 | 3.9 | 3.8 | 3.8 |
| Creatinine (0.05-0.11 mmol/L) | 0.19 | 0.13 | 0.18 | 0.11 |
| Urate (0.15-0.45 mmol/L) | 0.33 | 0.28 | | 0.23 |
| **Urinalysis** | | Mixed growth | | strep |
| pH | 8.5 | | | |
| Protein | 3+ | 1+ | | + |
| Glucose | Nil | nil | | |
| Blood | 3+ | | | |

# Urea

*Reference range*
Urea             2.5-8.0 mmol/L

Urea is a by-product of protein metabolism from the deamination of amino acids and forms the major route for nitrogen excretion. It is filtered from the blood at the glomerulus, but when the GFR is lowered, passive tubular reabsorption occurs. This can occur in either dehydration or when there is impaired renal function. Urea levels are increased in high dietary protein consumption or in catabolic states, and decreased in liver disease and on low-protein diets. Most patients on the Gerson treatment will have a slightly low plasma urea concentration, unless they have renal impairment or suffering from dehydration.

# Urate

*Reference range*
0.15-0.45 mmol/L

In the absence of any metabolic disorder (such as gout), hyperuricaemia will indicate increased formation of uric acid and/or decreased excretion. Uric acid is a breakdown product of purines (found in the nucleotides of the cell's DNA/RNA) and in advanced malignancy increased nucleic acid turnover may raise serum urate. Hyperuricaemia is also a feature in late renal failure, if the GFR falls below 20ml/min. High urate is also an indication of gout.

# Urinalysis

A urinalysis is performed routinely to screen for bladder/kidney infection (micro-organisms, blood, protein), glucose and metabolic disease. A 24 hour collection may also be requested in suspected protein-losing states due to nephropathy associated with uncontrolled diabetes, nephritis or hypertension.

**pH** (4.5 - 8.0) - the patient's pH will invariably be high on the Gerson treatment, due to the high volume of alkaline foods. The addition of a couple of tablespoons of organic wine or apple cider vinegar to the diet will reduce the pH.

**Specific gravity** (1.005 - 1.020) - indicates how dilute or concentrated the patient's urine is. A dilute urine (<1.005) could indicate diabetes insipidus, tubular necrosis or pyelonephritis. A high specific gravity would occur in SIADH (as found with specific malignancies), dehydration, nephrotic syndrome (renal protein-losing), acute glomerulo-nephritis, diabetes and shock.

**Proteinuria** - kidney/bladder infection

**Microalbuminuria** (<20 mg/L) - nephritis, renal failure, diabetes, hypertension. The 24 hour urine collection test is used to determine renal losses of albumin (microalbuminuria). Increased losses signify renal disease.

**Creatinine clearance** (8-16 mmol/L) - nephropathy, renal stenosis, congestive heart failure, high blood pressure. The 24 hour urine collection test is used to determine renal filtration capacity. A decreased creatinine clearance signifies renal disease.

**Glucose** - diabetes, Cushing's syndrome (ectopic secretion of ACTH)

**Blood** - infection, obstruction, trauma, current menses

**White cells** - infection

# Inflammatory Markers

These are used in conjunction with other tests to determine the presence of inflammatory disease. They provide useful markers for monitoring treatment efficacy and disease progression/regression. Elevation in cancer, if there is no other concomitant disease, can indicate a poorer prognosis.

## C-Reactive Protein

*Reference range*

< 5.0 mg/L

CRP is an acute phase protein that is released from the liver in response to both acute and chronic inflammation, as seen in infection or in chronic inflammatory disease (including autoimmune conditions) and malignancy, and also following tissue injury. Its role is to activate the immune system to clear the debris of inflammation, necrotic tissue and certain bacteria. This marker can be used to monitor disease progression or regression and the effectiveness of treatment. In cancer levels may be elevated when tumours are necrotising or when they are inflamed. This often occurs in late phase malignancy along with elevated neutrophils, and usually it is indicative of a poor prognosis.

CRP is a more sensitive and accurate reflection of the acute phase response than the ESR.

## Erythrocyte sedimentation rate (ESR)

*Reference range*

< 15 mm/hr

The ESR is a measure of non-specific inflammation which can stem from any cause, such as infection or an inflammatory disease process, including malignancy. In an inflammatory exudate red blood cells tend to form rouleaux stacks which have a higher rate of sedimentation; these are heavier and will sediment faster than red blood cells from a normal blood specimen. The sedimentation rate is measured in millimeters/hour and a range above 15mm/hr indicates inflammation.

# Tumour Markers

Tumour markers are substances that can be detected in the blood, urine or body tissues in higher than normal concentrations in patients with certain types of cancer. These substances are either secreted by the tumours themselves, or are antigens expressed on malignant cell surfaces, or are substances produced by the body in response to the presence of cancer.

Tumour markers are useful for monitoring disease and to detect recurrence. They are not diagnostic in themselves as they are not 100 percent accurate, and may be elevated during flare-ups. They should only be used as a guide. They can reflect the extent/stage of the disease and indicate how quickly the disease is likely to progress.

- α-Fetoprotein (AFP - a glyco-protein) - hepatocellular carcinomas, testicular teratomas, germ cell cancer of ovary and testis. Correlates well with tumour bulk.

- CEA (carcinoembryonic antigen). CEA is raised in 30-85 percent of patients with colorectal cancer, liver metastases, gastrointestinal tumours. It can be raised in other cancers, including breast and lung. Decrease does not indicate regression, but an increase can indicate recurrence. It may be moderately raised in non-malignant conditions, such as obstructive jaundice, cirrhosis, pancreatitis, diverticulitis, inflammatory bowel disease and renal failure. The half-life of CEA is about 6 days.

- hCG (human chorionic gonadotropin). Normally produced by the developing foetus. Raised levels found in trophoblastic disease (a rare cancer that develops from an abnormal fertilized cell) and germ cell cancers. May also be elevated in breast, lung, pancreatic, ovarian and gastrointestinal cancers. Benign conditions such as inflammatory bowel disease, ulcers and cirrhosis may also have elevated levels of hCG.

- PSA (prostate-specific antigen). Produced by both normal and abnormal prostate cells, therefore may be elevated in both benign and malignant prostate conditions. This marker is used to monitor the effectiveness of prostate cancer treatment. On the Gerson treatment PSA invariably rises in the initial stages of the therapy before it falls.

- Paraproteins - myeloma. They are detected in urine and serum and correlate well with tumour bulk. Bence Jones proteins (immunoglobulins) are measured in the urine in patients with multiple myeloma. The paraproteins are characteristic of the proliferation of B cells.

- CA (carbohydrate antigen)
  - CA 125     Ovarian cancer, occasionally breast and colorectal cancers. Also may be raised in benign conditions, such as endometriosis, ovarian cysts or fibroids, cirrhosis and hepatitis.
  - CA 19-9     Pancreatic adenocarcinoma, liver, stomach, colorectal and gastric carcinomas. In pancreatic cancers higher levels of CA 19-9 are associated with more advanced disease.
  - CA 50     Colorectal cancer.
  - CA 15-3     Breast. Raised in up to 20 percent of patients with localised breast cancer and 70-90 percent in those with metastatic breast cancer. It may also increase in cancers of the lung, uterus, stomach and other organs, and in patients with benign breast and liver disease.

- **Ferritin** - liver disease, certain cancers due to release of the protein from tissues, renal, bladder, breast and prostate cancers.

- **Enzymes as tumour markers**
  - Placental alkaline phosphatase - testicular seminomas.
  - Prostatic acid phosphatase (PAP) - disseminated prostatic carcinoma. May also be associated with multiple myeloma, osteogenic sarcoma and bone metastases.
  - Alkaline phosphatase (secondary, not tumour derived) - biliary obstruction, bony metastases. Ectopic production of ALP in bronchial carcinoma (tumour derived).
  - Lactate Dehydrogenase (LDH) - this enzyme is found throughout the body and therefore cannot be used for screening, but it can be used to monitor the course of a patient's cancer.
  - Neuron-Specific Enolase (NSE) - neuroblastoma, small cell lung cancer, medullary thyroid cancer, carcinoid, pancreatic endocrine tumours and melanoma.

# Malignancy: the metabolic complications

## Paraneoplastic syndromes

*Ectopic hormone secretion by non-endocrine tumours*

The paraneoplastic syndrome refers to a clinical picture which arises with specific cancers, whereby a non-endocrine tumour secretes a hormone or substance which has hormonal activity. This is referred to as ectopic hormone secretion by non-endocrine tumours. The most frequently encountered syndromes are dilutional hyponatraemia, hypercalcaemia and Cushing's syndrome (high concentration of glucocorticoids).

- **ACTH**: small cell carcinoma of bronchus, carcinoid tumours.
*Features:* glucose intolerance (high blood glucose), high sodium/low potassium, muscle weakness and wasting, truncal obesity, hypertension, bruising, thinning of skin and striae.

- **SIADH (vasopressin)** - small cell carcinomas of bronchus, carcinoid tumours (intestinal endocrine cells), pancreatic adenocarcinomas.
*Features:* dilutional hyponatraemia (water retention), drowsiness, confusion, fits and coma which may mimic cerebral metastases.

- **PTHrP (parathyroid related peptide)** - true ectopic secretion of PTH is rare: squamous cell carcinoma of head, neck, lung and oesophagus
*Features:* hypercalcaemia, muscle weakness, cardiac arrhythmias, polyuria and dehydration, abdominal pain, nausea, vomiting and constipation, mental changes (drowsiness, personality changes, concentration impairment, coma)

- **Insulin** (rarely by ectopic) or insulin-like growth factors (somatomedins): Fibrosarcomas, mesotheliomas, spindle cell sarcomas
*Features:* hypoglycaemia

- **hCG (human chorionic gonadotrophin hormone)**: bronchial carcinomas, hepatic tumours in puberty, choriocarcinoma, testicular teratomas.
*Features:* gynaecomastia

- **Erythropoietin** - uterine fibromyomata, cerebellar haemangioblastoma
*Features:* polycythaemia.

## Carcinoid syndrome

Although this does not fall under paraneoplastic syndromes, carcinoid tumours liberate vasoactive substances such as serotonin, histamine, kinins and substance P into the circulation. These compounds, if arising from tumours in the gut, are deactivated by the liver. Carcinoid tumours in the liver, ovaries or lungs liberate these products directly into the systemic circulation where they exert their effects. Elevated urinary levels of 5-hydroxy indole acetic acid (5HIAA) will confirm this syndrome.

*Features:* cardiac lesions, flushing, diarrhoea, nausea, vomiting, colicky pain, pulmonary stenosis, bronchospasm, wheezing, skin lesions (pellagra - dietary tryptophan is diverted towards serotonin synthesis and away from protein and nicotinic acid synthesis, so many of the symptoms relate to dietary deficiencies of B3).

# Cancer Cachexia

Cachexia is a common feature of advanced malignancy, the symptoms predominantly being weight loss, weakness, anaemia and fever. The weight loss may be caused by the increased energy requirements of the tumour (inefficient anaerobic energy metabolism) and/or due to fever. Additionally, many terminally-ill patients suffer anorexia. In many cases the production of cachectin (a cytokine: tumour necrosis factor-α) is responsible for the increase in BMR, hence increasing energy requirements.

# References

1.  *Hepcidin: Inflammation's iron curtain*, Oxford Journals, Rheumatology 2004;43:1323-1325, 27 July 2004; http://rheumatology.oxfordjournals.org/content/43/11/1323.full.pdf+html
2.  *Iron homoeostasis in rheumatic disease*; Oxford Journals, Rheumatology volume 48, Issue 11 pp1339-1344 http://rheumatology.oxfordjournals.org/content/48/11/1339.full
3.  Alexander, K; *Iodine, a century of medical fraud*; http://www.kathrynalexander.com.au/iodine-a-century-of-medical-fraud.html

# Recommended Reading

Marshall, William J.: *Clinical Chemistry*, Gower Medical Publishing
Macleod, Edwards and Bouchier: *Davidson's Principles and Practice of Medicine*, Churchill Livingstone
Murphy, Lawrence and Lenhard: *Clinical Oncology*, American Cancer Society
Edwards, C.R.W: *Endocrinology*, Heinemann

# Chapter 4

# Treatment - Medication Rationale

This section explains the rationale behind the specific treatments used in detoxification therapies for both the patient with a strong constitution who can undertake the full therapy, and for those in a weakened condition who have either received chemotherapy or have a concomitant or chronic disease.

Supplements to support the digestion, assist the potassium status and increase the metabolism are regarded as standard. Other supplements or adjunctive treatments that are regarded as therapeutically beneficial to the patient are also included in this program. When assessing a possible adjunct to a therapy, we must always ensure that it meets the following criteria:

- it must be non-toxic;
- it must support detoxification and not push the body too far (remember that detoxification is an aggressive therapy on its own);
- it must not stimulate but replenish;
- it must assist and support the healing mechanisms and not suppress them.

Some adjuncts singularly address the disease process and this is where the biggest mistakes occur as patients and other practitioners may ascribe greater importance to suppressive treatments over treatments that increase the patient's capacity for cure. Invariably, emphasis is placed on those treatments and the patient may forfeit others that build the healing potential. So it is important to assess where each treatment fits and how it will help to improve outcome.

## The Juices

On the full therapy 13 x 8 ozs (240mls) fresh juices are taken daily: 1 orange, 5 carrot and apple, 4 green, 3 carrot only. Liver capsules are taken along with the carrot only juices.

On a modified therapy 10 juices are taken daily. The 3 carrot only juices are generally the ones which are omitted.

Each juice is taken fresh, hourly. This ensures a constant hourly flushing of the body with nutrients, specifically potassium. Potassium compound solution (see later) is added to ten of the juices.

Carrots are very detoxifying; in juice form they are able to draw toxins out of the cells. In agriculture they are seen to have the same capacity; farmers will crop carrots to "clean" the soil (another reason to beware of juicing commercial carrots). In traditional Chinese literature carrots are regarded as a liver stimulant, or supporting Liver Qi. Dr. Gerson added carrots to the juicing regime when he observed one patient making better progress on the carrot juices rather than the traditional orange juice used at that time.

The green juices are tonifying and build the blood. They are rich in betaine, folate, vitamin K, iron and magnesium, along with other trace elements not found in carrots. The patient requires a broad spectrum of nutrients and therefore the green juice becomes essential. Many patients are extremely deficient and would not make good their deficiencies without the green juice. It is essential that you use only the greens that are allowed, and not be tempted to add other greens to the mix. Many green vegetables, particularly those of the brassica family, are goitrogenic, which means that they can inhibit the uptake of iodine by the thyroid gland. This becomes of greater consequence if you are not taking thyroid hormone, or when reducing it.[1]

The addition of apples to the juices is critical. Green, sour apples are the best for their high levels of malic acid and pectin. When the pulps of both the apple and vegetable are mixed together before pressing, the malic acid solubilizes and extracts a greater nutrient value from the vegetables than could be gained from the vegetables alone. Additionally, the pectin in apples is an immune-stimulant.

In general, it takes double the amount of vegetable/apple matter to produce the amount of juice required; i.e. 500g of vegetable will produce 250mls of juice. If the vegetables are very juicy, then you may require less but if they are dry (as old carrots tend to be), then you may require more.

# The carrot and apple juice

*Equal quantities of carrot and green apple to give 240mls (8ozs) juice*

# The green juice

*1 thin wedge red cabbage*
*1/4 green capsicum*
*1 leaf endive*
*1 leaf chard/silver beet*
*Beet tops (young inner leaves)*
*2 sprigs watercress*
*large handful of cos, green or red leaf lettuce (not iceberg)*
*1 medium green apple, cored*

NB: It is important to include as many of the above ingredients as possible. Do not substitute with other green vegetables when out of season, but use as many of the allowed ones as you can.

# The carrot and liver juice

During the 1940's, following the introduction of agricultural chemical fertilizers and pesticides, Dr. Gerson found that it was becoming increasingly difficult to achieve consistently good results with his therapy. It was at this point that Dr. Gerson introduced the raw liver juice to the therapy. He experienced better and more consistent results with this addition. We are unable to use the raw calves' livers now, due to cross-contamination of these livers from camphylobacter at the abattoir, and the difficulty in procuring fresh, organic calves' liver that is unfrozen and less than 60 hours old (max. weight, 4lbs).

If you are able to obtain organic calves' liver then, bearing in mind that it is cross contamination from the animals' entrails in the abattoir to the outer surface of the liver, you should be able to sterilize the liver by immersing it in water heated to 80°C for 10 seconds only. You may trim any discoloured outer flesh from the liver before juicing. The traditional method of juicing liver requires slicing the liver into strips and feeding these into the machine, alternating with carrot pieces.

# Standard Medications

## Potassium Compound Solution

The potassium compound solution is an equal mixture of potassium acetate, potassium monophosphate and potassium gluconate salts. It comes in airtight containers of 100g. Each batch of 100g should be dissolved in distilled water to make a 1L x 10% solution and stored in a dark glass bottle in a cool place.

### Dosage:

During the first 4 weeks, the patient on the full therapy should add 20ml of potassium compound solution to 10 of the juices (1 orange, 5 carrot and apple and 4 green). No potassium compound solution is added to the carrot only juice. After 4 weeks the amount of potassium compound solution is halved to 10ml in each of the 10 juices. This dose continues throughout the therapy until the patient is healed. Later in the therapy, patients are allowed to prepare some of the apple and carrot juices in advance and store them in a stainless steel/glass lined flask (for no longer than 2-3 hours). The potassium compound solution must be added to the juice prior to taking, not in advance.

On the modified therapy, the patient takes 10ml of potassium compound solution in each of the 10 juices and maintains this dose.

This medication raises cellular potassium, restores normal cell metabolism and reduces oedemas.

### Contra-indications:

- Any inflammatory condition/bleeding of the gastrointestinal tract, particularly of the oesophagus and stomach. The potassium compound solution may aggravate these conditions and must be introduced cautiously. Oatmeal gruel will help to alleviate inflammation and burning.
- Cardiac, respiratory and renal insufficiency. Do not prescribe potassium until blood work has been analysed. Then start with 5ml in 10 juices daily, increasing gradually if the patient is tolerating it well.

## Lugol's 1/2 strength solution

Lugol's is an iodine solution containing inorganic iodine and potassium iodide and is used at half strength. Each drop of Lugol's solution, half-strength, contains 3.125mg iodine. Iodine is taken up by the thyroid gland for the synthesis of thyroid hormones; by breast tissue (protective against breast cancer); by the ovaries (follicular development); it is postulated that it is required for the functionality of the hormone receptors for steroid hormones, insulin and the hypothalamus and pituitary stimulating hormones; for the production of hydrochloric acid in the stomach; and is required by the immune system during infection or inflammatory disease, and as an anti-infective in the destruction of pathogens (including Helicobacter Pylori).[2]

Dr. Gerson states that iodine at cell level is a decisive factor in cell differentiation, and nowadays it is believed to have a protective role against breast cancer and possibly ovarian cancer, and polycystic ovarian syndrome (PCOS).

In large doses iodine will suppress thyroid hormone synthesis. Lugol's solution must be prescribed along with the thyroid medication in the appropriate doses as stated. The larger dose at the beginning of treatment is seen to inhibit excessive growth of the cancer and accelerate healing. Many pharmacists will oblige and make this solution up for patients.

*Dosage:*

During the first 4 weeks: 18 drops daily; 3 drops in each of the following juices - 1 orange and 5 carrot and apple. Lugol's is not placed in the green juices or the carrot only juices. The green juices are very rich in enzymes and it is important that these enzymes are not disturbed. After 4 weeks the dose is reduced to 6 drops daily (1 drop in each of the 6 juices mentioned above).

On the modified therapy the patient takes a maximum of 6 drops of Lugol's daily. In the weakened patient this is further reduced to 1-2 drops daily.

Lugol's increases intracellular production of ATP and therefore controls the oxidation rate.

*Contra-indications:*
- allergy to iodine (cautiously add one drop after 5 days)
- use with caution in patients with autoimmune thyroiditis (both under and overactive thyroid) and monitor the TSH carefully
- in the weakened patient when thyroid is contra-indicated start with a reduced dose and monitor the thyroid (TSH). Under these conditions Lugol's is usually started at 1-2 drops daily.

# Thyroid

This medication is available in 1 grain and 1/2 grain tablets. It is dessicated pork thyroid gland. Thyroid is used to stimulate replication of the mitochondria and increase metabolism/oxidation/free energy (ATP).

It is very important to obtain thyroid supplements that are standardised to contain levothyroxine (T4) 38μg/grain and liothyronine (T3) 9μg/grain. There are many thyroid supplements on the market which contain no appreciable levels of T4 or T3. Many compounding pharmacies do sell natural thyroid at these potencies, but they may be in milligrams rather than grains. So it is important that you convert the milligrams to grains. Each grain = 60-65mg; therefore if the recommended dose is 2.5 grains, then the total milligrams required would be around 150mg. If, for any reason the patient cannot tolerate the natural thyroid, but requires thyroxine (which is T4 only) then 100μg of levothyroxine has the equivalent activity of 1 grain of natural thyroid.

*Dosage:*

During the first 4 weeks the patient on the full therapy takes 5 grains of thyroid daily. After 4 weeks the dose is halved to 5 x 1/2 grain tablets. The medication is taken at intervals throughout the day. Depending upon the patient's progress, the dose is gradually tapered down, although the patient may remain on a higher dose for longer than was recommended in Dr. Gerson's day. It is important to monitor the thyroid function through blood tests when reducing the medication. Increased thyroid toxicity (nutrition and environmental factors) can mean long-term use for many patients.

On the modified therapy the patient takes a maximum of 2 1/2 grains daily. In a weakened patient this may be reduced to 1/2 - 1 grain daily.

As thyroid has a long half-life (6-7 days), any alteration of the dose will take up to 10 days for clinical response to changes in medication to appear. Therefore it is important not to lower the dose too rapidly when making modifications to the treatment.

Dosages may be determined, in the absence of contra-indications (see below), by the axillary temperature test on waking. The normal temperature range is 36.7°C - 36.8°C (97.8°F - 98.2°F). Most cancer patients have a low temperature. Below or at this temperature medication is initiated. If the temperature rises above this, take for 3 consecutive days before reducing, but make sure that the temperature is not raised due to fever, infection, electric blanket, healing reactions or severe pain.

Instruct the patient to take his/her pulse and temperature before rising daily and to keep a record of the results. Many patients do complain of tachycardia from time to time. It is important to recognise if the tachycardia is from the caffeine of the enema or the thyroid medication. You may advise the patient to take the pulse after the enema to determine the cause.

### Contra-indications:

- Hyperthyroidism or symptoms of: tachycardia, tremors, anxiety, insomnia, high temperature, rapid pulse rate (over 120 beats/minute);
- Cardiac, respiratory insufficiency. Thyroid potentiates the action of catecholamines and increases cardiac output (tachycardia, arrhythmias, palpitation). These effects increase pulse rate, temperature and increased anxiety levels;
- Excessive weight loss due to over-prescribed thyroid hormone;
- Weakened patient; and
- Osteoporosis or bone metastases; a lower dose may be required in these patients

# Niacin

Niacin is the activated form of vitamin B3. You must make sure that the patient is using niacin or nicotinic acid and not nicotinamide, which does not have the same biological flushing effects on the body. Niacin acts as a vasodilator, through its effects on histamine release, which improves circulation and skin temperature. Niacin increases the capacity for cellular oxidation, as it plays an integral part in the shuttling of hydrogen atoms from the Krebs Cycle to the electron transport chain, where the hydrogen atoms are divested of their electrons. These pass down the chain to be taken up by oxygen, a process which results in the formation of ATP. (See diagram 3, p28). Niacin is also a co-factor for the enzyme system (GAPDH) that helps feed sugar into the energy cycle. Niacin becomes consumed under oxidative stress, and so by default the cycle will become interrupted, and when sugar cannot be fed into the energy cycle an accumulation of glucose upstream metabolites occurs. This is known as glucose toxicity which stimulates yet more free radical production resulting in major oxidative stress which compounds insulin resistance.[3, 4]

### Dosage:

6 x 50mg daily. It is often advised to take the tablets with meals or allow to dissolve under the tongue in order to minimise the flushing effects. When purchasing niacin, you must ensure that it is not a slow release tablet and that it is not complexed with calcium.

### Contra-indications:

- Any bleeding, haemorrhage
- Allergy to niacin
- Ulcers/gastritis in the gastrointestinal tract
- Corticosteroid therapy
- Blood thinning agent therapy
- Surgery: cease niacin 3 days prior to surgery and for 3 weeks post surgery.

# Acidol Pepsin

Acidol Pepsin is another digestive aid to assist protein digestion in the stomach. Many patients have low stomach acidity, and under these circumstances the first stages of protein digestion will not occur. Hydrochloric acid activates pepsin to begin the digestion of protein, and it aids in the absorption of iron, calcium, zinc and B12. Low stomach acidity is caused by a general lowering of the potassium status in the body. The parietal cells which secrete hydrochloric acid are stimulated by various controls - nervous and hormonal - which activate a proton pump which pumps out hydrogen ions in exchange for potassium ions.

A sufficient acidic response in the stomach will lower the pH to 1.5 which is critical for the ongoing digestion in the duodenum and small intestine. There is an optimum pH range within which digestive enzymes operate. An extremely acidic chyme will stimulate the release of the hormones CCK (cholecystokinin) and secretin by the duodenum. These hormones are essential for the release of alkalizing fluids from the liver (bile) and the pancreas (bicarbonate), which will raise the pH of the chyme to between 6 and 8. It is within this narrow range that the pancreatic enzymes can function. You can appreciate that if the pH of chyme when entering the duodenum is not sufficiently low enough, then it may fail to generate an adequate response from the liver and pancreas, leading to poor digestive capacity with fermentation, gas and bloating.

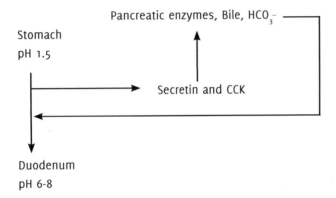

**Dosage:**
2 before each meal (6/day).

**Contra-indications**
- gastric ulcers
- gastritis, intestinal bleeding, oesophageal problems
- blood thinning agent therapy, NSAIDs and aspirin.

# Pancreatin

The pancreatin enzymes taken with meals are primarily for supporting the digestion of the patient. On a nutritional therapy healing is dependent upon the vigour of the digestion in accessing all the nutrients required by the body. In cancer the digestion of the patient is weakened, a fact that you will see highlighted in your patients on the high carbohydrate diet. Patients can experience tremendous amounts of painful gas and bloating which becomes progressively worse during the day. These patients may find that the addition of the pancreatic enzymes helpful, with an additional dose taken late afternoon with the 5pm juice, as the digestion may be severely taxed by this time.

Additionally, large quantities of pancreatic enzymes are required for the role they play in potentiating the immune assault on the cancer cell. As discussed earlier the digestive action of the pancreatic enzymes on the outer coat of the cancer cell membrane forms the primary immune response, and is fundamental to the unmasking of antigenic sites which renders the cancer cell vulnerable to the secondary response of immune attack and digestion. Until this occurs, the cancer cell can avoid detection by the immune system.

It is interesting to note that cancer does not usually occur in the first segment of the duodenum, the area where the pancreas first empties its enzymes and they become active. Of course pancreatic cancer occurs - but the enzymes are inactive within the pancreas. Chymotrypsinogen, the pancreatic precursor enzyme is activated to chymotrypsin by trypsin in the duodenum, and together they digest protein.

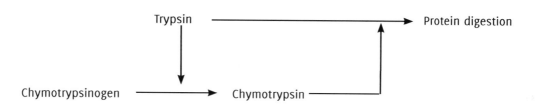

Obviously a diet that doesn't consume the bulk of the pancreatic enzymes for its digestion is going to favour the absorption of surplus enzymes into the system where they can perform their second role of keeping the system free of bacteria, fungi, parasites and any neoplastic cells. They start the digestion of tumour tissue and in the process expose the tumour to the white cells of the immune system. The nutritional program is not only one that is full of living food enzymes (in the juices), which assist their own digestion and therefore do not draw on the body resources, but is also low in protein. Excess dietary protein robs us of the protein-digesting enzymes, trypsin and chymotrypsin, and it is no wonder that the over-consumption of protein in our Western world is being blamed in many medical circles for the rise in incidence of chronic disease.

### Dosage:
Pancreatin 325mg x 3, 4 times daily to be taken after each meal and with the 5pm juice. If the digestion is very poor, then the dose can be increased by taking an additional 1,200mg pancreatin tablet with each dose. Dr. Gerson indicates "The administraion of digestive enzymes in digestive disorders has not fulfilled early expectations. Despite this fact, I found pancreatin in many cases a valuable help in the therapy. A few patients cannot stand pancreatin, the majority are satisfied to have less digestive trouble with gas spasms and less difficulty in regaining weight and strength. We use the tablets after the detoxication." (pp211-212)

### Contra-indications:
* Sarcoma patients. The reasons for this are not clear from Dr. Gerson's writings.
* Ulcerative colitis or inflammatory bowel disease. Pancreatin may worsen the symptoms so supplement with caution.

### WobeMugos enzymes
Additional enzymes are recommended in many cases, to be taken away from food, for their benefits on the cancer metabolism. A mixture of plant and animal enzymes have been found to have the best synergistic effect, and the studies on WobeMugos indicate the therapeutic range.

The WobeMugos enzymes were a combination of chymotrypsin, trypsin and papain, carrying high amounts of chymotrypsin. The levels of enzymes may be measured in milligrams and activity units, although you should ideally measure the strength of enzyme activity per unit (activity units). The milligram unit is confusing to the lay person as it may only be a reflection of the activity units (milligram equivalents) and not the actual weight so the milligram content may mean very little, if anything. For example, if a product has only 1 mg of chymotrypsin containing 1,000 units/mg in it, then the product labelling may state that it contains 1,000 mg of chymotrypsin with 1 unit per milligram activity. Similarly, if a product has 200 activity units per milligram and it is said to contain 120mg, then the total activity units would be 200 x 120 = 24,000 units. Most enzyme supplements do not contain appreciable amounts of chymotrypsin, but there are a few on the market today.

The dose of WobeMugos varied from 2-5, three times daily and the activity in each tablet contained:
- papain 100mg (270 units, total)
- chymotrypsin 40mg (12,000 units, total)
- trypsin 40mg (1,740 units, total)

# Liver capsules

Liver capsules are a replacement for the raw liver and are taken along with the carrot only juice.

**Dosage:**
2 x 500mg liver capsules to be taken at 11am, 3pm and 4pm. For those patients not taking the carrot only juices these capsules may be taken at this time with a little distilled water. They may be increased to 8/day if the patient is anaemic.

# CoQ10

CoQ10 is also used as a part replacement for the raw liver juice. Raw liver has quantities of CoQ10 which have been found to be an essential nutrient involved in cellular respiration. It is part of the electron transport chain involved in the shuttling of electrons, which imparts the energy for the formation of ATP.

**Dosage:**
300-600mg daily.
Start at the lower dose of 300mg and increase over a few days. Make sure that the CoQ10 is pure, that it does not contain soy, vitamin E, or calcium and magnesium as carriers.

**Contra-indications:**
- Cardiac, respiratory and renal insufficiency - proceed gently at 90-100mg daily and watch for any heart irregularities/tachycardia. Increase as tolerated.
- Start slowly in chemotherapy pre-treated patients

# Crude Liver and B12 Injections

The formation and maturation of red blood cells is dependent upon adequate supplies of B12 and folic acid. B12 governs DNA synthesis for cell replication, and the effects of deficiency will be found in tissues with a rapid turnover, such as all blood cells. Therefore any changes in the counts for red cells, platelets and granulocytes will all reflect B12 deficiency. The detoxification therapy is very low in B12 (mainly found in animal products) and additionally patients with pernicious anaemia or whose digestion is compromised may be unable to absorb this vitamin. Therefore, in the initial stages of treatment, low doses of B12 are given as an injection on a daily basis at 100µg per dose. Oral doses, as methylcobalamin, may also be recommended, if the patient is able to absorb this. The cyanocobalamin form of B12 is no longer recommended. Dr. Gerson recommended the incremental daily dosing rather than weekly dosing for B12.

The crude liver returns some nutrients and enzymes, also minute quantities of hormones, to the body. They have been found to be essential in the healing process. Obtaining the crude liver injections can be difficult.

*Dosage:*
0.1cc B12 + 3.9cc crude liver as an intramuscular injection. The B12 dose may be increased in anaemia, low RCC and low WCC. If you are taking oral B12, as methylcobalamin, then take 3cc of the crude liver, by injection.

# Flaxseed Oil

Flaxseed oil contains both the essential fatty acids (EFAs), linolenic acid and linoleic acid, but is particularly rich in the omega 3 series, linolenic acid. Although this is a non-fat program, flaxseed oil is included following the work of Dr. Johanna Budwig, which indicated the therapeutic role of flaxseed oil in cancer. The therapeutic effects of flaxseed oil (specifically linolenic acid) are the following:

- It attracts oxygen at the cell membrane and transports oxygen into the cell;
- By virtue of its chemical structure (grouping of its double bonds) an electrical field is created which is capable of storing energy in the cell and intracellular membranes. These membranes cover a huge surface area that acts as a workbench for much of the cells' enzymatic activity, which can tap into the stored energy on demand;
- It can detoxify the fat-soluble toxins. Studies proved that animals fed on flaxseed oil failed to develop cancer from being exposed to cigarette smoke. The oil detoxified the benzopyrin, the agent responsible for causing cancer in the smoker; and
- It is a carrier for Vitamin A (important for the immune system).

*Dosage:*
2 Tablespoons (20ml) of flaxseed oil daily for the first month, then reduced to 1 Tablespoon (10ml) daily for the remainder of the therapy. Occasionally, this amount may be increased to 1.5 Tbs daily if the patient is experiencing severe skin cracking, or 2 Tbs daily if the patient's cholesterol levels are high.

# Coffee Enemas

On the full therapy these are taken 5 times daily (6am, 10am, 2pm, 6pm, 10pm). They may be reduced later, depending upon progress and tumour bulk. With high tumour bulk they need to be maintained at this dose and even increased in times of flare-up. They can be taken at two hour intervals during the height of a flare-up, but this is not advised over a prolonged period. The general advice is usually 1-2 extra enemas in times of flare-up. Too many coffee enemas may create a disturbance in the patient's electrolyte balance (sodium/potassium).

On the modified therapy 2-3 coffee enemas are taken daily which may be reduced, in the weakened patient, to half-strength coffee/chamomile tea enemas.

### Contra-indications:
The contra-indications set out below are to be observed in the initial phase until the patient has stabilised. You would commence with just the chamomile tea enemas and then gradually introduce the coffee at 2 fl ozs (60mls), increasing until you have the full strength or as much as the patient can tolerate.

- Bleeding and/or ulceration in the gastrointestinal tract
- Hypertension, tachycardia
- Cardiac, respiratory or renal insufficiency
- Diarrhoea
- Dehydration
- Warfarin medication (it rapidly increases warfarin excretion)

# Castor Oil Treatment

On the full therapy the patient takes the castor oil treatment (by mouth and later followed by enema) on alternate days. The castor oil taken orally stimulates the liver to release larger amounts of toxic bile and additionally inhibits reabsorption of this bile. It also increases peristalsis and helps the patient to clear toxic residue from the whole length of the gastrointestinal tract. The elimination is very strong on this treatment. Dr. Gerson reduced the number of castor oil treatments to twice weekly after the first 4 weeks, but nowadays we observe the patient and only reduce further when the patient is responding positively to the therapy and the tumour masses are seen to be shrinking. You must not be too hasty in reducing the castor oil treatment. From alternate days the dose is reduced to 3/week, then 2/week, then once every five days. Don't hesitate to increase again if the patient is failing to heal at the expected rate. For many patients, their livers require this additional support in detoxification, and therefore the castor oil treatment remains essential. These patients will recognise the benefits of this treatment. Generally, the indication is that the more toxic you feel with this treatment, the greater the amount of toxicity you hold. Patients gradually feel less and less toxic following this treatment as they progress - which is a good indication of the reduction of toxicity.

Patients on the modified therapy do not take the castor oil treatments at the beginning of the therapy. The practitioner must be very cautious about introducing the castor oil treatment to patients who have undergone chemotherapy. The castor oil treatment may be introduced to a weakened patient or one that has received chemotherapy when they are seen to be strengthening and responding favourably (generally around 6 months). Initially only the castor oil in the enema is given, with 2 Tbs (20ml) castor oil increasing to 4 Tbs (40mls) in the enema. If the patient responds well, then you may start giving the castor oil by mouth, but starting with 1-2tsp (5-10ml). You may start this treatment once or twice weekly. It is not advised that these patients take the full amounts of castor oil by mouth.

### Contra-indications:
- Chemotherapy pre-treated patient
- Extremely weakened liver - hepatitis, liver disease
- Ulcers/bleeding/inflammation - anywhere in the gastrointestinal tract
- Diarrhoea

# Adjuncts

## Clay packs and Castor-oil packs

These packs are useful in alleviating pain either associated with tumour swelling, liver congestion/spasms in the liver/gall system, general muscle spasms or bone pain. Most patients will experience some pain associated with the healing inflammation during flare-ups, and the clay or castor oil pack can be a good first line treatment in alleviating pain.

**The clay pack** is used for "hot" inflammations around the joints, tumour swelling, and to reduce areas of fluid retention either through injury or general oedema. Clay packs are often administered twice daily over the liver area (liver metastases) where they actively draw out toxicity. They can be kept in place for 2-3 hours and cannot be re-used, as they have adsorbed toxins and therefore hold the toxicity. The use of clay packs is also effective in cases of brain tumour/metastases.

The type of clay used is a Montmorillonite clay (not a sea clay). The structure of this clay gives it both adsorbent and absorbent qualities. 1 gram of this clay has a surface area of around $800m^2$. This surface area is negatively charged and has the capacity to pick up and hold toxins and pathogenic micro-organisms. Toxins/organic matter will not only stick to its outer surface but enter the space between the layers and be absorbed into the inner layers. Montmorillonite clay is the best type of clay to use in any type of gastro-enteritis, cholera or general food poisoning. Gerson patients suffering diarrhoea are advised to take 1/4 tsp of this clay along with 1/4 tsp potassium gluconate in peppermint tea until symptoms are resolved.

Clay has been used for centuries by all the indigenous populations around the world to guard against dysentery. Most tribes had a practice of dipping their food in clay water before eating, to protect against "sour" stomach and dysentery. [5] Clay used to be a standard medication in the army to protect against cholera, as it reduced the mortality rate from 60% to 3%.

**The castor oil pack** is generally used for muscle pain/bone pain and to alleviate spasms and cramping. This warm pack increases circulation to the area, relaxes the muscles and disperses toxicity. During the initial stages of detoxification shifting toxins will often lodge in muscle tissue causing muscle contraction, stiffness and pain, particularly in the shoulder/neck area. The castor oil pack can also be used to shift mucous congestion in the lungs. It is also useful over the abdomen if the patient is suffering from intestinal spasms and cramps. In bone pain the muscles will tend to contract around the bone exacerbating the pain and the castor oil pack will prove invaluable. The castor oil pack can be re-used and kept in place for as long as required.

The castor oil pack has been used for centuries in most cultures from China to Africa, the Mediterranean and the Americas. Edgar Cayce raised the profile of castor oil both for internal and external use:

- Increases eliminations of the gastrointestinal tract
- Stimulates functional activity of the gastrointestinal tract
- Stimulates liver/gall bladder
- Heals lesions and adhesions/dissolves scar tissue
- Releases and disperses mucus congestion (lungs/abdomen/bowel)
- Releases and disperses congestion/acidity

- Relief of pain and inflammation: increases blood and lymph circulation to the area
- Reduces muscle spasms

Recent research has indicated that castor oil acts as an antitoxin agent and has an impact on the lymphatic system including the immune system. Test results in a blind study revealed an increase in lymphocyte production and increased activity of the T lymphocytes in the group using the castor oil packs.[6]

Patients will discover, through experimentation, which type of pack will provide the most relief from symptoms. Many patients have found that an initial 30 minute application of the warm castor oil pack followed by the clay pack has afforded the best relief.

# Vitamin C

The literature on the use of Vitamin C in cancer is very impressive. However, we do not supplement with Vitamin C on this nutritional program, as the fresh produce and juices supply ample amounts of it with all its co-factors. However, if the patient has had chemotherapy, has taken medical prescription drugs for any condition for a prolonged period of time, has smoked or taken recreational drugs, then Vitamin C may be used at a dose of 3-5g for a period of time. Vitamin C is used to limit the damaging effects of free radicals when the body is detoxifying these chemicals. Indeed, studies have shown that vitamin C reduces the effects of methotrexate (a chemotherapy drug), as it accelerates the detoxification of this drug by the liver. However, it was also found to potentiate the effects of the other chemotherapeutic agents.[7] Vitamin C would probably assist in the detoxification of a patient who has undergone chemotherapy, particularly during flare-ups.

It is through the work of Linus Pauling that we have begun to understand the role of Vitamin C in the control of infectious disease. This vitamin not only restores the bacteriocidal activity of leucocytes, but is a powerful antioxidant and therefore protects tissues against damage from free radicals. [8] In relation to Dr. Gerson's Therapy we must remember that the free radicals generated during an inflammatory response augment this response. Vitamin C can both amplify and neutralise the response in chronic inflammation and normal tissue, respectively, and perhaps this is where its value lies, as we have seen, in chronic or tumoural inflammation, but as an adjunct to the Gerson therapy on an ongoing basis, its role may be questionable. Dr. Gerson preferred to give the juice of six lemons daily to assist combating infection.

The role of Vitamin C in cancer is not conclusive. Studies have revealed an increase in survival time of terminally ill patients from 3 months expected survival to an average survival time of 261 days, and patients noted improvements, such as a reduction in pain, fewer withdrawal symptoms when narcotics/morphine were discontinued, and decreased volume of ascites and effusions.[9] The antioxidant effect of Vitamin C would account for reduction in pain and inflammation from necrotic and ulcerating tumours (hence reducing ascites and effusions), and the rapid detoxification of drugs such as morphine. These patients were taking 10g of Vitamin C daily.

## Three main arguments for the use of Vitamin C in cancer
1. Vitamin C inhibits the enzyme hyaluronidase, which is released by malignant cells and attacks the hyaluronic acid of the intercellular cement of surrounding tissues. This weakens the tissues and permits infiltration of the malignancy.
2. Vitamin C increases the synthesis of collagen in the intercellular cement, which strengthens the surrounding area, preventing tumour invasion and growth. Tumours may also be encapsulated by collagen, which inhibits metastasis.

3. Vitamin C forms hydrogen peroxide which is known to be toxic to cancer cells due to their low capacity for the enzyme catalase which would normally convert hydrogen peroxide to oxygen. Vitamin C's oxidant capacity is dose dependent and requires high doses taken intravenously, not orally. The dosage can range from 30g to 200g as an infusion. Many practitioners recommend twice weekly infusions, but the best results may be obtained by having these more frequently, even on a daily basis.

However, there is evidence that high intakes of oral Vitamin C may cause "over-healing", where too much scar tissue is produced.[10] Collagen is also laid down in blood vessels making them less distensible and harder.

Although there have been remarkable anecdotal outcomes with IV Vitamin C, the results do vary. It must be remembered that vitamin C is not seen to be curative but useful as an adjunct in the control of certain outcomes. "Vitamin C has been shown to be safe when given to healthy volunteers and cancer patients at doses up to 1.5 g/kg [oral dosing], while screening out patients with certain risk factors who should avoid vitamin C. Studies have also shown that Vitamin C levels in the blood are higher when taken by IV than when taken by mouth, and last for more than 4 hours."[11] It is worth noting that the activity of vitamin C will be limited by the dose given and the amount of time it is held in serum, which may be little more than 4 hours, which would underpin the requirement for more regular infusions at higher dosage.

Vitamin C has been used as an adjuvant in:
- radiotherapy, where it reduces the nausea thought to be caused by the sudden metabolic overload of the toxic breakdown products of dead tissues; and
- Chemotherapy, where it assists in the detoxification of drugs through enhancing the liver enzyme detoxification system. Vitamin C is withheld for 24-48 hours during intensive chemotherapy treatment that includes the drug methotrexate.

*If prescribing Vitamin C, do not use sodium or calcium ascorbates.*

# Charcoal

Ground charcoal tablets, available from any chemist, can be taken with juices to alleviate gas.

# Hyperthermy/Hydrotherapy

Many patients undergo hydrotherapy (immersion in hot water for a specified length of time) to increase body temperature. Hyperthermy (the raising of the body temperature either through hydrotherapy or microwave radiation) as a single treatment is ineffective against cancer. Less than 1 in 100 human cancers are destroyed by temperatures above 41.8°C (the maximum tolerance temperature of the human liver). The cytoplasm of certain tumour cells is only "poached" by hyperthermia (at 39°C) and dies at 46°- 47°C. Cancer cells are stimulated and grow faster with hyperthermy as a sole treatment, but when used in conjunction with chemotherapy and radiotherapy, by virtue of its capacity to synchronize cell division it can improve the killing power and result in lower doses of these treatments achieving improved response rates.[12] (See Chapter 6, p130 for a fuller explanation.)

Hydrotherapy (raising the body temperature to between 37°C and 40°C) used in conjunction with Laetrile and ozone ensures a 3-10 fold gain in effect of these treatments. It is not recommended that the patient undergoes more than two hydrotherapy treatments a week and is accompanied by a carer. The patient should maintain this temperature for around 20 minutes in a hot bath, keeping the head covered to avoid heat losses. As the blood pressure can drop, it is important that the carer helps the patient after the treatment and that they are kept warm and put into bed following the treatment in order to rest.

# Laetrile

Used as an adjuvant in prostate, breast and lung cancers and with bone metastases. Laetrile is also effective in alleviating bone pain from metastases.

Laetrile is the purified form of B17 (amygdalin) and was developed by Dr. Ernst T. Krebs Jr (Dr. Biochemistry, d. 1996). Dr. Krebs followed the philosophy of Dr. Beard and began a search for a nutritional factor that was hinted at by Dr. Beard for the control and cure of cancer. [13, 14]

B17 is composed of 2 units of glucose, one of benzaldehyde and one of cyanide, all tightly locked together. Locked in this natural state it is chemically inert and has no effect on living tissue. The enzyme beta-glucosidase can unlock the compound and release the cyanide and benzaldehyde. Together they are synergistically 100 times more poisonous than separately. The enzyme beta-glucosidase is found in high quantities in the cancer cell, so B17 is unlocked by the cancer cell and releases its poisons to it. The enzyme rhodanese, which is high in normal cells but low in cancer cells (rhodanese is also inhibited by hCG which is high in cancer cells), neutralises cyanide by converting it to the by-product thiocyanate. Furthermore, benzaldehyde is oxidized and converted to benzoic acid by normal cells which is known to have analgesic properties, so relieving the intense pain associated with terminal cancer. These compounds have a deadly synergistic action in malignant cells that do not have any oxidative metabolism, but are of no detriment to the normal cell and can have therapeutic effects with regard to pain management and the reduction of oedemas. Laetrile, whilst having no effect on normal tissue, will attack the cancer cell and raise the temperature of tumour tissue. Used in conjunction with hydrotherapy, its effects are amplified 3-10 fold.

B17 is also used for the production of B12 by the body. It is stated in most textbooks that B12 is only available from animal sources; however, the cyanide radical of B17 combines with hydrocobalamin to form cyanocobalamin (B12). Thus, laetrile can stimulate haemoglobin synthesis and increase the blood count of both red and white cells.

Apricot kernels do not contain any therapeutic levels of B17 and B17 is difficult to absorb. While they may have a role in prevention, they are classed as seeds and as such are too high in fat and anti-tryptic factors to be recommended on this therapy.

***Dose:***
Intra-venous 6cc/day (equivalent of 2 x 10cc ampules) for 21 days - helps to absorb fluids and increases the temperature in tumour tissue.[15] Using a peripheral venous catheter (PVC), or butterfly port, for quick and safe access over time, the IV "push" is done twice daily, morning and evening. Infections are always possible at these sites, so hygeine is important and also catheter replacement. Following IV, take 2g laetrile daily in tablet form for 3-6 months. Take on an empty stomach 1/2 hour before eating. If the laetrile upsets the stomach, it can be crushed with pancreatin and administered rectally as a paste.

# Bio-oxidative Therapies

Bio-oxidative therapy uses ozone and hydrogen peroxide. Ozone ($O_3$) is a form of energized oxygen, carrying additional electrons and hydrogen peroxide ($H_2O_2$) is converted to oxygen by the enzyme catalase. Both of these compounds are used to accelerate oxidative metabolism.

As early as 1856 ozone was used to disinfect operating theatres and in 1860 to purify water treatment plants (Monaco). In 1915 medical ozone was used to treat skin diseases and to disinfect wounds during the first World War, By the 1930's ozone was used in rectal insufflation to treat colitis. In 1945 it was used by intravenous injection and in the 1950's it was first used as a treatment for cancer.

We must remember that oxidation is the transfer of electrons and that ozone is a very reactive product in that it can donate or accept electrons; therefore it acts as a free radical and a free radical scavenger. Electrons hold potential energy, which can either be used destructively or constructively. Free radicals carry unpaired electrons, which means that they are always seeking electrons to balance their molecules and, if uncontrolled, will destroy healthy body tissue. The enzyme systems of the body can safely balance these reducing/oxidising reactions (donation/receiving of electrons) so that tissues are not destroyed by the body's production of free radicals. Superoxide dismutase (SOD), glutathione peroxidase and catalase, the three antioxidant enzyme systems involved in the shuttling of electrons from superoxide and hydrogen peroxide to molecular oxygen, require selenium, iron, manganese, copper and zinc as co-factors.

During inflammation the immune cells of the body will produce superoxide ($O_2^-$) and hydroxyl ($OH^-$) ions. These radicals will destroy bacteria, viruses, yeasts and abnormal cells. In 1974 Dr Joachim Varro revealed peroxidase intolerance in cancer cells, and that hydrogen peroxidase contributed to the lysis of tumour cells by macrophages and granulocytes in vitro. However, to the healthy cell, catalase will convert hydrogen peroxide to oxygen. Other effects noted are the dilatation of blood vessels (increasing blood flow); the increasing of cardiac output; increasing the immune response by stimulating the formation of granulocytes and monocytes; stimulating T-helper cells, and producing interferon and tumour necrosis factor (TNF).

### Application:
Ozone and hydrogen peroxide are added to a base of oxygen or water respectively.


## Ozone

### By rectal insufflation
1-5 parts ozone : 95-99 parts oxygen (1%-5% solution). It is important to achieve a therapeutic concentration as too high a concentration is immunosuppressive and too little is ineffective. 100 - 800mls of oxygen/ozone mixture is introduced through the rectum and absorbed via the intestines. This process takes 90 seconds to 2 minutes and the mixture is retained for 10-20 minutes.

On this therapy patients can take 30mls (cc) twice daily via rectal insufflation. We do not recommend this treatment if the patient suffers an inflammatory bowel condition.

### By injection
*Minor auto-haemotherapy* - 10ml of the patient's venous blood is treated with oxygen and ozone and given via intramuscular injection.
*Major auto-haemotherapy* - ozone and oxygen bubbled into 50-100mls of the patient's blood for several minutes and then the ozonated blood is re-introduced into a vein.

## Hydrogen Peroxide

### By mouth

With all the current literature on oxygen therapies, many patients add oral hydrogen peroxide to their therapy. However, accessing the food grade hydrogen peroxide can be difficult.

The 3% and 6% hydrogen peroxide obtained from chemists contains a variety of stabilizers (phenol, acetanilide, sodium stancite), which are contra-indicated for oral use or skin bathing on this therapy. This form of hydrogen peroxide may be used as a general disinfectant for the bathroom and of the enema catheter, providing it is rinsed thoroughly with distilled or reverse osmosis water.

For internal use the hydrogen peroxide concentration must not exceed 0.5%. The patient will need to obtain 35% food grade or 30% reagent grade hydrogen peroxide. The suggested oral ingestion by many authors is 10 drops, 3 times daily in 240ml distilled water. Owing to its very caustic action on the stomach, many people will start with 1 drop 3 times daily, and gradually increase. Many patients will be unable to tolerate oral hydrogen peroxide.

### By bathing:

In cases of infection, it is therapeutic to use hydrogen peroxide in the bath. The patient will need to run a hot bath and add 200mls of 35% hydrogen peroxide to it. Take two baths a day for 3 days and then one bath daily for the next 3 days. After bathing, while the skin pores remain open, the patient should rub a 2% solution of food grade hydrogen peroxide over the skin. If your water is from a municipal source and high in chlorine, then running a very hot bath and leaving the windows open for the steam to evaporate should suffice. The chlorine, being a volatile gas, will be driven off through the steam.

### *Dilution:*

Converting 35% hydrogen peroxide to 2% hydrogen peroxide:

1 part 35% hydrogen peroxide : 16 parts distilled water.

Converting 35% hydrogen peroxide to 0.5% hydrogen peroxide:

1 part 35% hydrogen peroxide: 69 parts distilled water.

**Important:** The melanoma patient should not have massage, hydrotherapy or hyperbaric oxygen treatment, as too much irrigation/stimulation accelerates the growth of the tumour. Ozone therapy, however, may be given and the patient may be instructed to use hydrogen peroxide packs on their tumour site.

# Colloidal Silver

Colloidal silver used as an external spray has proved of benefit in the treatment of exposed and ulcerating wounds/ tumours. Silver is a heavy metal and should not be taken orally by those following the Gerson Therapy.

# Polarizing Treatment - GKI

The history of this treatment dates back to the work of Dr. Sodi-Pallares, a heart specialist who became famous for his polarizing treatment in chronic heart failure and infarction. He proved that heart disease originates from the changes in metabolism of the myocardial fibres due to sodium retention, loss of potassium and an increase of lactic acid. In 1969 he presented his results to the NY Academy of Sciences, where he was able to demonstrate that his polarizing therapy (GKI: glucose, potassium, insulin) halved the death rate in those experiencing heart attack symptoms.

The polarizing solution given to heart attack patients was 1 litre 10% dextrose in water, 20 mEq K chloride and 15 units of lente insulin. A maximum of 3 litres was administered over 24 hours. The insulin increases the uptake of potassium into the cells, improving ATP production. Dr Sodi-Pallares also found that he could reduce the dose of defibrillating drugs to 1/4 of the usual dose.

The therapy was abandoned despite the results obtained. A recent editorial by Dr.Carl Apstein of Boston University, reviewed this treatment and estimated that the polarizing therapy could prevent 75,000 deaths from heart attack each year. The comparison he draws between the cheapness and effectiveness of the treatment (less than US$50.00 for an intravenous GKI) and the cost of anti-clotting/clot dissolving drugs is not lost on the reader. [16]

This treatment has been found to be of some benefit to the cancer patient, primarily in the reduction of oedema (ascites, oedema, effusions). The treatment differs slightly, as it has been found that it is better to administer an insulin injection (3 units) and add the potassium compound solution to the juices (20ml in each of the 10 juices), whilst increasing the fruit within the diet. This treatment can be done daily until the crisis is resolved. It has been found to be an effective treatment in the initial instance, but if the problem is a recurring one, then this treatment may cease to be effective.

# Spirulina

Spirulina as a powder, delivers 60% protein by weight and has been given when the use of soured milk products is contraindicated (allergy) to replace the protein that you would find in dairy. Spirulina is *not* a substitute for dairy as no studies indicate its value in improving patient outcome. If spirulina is recommended, It is essential to use an organic supply of spirulina, bearing in mind it is a food concentrate that is heavily processed. When supplementing spirulina, 5g dried spirulina delivers 3g protein which compares with 100g of non-fat yoghurt. When replacing dairy protein with spirulina, then a minimum of 10g spirulina daily will supply around 6g protein. Other heavily processed dried grasses have been recommended, such as green barley, which is preferred by some practitioners due to its lower sodium content. Wheat grass may be too high in protein and too strong for the patient on this treatment.

On a note of caution, spirulina is high in cobalamin (B12) analogues which interfere with the use of cobalamin proper by the cobalamin coenzymes. Therefore if there is a B12 deficiency or known problems with B12, then it would be wiser to source an alternate source of protein if dairy cannot be taken.

# Bee Pollen

Bee pollen is another alternative source of protein. The recommended dose is between 2-4 tsp daily. Please recommend caution with this product as allergic reactions may occur. It is best to start at 1/2 tsp and observe for allergic reactions. Again, it cannot be seen as a replacement for the dairy.

# Essiac Tea and Pau D'Arco Tea (Three Way Tea)

These herbs have been shown to have anti-cancer properties and may be used by patients.

**Dose for Essiac Tea:**
60ml morning and afternoon.

Occasionally other herbs may be prescribed for their positive effect on the nervous system (St. John's Wort), to aid sleep (lime flowers, jasmine flowers, skullcap, lavender, hawthorn berries, cowslip flowers), and to aid detoxification by the liver (milk thistle). Homoeopathic remedies may also be administered.

# Other Alternative Therapies

| Accepted Treatments | Prohibited Treatments |
|---|---|
| Reflexology | Aromatherapy |
| Vacuflex therapy | Swedish or deep massage |
| Manual Lymphatic Drainage | Colonics |
| Reiki | Swimming in the sea or in chlorinated pools |
| Counselling | Floatation tanks |
| Shiatsu (good for pain relief) | Exercise |
| Acupuncture | |
| Osteopathic or chiropractic treatment (be cautious in cases of bone metastases) | |
| McTimony chiropractic treatment | |
| Rebounding | |
| Homoeopathy | |

# General Modifications

This section covers general modifications for the diet, juicing, enemas and medications, for the various groups of patients. Although the medications have been covered previously, you will be able to see at a glance the contra-indications to the medications in the different groups. The practitioner is recommended to refer to Dr. Max Gerson's *A Cancer Therapy, Results of Fifty Cases*, and Charlotte Gerson and Beata Bishop's *Healing the Gerson Way* for further insight.

## Contra-indications to specific medications in the strong patient on the full therapy:

1.  Thyroid medication should be reduced/omitted if the patient is hyperthyroid (pulse and temperature increased), if there are heart irregularities, or if the patient is experiencing unacceptable weight loss. It may be temporarily discontinued during menstruation.

2.  Niacin should be omitted if there is any bleeding, ulceration, haemorrhage or suspected occult blood loss. Niacin may be temporarily omitted during menstruation or if the patient is suffering bleeding from haemorrhoids. Niacin should not be given to patients taking blood thinning agents, and niacin should be stopped a few days prior to surgery and resumed 3 weeks after surgery.

3.  Acidol pepsin should be omitted for patients who suffer from peptic, duodenal or intestinal ulcers.

4.  Potassium compound solution should be introduced carefully if the patient suffers from ulcers, cardiac, respiratory or renal insufficiency, or if the blood results indicate high serum potassium.

5.  CoQ10 should be introduced carefully if the patient suffers from tachycardia.

6.  Castor oil treatments should not be undertaken if the patient suffers from any bleeding or ulceration of the colon and digestive tract, inflammatory bowel disease or severe diarrhoea.

*These modifications apply to all patients.*

# Full Therapy

On the full therapy, during the first 4 weeks, the patient takes:

+ 13 x 240ml juices
+ 20ml potassium compound solution in 10 of the juices
+ 5 grains thyroid
+ 18 drops of 1/2 strength Lugol's (3 drops in each of the apple and carrot juices, and the orange juice)
+ 5 coffee enemas
+ Castor oil treatment on alternate days

- No cultured milk products (for the first 6-8 weeks)
- Flaxseed oil, 20ml daily

After 4 weeks, the doses of potassium, Lugol's and thyroid are reduced accordingly:
- 10ml potassium compound solution in 10 of the juices
- 2 1/2 grains thyroid
- 6 drops of 1/2 strength Lugol's (1 drop in each of the apple and carrot juices, and the orange juice)
- Flaxseed oil, 10ml daily

The number of coffee enemas and castor oil treatments will remain the same. Cultured milk products (non-fat yoghurt) will be added at 6-8 weeks unless the blood results indicate earlier.

Occasionally the patient on the full therapy fails to have a healing flare-up in the first few months. If this is the case then the patient may revert back to the original medication of 5 grains thyroid, 18 drops 1/2 strength Lugol's and 20ml of potassium compound solution in 10 of the juices for a period of 2-3 weeks. This often has the effect of stimulating a healing flare-up.

# Modified Therapy

## For the patient who has received chemotherapy but is fairly strong

- 10 x 240ml juices
- 10ml potassium compound solution in the 10 juices
- 2 1/2 grains thyroid
- 6 drops of 1/2 strength Lugol's (1 drop in each of the apple and carrot juices, and the orange juice)
- 2-3 coffee enemas
- No castor oil treatment
- No cultured milk products for the first 6-8 weeks
- Flaxseed oil, 2 Tbs (20ml) daily

This medication is not reduced after 4 weeks but maintained at these levels. The flaxseed oil is reduced to 10ml daily after 4 weeks.

The castor oil treatment may be introduced later by enema and then by mouth at the reduced dose of 5-10ml by mouth. The castor oil treatment may push an already damaged liver (from the chemotherapy) too hard and cause the release of too many dangerous chemotherapy toxins. The practitioner must bear this in mind if he/she wishes to introduce the castor oil treatment. It is wise to wait until the patient has been on the therapy for 6 months and has experienced the "six month flare-up" before ascertaining the safety of the castor oil treatment.

## For the weakened patient with or without chemotherapy pre-treatment

### Diet and Juices
These patients may start with the diet and up to 10 juices daily. The green juices are very strong and may either cause vomiting or "go straight through." Under these circumstances you may dilute the green juices with gruel. Depending on the volume of liquid your patient can tolerate, you may start with only 50ml per juice/gruel and

then increase. If lack of appetite is a problem then it is important to recommend the porridge (gruel is also very nourishing and soothing when there is toxic bile), stewed apple, Hippocrates soup and mashed potato. The diet, at this stage, is more important than the juices but no raw foods (other than the juices) or salads should be given until the patient is feeling stronger. Patients with effusions, ascites or oedemas may have to reduce the quantity of juices, as the high fluid intake will generally aggravate the situation. Dietary restrictions may have to be reviewed if the patient cannot eat the volume of food required for healing over a prolonged period, particularly if they start deteriorating. The diet is high volume/low nutrient density, so additional protein may be added under these circumstances.

### Enemas

Chamomile tea enemas can be used to clear the bowels, but this will not be strong liver stimulant. As the patient improves you can start adding a little coffee to the chamomile tea enemas.

No castor oil treatment.

### Medications

You may start with perhaps:
- 1-2 drops 1/2 strength Lugol's;
- 1/2 - 1 gr thyroid; and
- 5ml/juice of the potassium compound solution.

In the very weak patient these doses may remain at this level for some time; however, you may be able to increase the potassium to 10ml/juice, if the blood results indicate that serum potassium is normal and there is no renal or cardiac insufficiency.

It is important to remember that the detoxification therapy, with its high volume of fluids and potassium, Lugol's and thyroid medications, may tax the cardiac, respiratory and renal organs. Any patient with insufficiency in any of these organs must start slowly with the medications which may be gradually brought safely up to their maximum dose over a period of 1-4 weeks (or longer), depending upon the patient's condition. It is wise to have weekly blood tests taken to establish your patient's progress and appropriate doses for the medications.

The weakened patient's blood results may indicate reduced protein levels. Under these circumstances it is wise to include the soured milk protein at the outset of treatment. In patients who require tapping of effusions/ascites, the protein levels may become vulnerable and under these circumstances fish may be introduced into the diet.

# Non-Cancer Patients

Many patients, who do not have cancer, may wish to undergo a modified detoxification plan and will seek help and guidance when embarking on such a regime. The practitioner is urged to rigorously apply the philosophy behind detoxification when appraising the case and making recommendations.

## Diet

In order to initiate the healing and detoxification process, the same principles must be applied for any patient, whether they suffer from a malignant condition or a chronic degenerative disease. The four basic principles as applied to diet must be observed:

+ Organic and chemical-free foods, fresh (not canned/preserved, etc.)
+ No salt/high potassium diet
+ Reduction in protein
+ No fats, other than flaxseed oil

## Protein

It would be advisable to eliminate the animal proteins using only protein found in vegetables in the initial stages of the therapy. The patient's life-style would have to be taken into account, as many patients have to continue to work during their therapy. In autoimmune diseases protein intake usually has to be restricted on a more or less permanent basis, according to their response, as proteins are known to aggravate these conditions.

Protein may be gradually introduced as the therapy progresses. The general indications are:

+ soured milk products (non-fat yoghurt; non-fat, unsalted pot cheese)
+ Brown rice one - three times/week
+ Legumes one - three times/week
+ 2 eggs/week
+ Fish one - three times/week

Proteins are introduced gradually with firstly cultured milk products, then grains once/week; legumes weekly, eggs and then fish. At all times you will be observing the patient's progress, healing and regeneration. It is important to germinate (not sprout) the grains and legumes before cooking. If a patient wishes to remain vegetarian, then the combining of second class proteins should be observed, so that the patient maintains a healthy protein status for healing and maintenance. The Gerson Therapy, applied as the full therapy, does deliver sufficient protein for healing,[17] but any reduction in the volume of vegetables, both in juicing and at meals, will reduce the available protein and therefore one would have to address protein quality from other vegetarian sources, such as legumes and grains.

## Fats

Cooking with oils is never recommended. Fats are re-introduced cautiously, firstly as soaked nuts (almonds, hazelnuts and cashews have the lowest fat value) and later as a little unsalted butter. Oils are best avoided, other than flaxseed oil (recommendations at say 10-20ml daily) and unrefined cold-pressed sunflower or safflower oil as a salad dressing. Olive oil is not recommended for cooking. It can be used as a dressing, although the other oils mentioned contain the essential fatty acids, whereas olive oil is a mono-unsaturated oil and contains no essential fatty acids. Generally oils, other than those with the essential fatty acids must be regarded as empty calories, just like refined sugar. They are extracted from the seed leaving all the valuable minerals behind. High fat diets are expensive as they pull on the body's stores for their own metabolism. [18]

When the patient is well, they may occasionally cook in ghee which is non-toxic as a heated fat. The patient must remember that food cooked in oils heats to very high temperatures and distortion of the protein may render it a "non-food" of no nutritional value. In the case of allergic individuals and those suffering from autoimmune disorders, this can lead to a recurrence of the condition. Fats "heat" the liver, and any patient who has suffered from gastrointestinal ulceration, inflammatory disease of the digestive tract, gallstones or fat intolerance, or has past evidence of liver damage (viral, chemical, etc.) would be advised not to tax the digestion with additional dietary fat.

# Juices

I would recommend starting at 8 -10 juices daily (3-4 green, 4-5 carrot and apple, 1 orange). Orange juice should be omitted in arthritis and inflammatory/allergic conditions and also in conditions of mucus congestion/sinusitis/catarrh. As the patient progresses, the juices may be reduced to 6 daily (3 green, 3 carrot and apple) and then on an ongoing basis to between 3-4 daily.

# Enemas

The patient should start at 2 enemas daily (the same contra-indications apply as for the cancer patient) and depending upon the toxicity, these can be reduced to 1 daily. At 10 juices daily, if the patient is very toxic, then 3 enemas should be applied. Similarly, if a patient, who has reduced to 1 enema daily, experiences toxic build-up during the day, then a half strength coffee/chamomile tea enema should be enough to resolve the toxicity in the afternoon. The patient will learn to self-manage and recognise when additional coffee enemas are applicable.

The castor oil treatment is not generally indicated for non-cancer patients. A few exceptions may exist if the patient has had prolonged exposed to workplace chemicals.

# Medications

It is advisable to obtain blood work (full blood count, chemistry panel, liver function tests, thyroid function, vitamin D, B12 and folate assays, and iron status) before commencing with any medications. When a patient has a chronic degenerative disease, you may need to supplement with thyroid and Lugol's, and therefore it becomes imperative that you monitor the blood work each month.

- ◆ Potassium compound solution - 10ml in each juice, reducing to 5ml /juice with progress
- ◆ Niacin 50mg - 3 daily with meals
- ◆ Thyroid - 1/2 gr may be taken daily if the patient's basal temperature is below normal. Otherwise refer to blood results and medicate as appropriate.
- ◆ Lugol's 1/2 strength - use when supplementing with thyroid. In some patients Lugol's solution can block thyroid function. A urine iodine test can be used to determine iodine deficiency, and in patients with deficiency proceed with caution with the 1/2 strength Lugol's solution, regularly monitoring thyroid function.
- ◆ Pancreatin - 2-3 tablets with meals (maximum 9 daily)
- ◆ Acidol-pepsin/betaine hydrochloride - 1-2 before meals. Both the pancreatin and acidol-pepsin can be reduced as the patient progresses. Flatulence and bloating will contra-indicate any reduction of these medi-

cations. There are various digestive enzyme products on the market and it may be possible to substitute these with locally available supplements.

+ Liver capsules/tablets - 2 with each meal

**Vitamins A, E and C along with zinc and selenium** will support the immune system and may be taken if the immune function is deficient. Oily fish such as salmon, herring, tuna and cod's roe are rich in Vitamin A. The fresh juices are rich in vitamin C. Vitamin E may be found in nuts and the germ of grains (wheat germ). The practitioner must use his or her discretion when supplementing with nutrients. It must always be born in mind that we are looking to achieve nutritional status from the diet, and it is only if a patient has known nutrient deficiencies that are unable to be made good from the diet that we look to supplement with nutrients that may become at risk.

**The B12** status may become lowered on the vegetarian diet and therefore oral B12 may be taken on a daily basis. If the patient cannot absorb B12, then it is advisable to give it by injection. It is always worthwhile asking for a B12 assay prior to the patient commencing treatment and afterwards every 6 months (if they are not taking supplemental B12).

**Vitamin D** may also be deficient on the vegetarian diet. It is important to have some sunlight, which will instigate the conversion of cholesterol in the skin to vitamin D. Vitamin D deficiencies lead to poor calcium absorption and osteoporosis. Vitamin D is found in oily fish and in minimal amounts in dairy products.

**Iron** is generally not a problem if the patient continues with the green juices. The red beans (kidney and adzuki beans) are high in iron, as is dried fruit (dates, prunes, raisins), green leafy vegetables and herbs, such as parsley.

**Iodine** is found in sea food and seaweed. Kelp is a useful source of dietary iodine. Although kelp is contra-indicated in cancer treatment (too high in salt), it may be used in the less intensive treatment as part of a maintenance plan.

**Do not supplement with calcium.** Calcium can block the thyroid (opposes the uptake of iodine) and could exacerbate a hypothyroid condition. Calcium also acts in a similar manner to sodium in that it can adversely affect the healing process.

**Apply caution with magnesium.** It can have a stimulating effect on detoxification. It can tax the kidneys which could push the body too far on such a strong detoxification therapy as this.

Do not attempt to reduce any prescribed medication by the patient's doctor. The patient will usually confer with their doctor and reduce at a safe rate as their general health starts to improve.

## The Clay Pack

This is a cold pack used for hot inflammatory swellings, particularly useful for reducing oedema from these areas. You need enough clay and water to make a smooth spreadable mixture to cover the area at a thickness of about 1cm. Pour the clay into a glass bowl and add hot, distilled/RO water to make a smooth but not stiff paste. You need to use wooden and/or glass utensils (not metal or plastic) when handling clay.

Cut two pieces of flannelette the size of the area to be covered. Spread the clay mixture (with your wooden spoon) on the top layer of flannel and lay it over the area. Secure the pack with a wide elastic bandage (no plastic should be used, as the pack needs to "breathe"). Some authors state that a piece of thin gauze should be placed between the pack and the skin. However, other authors state that the clay should be applied directly onto the skin. Either is applicable, however, it is probably easier and less messy to use the gauze layer with the clay pack, particularly if the skin is broken.

The pack can be left in place for up to 2 hours or until it has dried out. It must then be thrown away as it cannot be re-used.

## The Castor Oil Pack

This is a warm pack for relieving spasms and cramping, whether in the muscles or in the internal organs, such as the liver and digestive system. It can also be used to shift mucus congestion in any area of the body, including the lungs.

1.  Soak a piece of flannelette, the size of the area to be covered, and then squeeze dry. Flatten out and place on a plastic bag/plastic sheet
2.  Cover with a second piece of flannelette.
3.  Spread a generous layer of castor oil over the cloth and spread over the area. Repeat with a third layer.
4.  Lay this, castor oil side down, over the body, keeping the plastic in place, and secure with a bandage.
5.  Place a heated pad (not electric) or a hot water bottle over this. If this is too hot, then you may cover the castor oil pack with a towel and remove this as the heat pack cools.
6.  Leave in place for as long as desired, minimum one and a half hours.
7.  If you wish to re-use the pack fold over in half, castor oil side facing inwards, and roll up after use to store until the next day.

## The Coffee Enema

The use of coffee in enemas for detoxification purposes has been a well known and practiced for many decades. There is no better stimulant for bile production and its subsequent flushing out than coffee, taken as an enema. This is due to a number of pharmacologically acting substances in the coffee. The combination of theobromine, theophylline and caffeine stimulates the relaxation of smooth muscles, causing dilatation of blood vessels and bile ducts. Hence bile flow is increased. Also increased are the number of toxins which are conjugated in the bile. This is due to the activity of the palmitates, which activate the enzyme system, glutathione-S-transferase, seven fold. This enzyme system, which is selenium-dependent, is responsible for conjugating toxins and quenching free-radicals and delivering them to the bile via the glutathionation pathway, where they are carried out via the common bile duct to the small intestine. The neutralization of free radicals effectively prevents oxidative damage and therefore this enzyme performs a protective role against hepatic damage due to toxins. There are six major detoxification pathways in the liver, of which glutathionation is but one; the other five pathways are not stimulated by the coffee enema.

The coffee enema is unsurpassed in its capacity to stimulate the flushing of toxic bile and without the coffee enema cancer patients would not be able to detoxify at the rate required for cure.

The effects of taking a coffee enema are not the same as drinking coffee. The coffee is absorbed by the mesenteric veins that serve the colon, and these flow directly into the portal vein which enters the liver. The enema is retained for 15 minutes, during which time it stimulates the hepatocytes to cleanse the blood, removing toxins. The entire blood circulation will be recycled through the liver about five times during this period, enabling a thorough cleanse. With the bile ducts open, a flushing of toxic bile is encouraged which enters the gastrointestinal tract. The large volume of fluid retained in the lower colon stimulates peristaltic activity, which ensures the propulsion of bile through the intestine to the outside. It is important to remember that the enema is given for the stimulation of the liver and not for the functioning of the intestines.

**Preparation of the coffee enema**

The coffee enema is prepared by putting 3 rounded tablespoons (or 1/4 cup) of organic, mild roast (higher caffeine content) ground coffee into one litre of distilled water which has just been brought to the boil. Continue on the boil for 3 minutes, uncovered, and then simmer on very low heat for 15-18 minutes, covered. Cool, strain through a fine mesh (not filter papers) and make up the quantity with distilled water to 1 litre. Straining the coffee in this way will ensure that you retain some silt in the enema which is high in palmitates. Pour the enema, lukewarm or body temperature, into the enema bag or bucket, and either hang it or place it on a flat surface (make sure the nozzle end is closed and the enema kit is not too high from the ground – 60–90 cm is sufficient). The patient must lie on their right side and the catheter placed into the rectum, before releasing the flow. Insert the catheter about 15-20 cm, or as comfortable as you can manage, as this will avoid uptake of the enema by the haemorrhoidal vein via the rectum, which will give a systemic effect. The bulk of the enema can then pass into the large colon and be absorbed by the mesenteric veins which deliver the coffee directly to the liver. Inject and retain for 15 minutes in the lying position. Pass the enema after 15 minutes. The bowels can continue operating independently even when taking the enemas and start functioning on their own after the enemas are discontinued.

Many patients at the beginning of the therapy experience problems in retaining enemas for the full 15 minutes. This occurs when the body is low in potassium and the musculature of the colon becomes hypersensitive. It will either contract and spasm making retention impossible because of the strong peristaltic waves, or it will clutch the enema so that the patient cannot release it. If the patient retains the enema and cannot release it, then the fluid will be absorbed into the circulation and passed via the kidneys.

*Tips to facilitate the enema procedure if difficulties are experienced:*
- *Take a 0.5 L Chamomile tea enema before the coffee enema. Do not retain. Chamomile will soothe and relax the muscles prior to your coffee enema and assist in the elimination of any bulk matter in the colon.*
- *Take a chamomile and coffee enema mixed (0.5L coffee:0.5L chamomile tea), or add some chamomile concentrate to the full-strength coffee enema.*

- *Take the enema in two smaller doses (this will take twice the time, as each enema must be retained for the full 15 minutes).*
- *Make sure the enema bucket is not placed too high. If the enema feeds into the rectum too quickly, this can set up counter spasms in the intestine.*
- *If you cannot release the enema - take another one back to back.*
- *Add 10ml of the potassium compound solution to the enema. This should be done for no longer than a few days, as the solution can be an irritant.*
- *Add 100ml Aloe Vera to the enema when there is inflammation in the bowel*
- *Make your total day's coffee enema requirement at one go and keep as a concentrate in the refrigerator. Dilute before use.*

# The Coffee/Chamomile Tea Enema

### Chamomile concentrate (4 full-strength enemas or 8 half- strength enemas)

- 1 cup chamomile flowers (dried)
- 1 litre distilled water

Simmer 30 minutes, strain and press. Add distilled water to make 1 litre. Keep refrigerated. To use, pour 250 mls into the enema bucket and add 750ml distilled water. Administer at body temperature.

### Coffee concentrate. (4 full-strength enemas or 8 half- strength enemas)

- 1 cup organic coffee, mild roast and finely ground
- 1 litre distilled water

Boil for 3 minutes and simmer for 20 minutes. Strain. Add distilled water to make 1 litre. Keep refrigerated. To use, pour 250ml into the enema bucket and add 750ml distilled water. Administer at body temperature.

**To make 1/2 coffee and 1/2 chamomile enema**, take 125ml of the chamomile concentrate and 125ml of the coffee concentrate, pour into the bucket and add sufficient distilled water to make 1 litre. Administer at body temperature.

# The Castor Oil Treatment

The liver of the cancer patient is very damaged and toxic. Dr. Gerson first introduced the castor oil treatment as he found that it gave the liver the additional support that was required for the intense detoxification at the beginning of treatment. It is through this treatment that very noxious substances and chemicals are effectively released from the liver. Although Dr. Gerson was able to reduce the frequency of this treatment after the first month, nowadays we find that patients continue to require this additional support for a longer period. It is important for the practitioner to observe the healing and detoxification of the client and to respond adequately to the requirements. It is important not to reduce the castor oil enemas prematurely, as this can affect the patient's progress negatively.

*Function:*

Castor oil is not metabolised/absorbed in the gut. The patient takes 20ml of castor oil on an empty stomach, first thing in the morning, aided by sweetened black coffee which stimulates the stomach to clear the castor oil and move it through to the duodenum. If the patient cannot tolerate black coffee, then a strong peppermint tea brew can be taken, but this is not as effective a treatment as the coffee. Once in the duodenum, the oil creates a huge stimulus to the gallbladder to release large quantities of bile (in the case of the cancer patient - toxic bile). So the castor oil by mouth effectively exploits the role of the bile in fat digestion and it has a far greater stimulatory effect than the coffee enema. Once the toxic bile is released, it binds with the castor oil, but as the oil is not digested and absorbed, it traps the toxins, inhibiting their re-circulation back to the liver. Consequently toxins (and bile acids) are removed from the body more effectively with the castor oil treatment. We must not forget that we are not just getting rid of toxins from the liver, we have to get them out of the body. Under normal circumstances a proportion of the toxic bile is reabsorbed in the small intestine, but the binding capacity of the castor oil inhibits this. The strength of the castor oil treatment in removing toxicity has been well documented, as it is on the castor oil days that you can smell the toxic fumes that are released with the enemas.

The castor oil by mouth is followed by a normal coffee enema. At 10am, 4 hours later, add 40 ml of castor oil to the next coffee enema, plus 1/4 teaspoon of ox bile powder and some castile soap (ox bile and soap help to keep the castor oil in suspension in the coffee enema). Although difficult to retain (especially if you have used too much soap) it will still create a very strong peristalsis which helps to clear any toxic bile from the small intestine and colon.

## Regime

5.30 am   20ml castor oil by mouth followed by a cup of black coffee sweetened with sugar.
6.00 am   normal coffee enema
10.00 am  castor oil enema

*To make the enema:*

> One prepared coffee enema
> 40ml castor oil
> 1/4 - 1/2 tsp ox bile powder
> Vegetable soap (castile)

Various methods have been tried, but the following works well:

Warm the castor oil in its bottle (place in pan of boiling water). Pour 4 tablespoons into a warm bowl and add the ox bile powder and the liquid soap. Mix thoroughly and add the prepared warm coffee enema, whisking as you go.

*Dose and contra-indications*

At start of treatment, take on alternate days. Dr. Gerson stopped this treatment after a few weeks. However, nowadays it is recommended to continue while observing the healing process. From alternate days gradually reduce to 3/week, then 2/week, then once every five days. Don't hesitate to increase if the patient is failing to heal at the expected rate.

*Contra-indications*

- ▸ Chemotherapy pre-treatment
- ▸ Extremely weakened liver - hepatitis, liver disease
- ▸ Ulcers - anywhere in gastrointestinal tract

# References

1. Alexander, K; *Dr. Gerson's green juice*; http://www.kathrynalexander.com.au/gerson-therapy/dr-gersons-green-juice

2. Alexander, K; *Iodine, a century of medical fraud*; http://www.kathrynalexander.com.au/iodine-a-century-of-medical-fraud.html

3. Alexander, K; *Insulin resistance, a natural protection against oxidative stress*; http://www.kathrynalexander.com.au/health-topics/insulin-resistance-a-natural-protection-against-oxidative-stress

4. Alexander, K; *Insulin resistance, some basics for helping yourself*; http://www.kathrynalexander.com.au/uploads/2/6/0/7/26077117/insulin_resistance.pdf

5. Price, Weston A.: *Nutrition and Physical Degeneration*, 1998, pp 266 - 267

6. Grady, Harvey: *Castor Oil Packs: Scientific Tests Verify Therapeutic Value*, Venture Inward, July/August 1988

7. Cameron, Ewan, Pauling, Linus: *Cancer and Vitamin C*, 1981, p193

8. Ibid. 1981, p114

9. Ibid. 1981, pp 129-139

10. Ibid. 1981, pp 113

11. National cancer Institute; *High dose vitamin C*; http://www.cancer.gov/cancertopics/pdq/cam/highdosevitaminc/patient/page2

12. Alexander, K.: *Far infra red saunas and the Gerson Therapy*; http://www.kathrynalexander.com.au/gerson-therapy/far-infra-red-saunas-the-gerson-therapy

13. Krebs Jr., Ernst T.:*The Nitrilosides in Plants and Animals*, http://users.navi.net/~rsc/nitrilo1.htm http://users.navi.net/~rsc/krebs3.htm

14. Gurchot Ph.D., Charles: *Suggested Mechanisms of Action of Vitamin B-17*, http://users.navi.net/~rsc/gurchot.htm

15. Krebs Jr., Ernst T.: *The Extraction, Identification and Packaging of Therapeutically Effective Amygdalin*, http://users.navi.net/~rsc/isomyg.htm

16. Gerson, Charlolotte: *Heart Disease*, Gerson Healing Newsletter, May - June 1999 (Vol 14, No.3)

17. Alexander, K; *Protein and the Gerson Diet*; http://www.kathrynalexander.com.au/gerson-therapy/protein-the-gerson-diet

18. Alexander, K; *Fats, creating a nutrient debt*; http://www.kathrynalexander.com.au/health-topics/fats-creating-a-nutrient-debt

# Recommended Reading

Alexander, K.: *Dietary Healing, the complete detox program*, ISBN 9780980376289

Erasmus, Udo: *Fats that heal and fats that kill*, 1986: Alive Publishing

Budwig, Johanna: *Flax Oil as a True Aid Against Arthritis, Heart Infarction, Cancer and Other Diseases*, 1992: Apple Publishing Co.

Knishinsky, Ran: *The Clay Cure*: Healing Arts Press

Dextreit, Raymond: *The Healing Power of Clay*: Editions Vivre en Harmonie

Cameron, Ewan, Pauling, Linus: *Cancer and Vitamin C*

Altman, Nathaniel: *Oxygen Healing Therapies*, Healing Arts Press

# Chapter 5

# PATIENT FOLLOW-UP & MANAGEMENT

In the 1950s many of Dr. Gerson's patients were cured within 18 months of starting his therapy. The general schedule of that time indicates how quickly Dr. Gerson was able to reduce the medications, and some of his case histories show the addition of certain protein foods to the diet. Due to the increased decline in the nutritional status of patients along with increased toxicity, we find that patients now have to remain longer on the diet (2 or more years), and the medications are reduced more slowly. For patients who have had chemotherapy it many be necessary to adhere to the therapy for up to 3 years and then to live closely by the diet for the rest of their lives. Under these circumstances the body needs this continued support, and any toxic burden appears to be to its detriment. However, the governing factors to the medication and dietary prescription remain the same:

- shrinking of the tumoural masses
- healing reactions/toxic eliminations
- stable blood results/tumour markers
- regeneration of tissue
- the return of energy and vitality to the patient

We need to see evidence that the therapy is working and assess how near the patient has come to total healing and cure. If the medications are reduced prematurely, or dietary protein is added too quickly, then the patient may go backwards or forfeit the opportunity to heal. As a practitioner you must observe and learn. If you add protein and the tumour starts growing, you know that you need to revert to previous levels, and if your patient did not experience a flare-up in the first few months of treatment, you may decide to place that patient on the full initial medication again to try and induce a flare-up.

The practitioner must always be acutely aware that in the seriously toxic patient and/or the patient who has undergone chemotherapy, pushing detoxification too fast can cause very serious and dangerous healing reactions. It is the serious toxic side-effects from the release of chemotherapy residues which can damage the patient further and lead to a rapid deterioration. For these reasons the castor oil treatment is used with great caution, and the liver and carrot juice (if the patient has access to fresh, organic veal liver) may be contra-indicated, or introduced slowly, for the patient who has had chemotherapy.

There are many variables to the prescription and diet, and it is the responsibility of the practitioner to apply the therapy, with a full understanding of the philosophy and the working of the therapy, but within the context of a medical understanding of the patient's case. The protocol will vary to take into account the following:

- strength/weakness of the patient
- ability to tolerate the diet and/or medications
- digestive capacity
- degree of toxicity
- capacity of the liver to eliminate safely

- concomitant illnesses including cardiac, renal or respiratory insufficiency
- current prescriptive medications
- metabolic and physical complications of malignancy.

It is unfortunate that many patients come for treatment when they have tried the orthodox route only to suffer a recurrence of the cancer which, by the time they come for help, many have metastasised and the patient's own resistance (immune system) is severely taxed. The practitioner, far from being able to start the patient on the therapy, has to introduce the diet and medications slowly, dependent upon blood results and the patient's symptoms, and very often the patient requires crisis management procedures which may indicate surgery, and/or drug/radiotherapy intervention. Under some circumstances the practitioner has to restore the patient slowly over a period of time before he/she can confidently introduce or increase the medications.

The guidelines set out below, along with the various case studies, should provide enough insight into case assessment and determination of the detoxification protocol. You must remember that each patient is different and treatment will vary. It is only through clinical practice and observation that you will become a skilled practitioner and able to interpret each situation and meet the specific requirements at any time to enable the patient to detoxify and heal adequately. As you become more qualified and practised, your interpretation of signs and symptoms will be more accurate, and your treatment more applicable and successful. You will become aware of the clinical effects of the therapy in a given situation, and how even subtle variations in the doses of medications/number of enemas will alleviate and facilitate healing.

# Patient Follow-Up

It is essential that patients are encouraged to keep their monthly appointments, particularly during the first 6 months. Careful note taking by the patient can be translated onto the patient follow-up consultation form and sent to you prior to their appointment, along with their blood results which must include the complete blood count, blood chemistry panel, thyroid function and urinalysis. It is important that you take practitioner notes and add these to your follow-up consultation form. You will need to make comments on the blood results and the patient's symptoms and detail changes in medication/diet to accommodate the overall situation. You will also need to check that the patient has been taking all the medications in the amounts prescribed and is following the diet rigidly.

Many patients make the mistake of thinking when "nothing is happening" that they do not need a consultation. To most people, our modern health culture indicates that we only need appointments when we have adverse symptoms. However, on the detoxification therapy, if the patient is having no detoxification symptoms, no toxic reactions or healing flare-ups, then we may need to re-evaluate whether the given treatment is enough to bring about a healing inflammation. If the patient is having flare-ups and detoxification symptoms and has learned how to self-manage, then after 6-9 months it may be agreed that a 2 monthly appointment is kept.

A major part of your role will be to teach the patient self-management, how to interpret the different reactions and how best to alleviate them. This will ensure that the patient does not make mistakes with the therapy. For example, a patient may be having toxic reactions and decide to reduce the coffee enemas because they panic and a well-meaning friend or relative has cast some doubt on this particular aspect of the therapy. If patients can be educated to understand what and why various symptoms are occurring and how to manage them, then they start to have greater confidence in the therapy and enjoy a greater degree of success.

# General Schedule Throughout the Therapy

If you compare the two charts on long-term follow-up (pp 193, 194) which indicate general guidelines as applicable in Dr. Gerson's time and the general guidelines as applied today, you will assess at a glance the major differences in protocol. The chart below details the main changes.

| Medications | Protocol in Dr. Gerson's Time | Current Guidelines |
|---|---|---|
| K compound | 10ml x 10 for 9 months, then reducing gradually | 10ml x 10 for 18 months, then reducing gradually |
| Thyroid | Reduced to 1.5 grain at 3 months | Remaining on 2.5 grain for at least 1 year, then reducing gradually |
| Lugol's | Reduced to 3 - 6 drops by 3 months | Reduced to 4 drops at 6 months; 3 drops by 9 months |
| Niacin | Reduced at 6 months | Reduced at 15 months |
| B12 + crude liver | Ceased between 4-6 months | Reduced to once/week at 1 year |
| Castor oil treatment | Ceased at 2-3 months | Reduced to once every 2 weeks at 18 months |
| Coffee enemas | Dependent on tumoural mass | Dependent on tumoural mass. Reduced to 4 at 6 months and 1 at 21 months. |
| Protein | Protein was added much earlier into the diet | At six months, depending on progress, introduce lentils once/ fortnight; fish at 15 months |

# Monitoring the patient's progress

Any changes in medication or diet are dependent on the patient's continuing progress which is assessed from two aspects, clinical studies (blood work/scans) and the patient's response to the therapy (flare-ups, etc.).

# Clinical Indications

## Blood Analysis

Blood work which indicates a healthy:

- red cell count
- haemoglobin status
- lymphocyte count
- white cell differential
- blood chemistry panel
- liver function tests
- kidney function tests
- tumour markers (if applicable).

Improvement in the status of the above, particularly the white cell differential and lymphocyte count, will indicate that the patient is progressing well. However good the blood work appears to be, any decision to modify the therapy must be taken in the light of other positive indications, such as scan results and general observation of the patient's healing reactions. Single readings of tumour markers are often unreliable indicators of disease progression, however, if there is an increasing trend, then this can be an ominous sign.

## Scans

After 6 months it is wise to request a scan (MRI, CT, PET or bone scan as applicable) to assess the progress (shrinkage of tumour, development of new lesions). In order to make a true comparison it is advisable to request the same type of scan as the one used for the original diagnosis. In general CT scans are better for the body tissues and MRI scans for the brain and spine. If there are bone metastases, it is wise to request a whole body bone scan to ascertain the degree and severity of metastases. Ultrasound scans can be unreliable, but for gastrointestinal tumours the colonoscopy or endoscopic ultrasound are the only reliable methods for diagnosing cancer. Although many patients feel unwilling to have CT scans, as the contrast media is toxic, the imaging is poor without it. The patient is encouraged to do an additional enema and take a few extra juices during the days following the scan to detoxify the added burden. If the scans indicate no progress, but no deterioration either, you may revert to the full therapy in the strong patient with no chemotherapy, particularly if that patient has not experienced any flare-ups. If the scans indicate significant progress, you may consider making slight modifications to the diet and reducing the enemas to 4 daily (depending on the amount of tumoural tissue) and reduce the frequency of castor oil treatments. The other medications will remain at a high level for at least the next 6-9 months.

# The patient's response to therapy

## Flare-ups

Reactions include toxic reactions, detoxification reactions and healing inflammations, and very often the three will occur together. As the body is building a momentum towards a flare-up (healing inflammation), the patient may notice strong reactions in the gut (detoxification of toxins irritating the gut) which often involve digestive problems, nausea, diarrhoea, inability to hold the enema and general feelings of systemic toxicity – headaches, irritability/irrationality, nervousness, soreness in the joints and muscles, and general malaise. These symptoms may occur with the healing crisis, which is quite distinct and often involves a general response (fever) along with a local response, such as the re-surfacing of old symptoms/injuries or pain and inflammation at the site of the tumour. At these times the patient may need to take more enemas to assist the liver in releasing the toxicity.

When assessing the patient's progress, you will be evaluating from past case notes and the symptoms described, whether the healing mechanism has been reactivated and how the patient is progressing.

The first crisis may occur within the first 5-10 days of the program and probably last around 2-3 days. A strong crisis is likely to occur in the $6^{th}/7^{th}$ week. In most patients the heaviest reaction will be in the $3^{rd}/4^{th}$ month. In pretreated chemotherapy patients you are not looking at a reaction until around the $5^{th}/6^{th}$ month and then again between 9-15 months. I have had patients who have had toxic and detoxification crises during the first year of the program but have not had their first healing crisis until around 15 months.

These cycles are only general and not golden rules. Also some patients have much stronger healing reactions than others; this does not mean that the patients with the strongest reactions are making the best progress. Each person is different and you are simply looking for that initial healing inflammation and symptoms of detoxification in order to assess the progress of the case.

You will also find that the cycle of reactions varies from patient to patient and each patient will become accustomed to their cycles and the types of reactions to expect. As the treatment progresses, the frequency and severity of the healing reactions lessen. The patient will be able to anticipate the reaction and learn how to alleviate some of the symptoms, so that they can remain on the therapy.

If your patient's blood work is good, the scan results are good and they have been experiencing healing reactions, then you may wish to adjust the therapy. The modifications to the medications within the first year will be minimal and also to the enemas and castor oil treatment. You will not be able to confidently reduce the main medications until 18 months into the therapy. The dietary modifications can begin at 6 months, if the patient is progressing well.

# Dietary Modifications

Specific dietary modification may be made when the patient has low iron, low sodium (<123), is allergic to any product, or suffers from diabetes.

- **Low iron/haemoglobin:** you may increase the green juices to 6/7 per day (replacing the carrot only juice). In the pretreated chemotherapy patient you may increase the green juices to 5/day and reduce the carrot and apple by one juice. Also recommend liberal use of organic dried fruit (stewed) such as prunes, apricots, raisins, and other iron-rich food such as spinach, beetroot, parsley and silver beet. Encourage the patient also to take some molasses daily (1 tsp).
- **Low sodium:** occasionally the sodium levels will fall to below normal. You may encourage the patient to increase the celery (not juiced), radish and silver beet in the diet. You may also need to reduce the number of enemas.
- **Low albumin:** this may occur if the patient is not consuming all the dietary recommendations or is suffering from ascites, nephrotic syndrome or advanced diabetes with renal involvement. You may encourage the patient to take more potatoes, increase the non-fat dairy, or even add fish.

- **Allergies:** these invariably occur with milk products and gluten. The patient may have a raised eosinophil count and present with allergic reactions such as eczema. You will need to remove the milk protein and replace with spirulina or bee pollen. If there is a gluten allergy you may need to remove the oats and rye and replace with quinoa.
- **Diabetes:** the fruits and sugars must be removed from the diet and the patient is given 6-8 green juices (without apple) and carrot only juices at the beginning of treatment. The blood sugar levels have to be monitored frequently.
- **Urine pH high** (over 7.5): introduce 20ml of organic wine vinegar or apple cider vinegar to the diet daily.
- **Nausea/poor appetite:** if the patient is having difficulty in eating all the foods, or having digestive difficulties, try to encourage porridge, Hippocrates soup, mashed potato and stewed apple. The diet, at this stage, is more important than the juices. This often occurs during a heavy detoxification crisis.

## Protein

There is sufficient protein in the diet not only to maintain tissue integrity but also to rebuild and regenerate. The practitioner must not be eager to increase protein prematurely, as protein feeds tumours. If the albumin levels appear to be below normal, you must question your patient thoroughly and find out how much porridge and potato they are taking. If you find that the patient is not eating a good bowl of porridge and only eating small amounts of potato then you must look to increase these foods before making any other dietary changes. Carrot juice is also a good source of protein.

Milk protein (soured milk products, no fat, no salt) is added to the regime at 6-8 weeks. Start with just a couple of tablespoons and then increase to a maximum of 1 cup of soured milk product such as yoghurt or 1 cup of salt-free quark. If the patient is allergic to milk products, then spirulina or bee pollen can be added to provide some protein value. Brown rice is allowed once/week from the beginning of the therapy. With the high arsenic levels now found in rice, quinoa is often recommended as a substitute.

If the patient's signs are looking good, then vegetable protein is added cautiously at around 6-9 months. Legumes may be introduced once a fortnight; then watch to see how the patient responds. If there are any adverse signs, then remove the legumes. If the patient continues to progress, legumes may be increased to once a week, then twice/week, brown rice twice/week, and at 18 months fish may be introduced. Remember, be cautious when increasing the protein.

If the patient is weak, has either been unable to eat, or is suffering effusions/ascites, which require tapping, nephrotic syndrome or advanced diabetes with renal involvement, then the protein albumin levels may fall to very low levels. You will need to advise increasing the daily protein, possibly adding fish to the regime until the patient is stable.

## Flaxseed oil

Flaxseed oil is reduced from 20ml/day to 10ml/day after the first 4 weeks. Occasionally, if the patient has dry, cracking skin or high cholesterol levels, the dose may be maintained at between 15ml-20ml daily.

# Juice Modifications

The juices remain at the same level for many months. The patient on the full therapy takes 13 x 240ml juices daily. It is not recommended to reduce the juices too early, and is preferred that the patient remains on the full number of juices until at least 18 months into the therapy. If the patient is making good progress, then they may be reduced to 10/day at 18 months until the end of the therapy. After the therapy the patient is advised to drink 3-4 juices daily. The pretreated chemotherapy patient, who starts with 10 juices, will generally be on the therapy for much longer and will maintain the 10 juices for that time. If this patient is doing well and tolerating the diet, coping with the sometimes heavy healing reactions, then they may be prescribed the full 13 juices. This will not occur at the beginning of treatment.

# Enema/Castor Oil Treatment Modifications

**Coffee enemas:** 5 daily for many months, depending on the amount of tumoural tissue. It is important not to reduce these prematurely and to even increase the number (up to 6-7/day) during flare-ups and toxic crises. You may advise the patient to take additional juices when increasing the enemas. If the patient awakes feeling very toxic in the morning, or suffers a bad night due to digestive pain/flatulence, then it is advisable that the patient does an additional enema during the night. Patients will generally know when they need to increase the enemas for toxic relief.

If the patient is progressing well and the tumoural masses are reducing, the enemas may be reduced to 4/day at 6 months; 3-4/day at 9 months; 3 daily at one year, and gradually reduce to 1 daily by 21 months.

**Irrigation through a stoma:** post bowel resection surgery, a temporary or permanent stoma may be created. It is possible to do the coffee enema via the stoma allowing the enema solution to flow in very slowly. Use an irrigation cone to help hold the liquid in the colon. There are some helpful YouTube clips on this procedure which can be found here:

| | |
|---|---|
| Part 1: Stoma Enema - Preparation | http://youtu.be/L2REtTdJ5XQ |
| Part 2: Stoma Enema - Putting Enema liquid into Stoma | http://youtu.be/878ga1tuyxc |
| Part 3: Stoma Enema - Soaking Stoma | http://www.youtube.com/watch?v=eS65aa093V8 |
| Part 4: Stoma Enema - Ending Enema & clean up | http://youtu.be/F5A1_505Ylw |

**Castor oil treatment:** this is a critical part of the therapy and should not be omitted except by chemotherapy patients or patients suffering inflammatory bowel disease/gastrointestinal bleeding/ulceration. The liver needs this additional support and the effectiveness of this treatment should never be underestimated. The castor oil treatment starts at every other day for 4 weeks, then it may drop to twice/week for the next 5 months. From this time on you can reduce very slowly to 1 every 5 days, then once/week at nine months, gradually reducing to once/fortnight and then phasing them out at around 18 months. Don't be afraid to increase them if the patient is very toxic.

With chemotherapy patients you may introduce the castor oil by enema at around 6 months. Then you may try the castor oil by mouth, but start with 5ml by mouth and observe how the patient reacts. You must be careful not to overstimulate the liver, which would cause extremely toxic side-effects from the elimination of the chemotherapy. The castor oil treatment should not be applied too frequently or at full strength in the chemotherapy pretreated patient.

Sometimes the castor oil treatment makes the patient nauseous with vomiting and diarrhoea. Under these conditions the castor oil treatment has to be reduced or stopped altogether because it inhibits the patient from doing the therapy. Under these circumstances it is wise to recommence the treatment, starting with 5ml only by mouth and gradually increasing as the patient can tolerate. Some patients cannot drink the coffee. You may then advise them to take very strong peppermint tea; although not as effective as the coffee in stimulating the stomach to clear the castor oil, it will exert a similar effect.

You will find that when the patient is very toxic, then the reactions from the castor oil treatment are very strong. As the patient improves, these reactions will lessen. Many patients, although not "liking" the castor oil treatment, do feel and are aware of the benefits.

# Medication Modifications

**Potassium:** on the full protocol, the initial dose of 20ml x 10 juices is decreased at the end of the first month to 10ml x 10 juices, and remains at this level for many months. When the serum potassium levels remain border-line, then I have known the potassium compound solution to be taken at 20ml x 10 for many months. The patient needs to stay on this high dose for at least one year. If the patient is progressing well, then at 18 months the potassium compound solution may be reduced 10ml in each of the 8 juices (around 80 ml/day) and gradually decreased until the end of the therapy. Many patients will continue with a small amount of the potassium for life. Pretreated chemotherapy patients will remain on the higher dose of 10ml/juice until the juices are reduced, possibly not until they have been on the therapy for 2 1/2 years.

**Lugol's 1/2 strength:** the initial dose for the patient on the full therapy is 18 drops, to be taken at 3 drops in each of the 5 carrot and apple juices and in the orange juice. At the end of the first month it is reduced to 6 drops (1 drop in each of the above juices). The chemotherapy patient will start at the lower dose and maintain this for many months. Lugol's is taken along with the thyroid medication and as this is reduced so, too, is the Lugol's. At six months, if the patient is progressing well, then the Lugol's may be reduced to 4 drops daily, at 9 months to 3 drops and by 12 months to 2 drops daily. At 15 months the dose may be reduced to one drop daily and will remain at this level until the end of the therapy. The chemotherapy pretreated patient or weakened patient will never take more than 6 drops daily. If they are started on a lower dose then, pending improvement, you may increase gradually to 6 drops daily. These patients will need to stay at this dose for at least one year.

**Thyroid:** on the full therapy the patient takes 5 grains daily for one month, which is then usually reduced to 2.5 grains. Monitoring of the thyroid function will dictate the amount of thyroid to be supplemented and very often the prescribed amount of this medication does fluctuate during the treatment. The patient needs to maintain this dose (2.5 grains daily) for at least one year, and over the second year it is gradually reduced: 12 months, 2 grains; 15 months, 1.5 grains; 18 months, 1 grain; 21 months, 0.5 grain. Many patients maintain 0.5 grain thyroid daily after the therapy. However, the thyroid will resume normal function after the medication ceases.

**B12 + crude liver injections:** B12 injections are prescribed at 0.1cc daily (depending on blood work) or the equivalent of 100µg/day. It is drawn up with the crude liver extract (2.9cc) so that the total injectable amount is 3.0cc. In some cases where there is a low red and white cell count with anaemia, the B12 may be increased to 0.5cc for a period of time. It is useful to request a B12 assay in these patients. When taking larger amounts of B12, reduce the crude liver extract accordingly (0.5cc B12 + 2.5cc crude liver). These injections are taken daily for 3 months and then, depending upon the progress of your patient, may be reduced at 3 months to alternate days; 6 months, twice weekly; 1 year, once weekly; 18 months, once every 2 weeks; 21 months, once monthly. We now generally prescribe oral methylcobalamin at around 500μg/day provided that the patient does not suffer pernicious anaemia, and then the injectable form needs to be taken.

**Digestive enzymes** - both the acidol-pepsin and the pancreatin are taken throughout the therapy. They may be slowly reduced after 9 months if the patient has a good digestion. By the end of the therapy the patient may be taking 1 pancreatin and 1 acidol-pepsin with each meal.

**Liver capsules** - are taken throughout the therapy and may be reduced to 3/day at 18 months.

# The Maintenance Plan

The patient who has made a good recovery within the two years and has not had chemotherapy pretreatment may resume a more normal eating pattern. However, patients should observe the laws of keeping a healthy body healthy and not introduce the very factors that led to the disease in the first place. The following guidelines may be useful:

- Eat only organic whenever possible;
- High potassium/low sodium diet;
- Low fat - use flaxseed oil; do not fry food - steam, grill or bake instead;
- Cook food at low temperatures;
- Follow a vegetarian regime, but if animal protein is introduce then limit this to fish 2-3 times weekly;
- Eat organic grain and legumes daily;
- Take 3-4 juices daily (1 orange, 1 green, 2 carrot and apple);
- Continue with a little potassium compound solution;
- Take a coffee enema if you feel toxic; and
- On-going thyroid medication will depend on basal temperature.

Patients who have been weakened or had chemotherapy may find that they have to stick very closely to the diet for life. The type of diet they must follow will become apparent to these patients if they listen to their body. They do not have the reserves that the stronger patient has and therefore require the continual support of a good dietary healing program.

Remember, that once you have reduced the volume of vegetables due to reducing the juices, you will need to ensure that you are meeting both protein and energy requirements for regeneration. Failure to eat sufficient carbohydrate to meet energy requirements will mean that you draw on your protein for energy, and regeneration will suffer. Failure to eat sufficient protein for tissue renewal will lead to a slow deterioration of tissue integrity and organ function and you will see symptoms of chronic degeneration. The body is like a vehicle; it needs to have adequate fuel and it needs to be maintained. So the maintenance program needs to follow the principles of Dr. Gerson's therapy by keeping the burden to a minimum while maintaining quality input, and also ensuring cellular health through the low sodium/high potassium approach.

# Dosages for the weakened patient

When determining the potassium, Lugol's and thyroid doses for the weakened patient or the patient with concomitant disease, you will need to refer to the blood results and the general condition of the patient. These three medications, along with the volume of juices, place a fair amount of pressure on heart, lungs and kidneys, and the kidney function tests, serum potassium, heart/lung performance and blood pressure should be monitored closely, with follow-up blood tests taken at weekly intervals until the situation is stable. If there are pleural or pericardial effusions present, then the heart and lungs will be working against pressure and you will need to reduce the volume of juices and the potassium, Lugol's and thyroid.

*Juices* may start at half the dose, still taken at hourly intervals (120ml x 10). If the patient cannot tolerate this amount, it may be reduced further.

*Potassium* may start at 5ml/juice. As you increase the juices, so too will the potassium increase to bring it to the maximum the patient can tolerate. Very often the patient will not experience difficulty with the potassium compound solution and you may find that once the patient is stable you can prescribe at 10ml/juice. The potassium medication can help to resolve effusions and ascites.

*Lugol's, 1/2 strength* may start at 1-2 drops daily. Lugol's is taken with thyroid. If the patient can only tolerate the minimum thyroid dose, then he or she may remain at this level for many months. If the thyroid can be increased, then Lugol's will be increased accordingly at a ratio of 2.5 grains thyroid to 6 drops Lugol's, 1/2 strength. It is always important to monitor the fT3 and fT4 to calculate your dosages.

*Thyroid* may start on 1/2 - 1 grain daily. Patients who are very ill may remain on this dose. The stable patient may gradually increase their dose to 2.5 grain daily. In cardiac insufficiency it is important to maintain the lower dose. Once again it is important to monitor the blood work. Thyroxine can be replaced safely with the thyroid medication in those patients suffering from hypothyroidism.

*Coffee enemas* may start at only 500ml of chamomile tea enema and increase gradually to 1 litre. Introduce the coffee in small amounts and monitor the progress of the patient. The caffeine and increased fluid volume may create an additional strain on the cardiac/respiratory/renal system. If the patient is dehydrated (low sodium levels) they you would need to reduce or replace the coffee enemas with chamomile tea enemas as they can exacerbate the crisis.

### Example 1
This lady was admitted to the Meridien hospital, Mexico, May 1999. She was very ill and in poor condition, and had bilateral nephrostomies due to pressure from a tumour on the L ureter. Her kidney function tests (urea and creatinine) were abnormal. Her potassium level was low. During her stay she had a blockage in the catheter and a urinary tract infection with high temperature. She was started on the 10 juices and her potassium medications were increased to 20ml per juice, but her level of tolerance was maintained at 180mls x 10 juice; 5ml K compound solution/juice; Thyroid x 1 grain; Lugol's 1/2 strength x 2 drops. During her 3 weeks stay the urea levels normalized (low protein diet), but the creatinine remained high. By July (2 months) her kidney function tests were stable and she was tolerating 10 x 240 mls juices with 10ml of potassium compound solution/juice. The nephrostomies were removed and she continued to improve. This was a very difficult case as she had been "burned" so extensively, due to previous radiotherapy to that area, that it was impossible for her to hold the enemas and therefore do the therapy. However, the quality of her life was much improved and she lived around 18 months after starting the therapy, for much of this time in positive spirits.

*Female aged 52. Advanced cervical carcinoma. Radical hysterectomy followed by 7 weeks radiotherapy, leaving patient with bowel and bladder incontinence. Three years later invasive tumour from the bladder pressing on L ureter causing obstructive nephropathy. Both kidneys enlarged and ureters dilated. Treated with bilateral nephrostomies and self-catheterisation.*

| Date | Juices 240ml each | Diet | Potassium compound | Lugol 1/2 Strength Drops in juice | Thyroid 1 grain tab | Niacin 50mg | Coffee enema | Other | Tests |
|---|---|---|---|---|---|---|---|---|---|
| 7/5/99 | 10 | No milk protein | 10 x 5ml inc to 10 x 20ml | 6 | 2 1/2 | 6 | 3 | | K 3.5 Urea 33 Creatinine 2.3 |
| 4/6/99 | 10 x 180ml | | 10 x 5ml | 2 | 1 | 3 | 2 | Imugen x 9 Essiac tea Nerve drops | K 3.9 Urea 13 Creatinine 2.3 AST 49 ALT 46 Hb 10.7 |
| 24/6/99 | 6 x 180 ml 4 green x 240 ml | Add milk protein - non-fat yoghurt | 10 x 5ml | 2 | 1 | 3 | 2-3 x 1/2 strength | Imugen x 9 Essiac tea Nerve drops | Creatinine 0.13 Hb 9.4 RCC 3.0 Lymphocytes 0.8 |
| 30/7/99 | 10 x 240ml | As above | 10 x 10ml | 2 | 1 | nil | 2-3 full-strength | Imugen x 9 Essiac tea Nerve drops | Hb 13.4 Lymphocytes 0.9 |

| In Hospital  General chemistry | 7/5/99 | 14/5/99 | 22/5/99 | 28/5/99 |
|---|---|---|---|---|
| Sodium (133-145 mmol/L) | 139 | 134 | 127 | 135 |
| Potassium (3.3-4.9 mmol/L) | 3.5 | 4.6 | 3.3 | 3.9 |
| Urea Nitrogen (8-25 mg/dl) | 33 | 19 | 18 | 13 |
| Creatinine (0.9-1.6 mg/dl) | 2.3 | 0.8 | 1.7 | 2.3 |

| | | 15/6/99 | 6/7/99 | 20/7/99 |
|---|---|---|---|---|
| General chemistry | | | | |
| Sodium (136-146 mmol/L) | | 139 | 141 | 141 |
| Potassium (3.5-5.2 mmol/L) | | 4.5 | 4.3 | 4.7 |
| Urea (2.5-8.0 mmol/L) | | 3.9 | 3.8 | 3.8 |
| Creatinine (0.05-0.11 mmol/L) | | 0.13 | 0.18 | 0.11 |

## Example 2

*Male - 78 yr. Diagnosed 20 years ago with choroidal melanoma - no treatment undertaken. 3 years ago diagnosed with multiple myeloma, with squamous cell carcinoma to base of tongue; metastases to lymph node in L axilla. Past history includes pernicious anaemia diagnosed at 34 yr; 69 yr, heart bypass; 72 yr, pacemaker fitted; 73 yr, mild diverticulitis and gallstones; current Hashimoto's thyroiditis, giant cell arteritis, fibrosis of R lung with small pleural effusion, L ventricular failure (heart enlarged) and secondary amyloidosis. Current medications included heart medications and diuretics along with potassium supplementation; thyroxine; chemotherapy every 6 weeks.*

This was an extremely difficult case, and between the May and July you will see that his level of tolerance for the juices was only 940ml daily; potassium gradually increased to 5ml x 8; we replaced the thyroxine with the thyroid medication and the dose eventually required was 3 grains/day. I did not medicate niacin or CoQ10. His RCC and haemoglobin did improve and his wife was able to look after him at home for many months.

| Date | Juices | Diet | Potassium compound solution | Lugol's 1/2 str | Thyroid grains | Infla-Zyme tabs | Injection B12 0.5cc with 2.5cc liver | Coffee enema | Blood tests |
|---|---|---|---|---|---|---|---|---|---|
| 11/5/99 | 10 x 125ml | No dairy | 10 x 2.5ml | nil | 1 | 9 | Daily | 2 x 1/2 strength | |
| 26/5/99 | 4 green x 250 ml 6 a/c x 125ml | | 10 x 2.5ml | nil | 2 | 9 | Daily | 2 x 1/2 strength | |
| 16/6/99 | 6 green x 250 ml 4 a/c x 125ml | + non-fat milk yo-ghurt | 6 x 5ml 4 x 2.5ml | nil | 2 | 9 | B12 x 1.0cc Liver x 2cc | 2 x 1/2 strength | Albumin 33 Hb 10..9 RCC 3.1 |
| 14/7/99 | 2 green 6 carrot/ apple 125ml | As above, + rice x 1/ wk fish x 2/ wk | 8 x 5ml | nil | 3 | 9 | B12 x 1.0cc Liver x 2cc | 2 x 1/2 strength x 500ml | Albumin 33 Hb 12.2 RCC 3.5 TSH 4.4 FT4 10 |

| | 23/04/99 | 04/05/99 | 7/6/99 | 21/6/99 | 5/7/99 |
|---|---|---|---|---|---|
| **General chemistry** | | | | | |
| Sodium (136-146 mmol/L) | 137 | 138 | 133 | | 137 |
| Potassium (3.5-5.2 mmol/L) | 4.3 | 4.4 | 4.5 | 4.4 | 4.3 |
| Albumin (35-50 g/L) | 39 | 40 | 33 | | 33 |
| | | | | | |
| **Haematology** | | | | | |
| Haemoglobin (11.5-16.5 g/dL) | 11.3 | 11.2 | 10.9 | 11.3 | 12.2 |
| RBC (3.8-5.5 x10$^{12}$/L) | 3.4 | 3.3 | 3.1 | 3.3 | 3.5 |
| TSH (0.04-4.0 mIU/L) | | 4.0 | 4.3 | 3.7 | 4.4 |
| FT4 (10-20 pmol/L) | | | 11 | 10 | 10 |
| **Urinalysis** | | | | | |
| Protein (0-150 mg/24hr) – Bence Jones | 110 | | 220 | | 230 |

# Chapter 6

# MEDICAL INTERVENTION: COMPLICATIONS OF MALIGNANCY

It is important that the practitioner learns to recognise when a crisis represents a medical emergency as opposed to a general flare-up. Careful case taking, type, location and size of tumours along with blood results will usually give a clear enough indication of the nature of the crisis.

The metabolic complications, which include the paraneoplastic syndromes leading to imbalances in electrolytes and fluid volume, the sick cell syndrome (low serum sodium), dehydration, elevated calcium (either a consequence of a paraneoplastic syndrome or due to bone metastases), cachexia, liver failure leading to ascites (low albumin), will all require medical intervention.

- The patient may be admitted to hospital if suffering with dehydration and be given an IV drip (Hartmann's solution).
- In the case of bone metastases (confirmed by body scan and elevated levels of ALP), a biphosphonate drug may be prescribed.
- In cachexia sometimes the drug Hydrazine Sulphate is prescribed. As tumours derive their energy from the anaerobic metabolism of glucose, they require vast amounts of glucose which is usually made available by the re-conversion of lactic acid (waste product of anaerobic metabolism) to pyruvate. Hydrazine Sulphate effectively shuts down the energy supply to the tumour by blocking the conversion of lactate to pyruvic acid.[1]
- Patients with metastasised carcinoid tumours who present with the clinical features of the carcinoid syndrome may require medication to control diarrhoea, cardiac and lung symptoms.
- Any paraneoplatic syndrome that leads to an electrolyte imbalance will require medical treatment.

The physical complications will include:

- Blockage or obstruction from the tumour pressing on vital organs or occluding tracts/ducts (bile ducts, ureter, gastrointestinal tract, bronchi) through external pressure. Under these circumstances local or general surgery may be required.
- Pleural effusions, ascites, brain oedemas - local inflammation from tumoural activity (pleurae, pericardia, peritoneal) and ascites from liver failure. Both these conditions may require tapping.
- Bleeding - tumours may ulcerate, become necrotic and bleed. In some cases blood transfusions may be required.
- Crises from concomitant disease - diabetes, hypertension

## Blockage in the Gastrointestinal Tract

Many patients are very constipated and it is important to remember that when the potassium status is generally low, then peristalsis is sluggish. If you can rule out any tumours within the gastrointestinal tract or in the adjacent tissues (enlarged liver, adjacent lymph nodes), then medications may be prescribed by the patient's doctor to accelerate peristalsis. If the blockage is caused by a tumour, then it may have to be removed if possible, through resection. Unfortunately many tumours are invasive and inoperable and the patient requires medical management. It is inadvisable to prescribe the niacin, potassium, thyroid and Lugol's medications immediately after surgery. The patient should be monitored and upon satisfactory progress these medications may be introduced. Niacin should be omitted prior to and up to 3 weeks after surgery, depending on the patient's recovery.

Obstruction of the gastrointestinal tract causes severe nausea and vomiting. It is not wise to give analgesics to the patient as the pain needs to be diagnosed.

## Blockage of the Bile Ducts

Tumours arising in the liver or the pancreas may press on the bile ducts. It will be clear from the blood work and the colour of the patient (jaundice) if this is occurring. Very often a stent can be placed within the affected bile duct to allow the functioning of the liver. This is a very effective treatment and can be done as a day patient. However, if the tumour is growing within the bile duct, then this treatment would not be feasible.

## Blockage of the Renal Ureters

Stents may also be placed in the ureters if these are occluded from external pressure. These too are effective and allow the patient to continue with the therapy.

## Bleeding in the Gastrointestinal Tract

Bleeding in the stomach is the most common occurrence and may be caused by ulcers, gastritis, or tumour.

- discontinue medications (potassium, thyroid, niacin, acidol). You may be able to keep some pancreatin and liver capsules. Potassium compound solution may act as an irritant. Although not specifically contra-indicated with bleeding, It may be wise to discontinue the Lugol's if you are reducing or ceasing thyroid medication;
- enemas - coffee : chamomile tea enemas or none at all. Coffee enemas may cause the flushing of alkaline bile into stomach, increasing nausea, diarrhoea, and general irritation;
- do not administer the castor oil treatment;
- juices: mix juices with gruel. You may have to discontinue the juices entirely and advise just gruel, chamomile tea or apple juice. Do not take peppermint tea, as this increases stomach acidity. Alternatively the patient may take half gruel/half juice in the morning but stop the juices in the afternoon and take gruel only;
- solid food: soup, mashed potato, apple sauce. No garlic, onions, tomato, raw vegetables or salad; and
- watch the haemoglobin and red cell count, as if the bleeding is extensive, the patient may require a transfusion. Dr. Gerson indicated that the prognosis was poor for patients who had received more than three blood transfusions.

## Brain Oedema

It can be difficult to manage the patient who has brain metastases, as the very nature of the therapy causes inflammation during the healing process. Inflammation and oedema in the brain can give rise to extreme vomiting, headache, blurred vision and seizures. Usually these patients are already taking steroids and anti-convulsants to guard against inflammation and seizures, and it is inadvisable to withdraw the medications. The situation has to be monitored and in the event of a crisis you may reduce the treatment (K, Lugol's and thyroid), lower the volume of liquids (contributes to oedemas) and reduce the enemas. An experienced practitioner may increase the enemas during a toxic crisis and this may help to alleviate the situation. In this situation the practitioner/doctor must be competent in the management of patients who are likely to suffer seizures and be able to take appropriate measures. Intravenous administration of mannitol may also help to alleviate the oedema.

Patients with primary astrocytoma may respond to the Gerson treatment, particularly if no drugs (anti-convulsants, steroids) are being taken. However, the risks of seizures and other complications may far outweigh any perceived benefits, particularly as the therapy cannot give immediate results  Once again, skilled management is required when treating these patients as the condition is difficult to treat and close monitoring is essential.

# Hypertension

This can give rise to severe vomiting. You will need to ascertain the blood pressure before and after the coffee enema, or if the patient has recently taken the thyroid medication. The episode may have been transient, caused by either the caffeine or the thyroid. Do not panic into immediately giving orthodox treatment but rather ascertain the cause. If the blood pressure remains high, you may need to recommend orthodox treatment to help the patient through the crisis, but then aim to reduce the medication.

# Hyperglycaemia

This is often a complication of cancer of the pancreas or diabetes. It is important not to stop conventional medications. You will need to work with the diet first by removing the apple and stewed fruits. Monitor the glucose daily, before and after meals. In a healing crisis the blood sugar can go up and, after the crisis, go back down. If the patient develops hypoglycaemia at night, you will need to recommend that the patient adjusts the insulin medication under the guidance of his/her doctor.

# Bone Metastases

As discussed, when the patient has advancing bone metastases, they may be recommended a biphosphonate or monoclonal antibody. The bones become very fragile and may disintegrate. Radiotherapy may also be advised particularly if there is risk of fracture or vertebral column collapse which would negatively impact the spinal cord and cause nerve compression. The patient needs to be careful with any manipulation, and even strong massage may fracture the bone. You will need to introduce the cultured milk protein into the program much sooner.

# Pleural Effusions

Lung cancer often results in metastasised tissue in the pleurae.  This causes inflammation and effusion. You must be careful with the fluid volumes on the diet (juices and enemas) during the first week, to determine how much of the treatment the patient can safely handle. A high fluid volume will exacerbate and increase the effusion. It is best to give small quantities at hourly intervals. The patient may find it difficult to breathe and if the situation deteriorates may require tapping. The polarizing treatment (GKI) may be used, but this must be administered by a doctor. Pleural sealing may be an option, the tetracycline talc is the preferred option, or a chemotherapy. Laetrile at 6g IV daily for 21 days helps to absorb fluids.

# Ascites

Ascites often occurs as a complication of ovarian cancer or liver failure. You will need to reduce the juices and adjust the program. Tapping may be required, or the polarising treatment. Unfortunately, after tapping the patient often fills up with fluid within a few days. Repeated tapping is untenable as the patient will lose a lot of protein and plasma and will deteriorate. You will need to replace the protein via the diet and may have to incorporate fish, sooner than with other patients. Generally the prognosis is poor, as the disease is far advanced by this time.

# Chronic anaemia

Chronic anaemia occurs in patients with chronic inflammatory disease and with malignancy. This type of anaemia is refractory to treatment. These patients have low serum iron, low iron saturation, low iron binding capacity, but high ferritin. Prescribing iron under these circumstances will not resolve the anaemia, but will increase the ferritin levels which becomes a risk factor for oxidative stress; in short, it fuels the inflammation.

The regulation of iron uptake and distribution is governed by an acute phase protein, hepcidin, that is made by the liver and levels are increased during inflammation and infection. It inhibits intestinal absorption of dietary iron and sequesters iron from the serum into macrophages to rob bacteria of this element which is essential for their survival.

As the cause of the problem is inflammation, then reducing the inflammation should restore the iron levels, by default. Prescribing iron in an inflammatory situation invariably results in an increase of hepcidin and sequestration of this supplemental iron which can be stored in any inflammatory tissue, such as the synovium in rheumatic joint disease, and will generate free radical activity which will increase the chronicity and destructive path of the disease. Iron injections, which bypass the tightly regulated pathways for iron absorption, are dangerous and can generate widespread oxidative stress.[2]

# Emotional Problems

Some patients have severe emotional problems and most will have emotional crises during the therapy. You will need to be able to recommend to your patient a counsellor who is sympathetic to the therapy. You have to remember that stress totally negates the healing process and causes organic problems. Stress activates the sympathetic nervous system (fight and flight) and deactivates the parasympathetic nervous system (rest and digest) which compromised the efficacy of the digestive system. As restoration of the digestive system is a prime requirement on therapies where food is your medicine then stress will be counterproductive to one's healing. When patients remain negative the prognosis may be poor. Counselling and homoeopathic treatments may go a long way to helping your patient alleviate their stress.

# Cardiac/Respiratory Insufficiency

This is often encountered with metastases to the lung, where the heart tries to compensate against a reduced pulmonary blood flow and increased pressure within the lungs. The patients will experience difficulties in respiration. You must manage volumes of fluid and adjust the medications (K, Lugol's and Thyroid) and coffee enemas. Medical treatment may be required to help resolve a crisis.

# Irritable Bowel Syndrome

This will resolve on the Gerson treatment, but these patients should not have the castor oil treatment. In the initial phases of the therapy use chamomile tea enemas and later introduce the coffee enema. These patients should not have ozone by rectal insufflation and it may be wise to omit pancreatic enzymes.

# Infections

Infections determined by patient symptoms, blood results or a culture must be treated by antibiotics. If the infection is left untreated, the cancer can progress. Tumour tissue hijacks inflammatory chemicals which it uses to promote its own growth. Dr. Gerson never left an infection unchecked during the first nine months of the therapy due to the negative effects on tumoural growth.

# Surgery

Surgery may be recommended when it offers a better prognosis and a chance to heal. A simple lumpectomy, where the tumour is defined and non-invasive, will decrease the toxic burden on the system and reduce the demand on the healing resources of the body which gives the patient an increased opportunity to rebuild defence systems and integrity into the tissues. Radical or wide excisions are not normally recommended. The concern for many patients is that growth factors are released from tissues damaged through surgery which not only stimulate healing (formation of scar tissue), but can also stimulate neoplastic growth. There is also the added risk of spreading the tumour by breaching any natural defences through surgical trauma. However, the patient has to weigh up the benefits versus the risks of surgery for their individual case, against their own criteria.

# Radiation

Radiotherapy is never curative. It is given to improve local tumour control, but will not affect widespread cancer nor will it improve survival time. Radiation may be used to halt the progression of bone metastases particularly when there is a risk of fracture in say the vertebral column. The practitioner should understand that the bone marrow in the adult does not recover when irradiated. If large areas, such as the pelvic area, are irradiated the immune system and the red cell count will be negatively affected and it may not be possible to stimulate immune activity. It's a question of weighing up the risks versus the benefits particularly if there is risk of fracture, compression of the spinal cord and nerves or vertebral collapse.

Radiation may also be used to shrink tumours, and this is often a prerequisite to surgery (as may be chemotherapy) for many patients. Some tumours remain resistant, while others require such large doses of radiation that the risk to surrounding tissue and organ function is great, although radiation procedures have improved in their capacity to target tissues more precisely, as with steroetactic techniques (gamma knife) for non-resectable brain tumours. The patient should check the possible side effects (incontinence, loss of saliva, etc.) before embarking on radiotherapy. In some cases it may be the only viable option to buy the patient time and quality of life. Unfortunately, radiotherapy also has the potential to accelerate/stimulate tumour regeneration, so the initial response may be good but tumoural growth may recur.[3]

In the case of breast cancer, women who are treated with radiation therapy have a higher risk of lung cancer, osteosarcoma, angiocarcinomas and cancer of other connective tissues. These cancers occur in the area that was irradiated and the risk increases over time. This means that the risk remains high even 30 years after treatment. Now that women are surviving longer with the newer targeted treatments, this may become a real risk factor for long-term survivors and therefore the benefits of radiotherapy should be carefully weighed against the risks, particularly if the overall survival remains good without having adjunct radiotherapy.

If radiotherapy is required it can be advantageous to prescribe N-acetylcysteine (NAC) during treatment as this supplement, which contains sulphur, has been found to selectively protect normal cells from chemotherapy and radiation toxicity, but not malignant ones. Of particular note is sulphur's anti-mutagenic and anti-carcinogenic effects. Sulphur, either as purified sulphur or as NAC, can limit radiation damage during radiotherapy as in advanced cancer. Thiols protect against radiation poisoning as they are able to concentrate in the micro-environment of the cell nucleus which houses our DNA, and scavenge free-radicals protecting against DNA mutation.[4]

# Chemotherapy

When deciding on chemotherapy, we return to the equation that the resistance of the body must be greater than the resistance of the tumour. Sometimes when the cancer is aggressive, or refractory to the therapy, the patient may opt to take some form of chemotherapy. This is to reduce the tumoural burden on the system and to buy the patient time. However, chemotherapy is extremely liver toxic and depresses the bone marrow, hence the immune system. So what you gain on the one hand, you may lose on the other. The patient has to weigh up the advantages and disadvantages in their specific case. A few patients who have opted to take some form of chemotherapy alongside the Gerson treatment have had encouraging results, and with the constant detoxification and nutritional replenishment that the therapy has provided, they suffered fewer side effects than normally expected.

It is useful for the patient to discuss less toxic chemotherapeutic agents with their oncologist. Although the consultant may be reluctant to prescribe a less toxic treatment on a procedural basis (he/she may not wish to prescribe a drug that is proved to be not as effective as a more toxic drug, or that is contraindicated with the specific procedure), we have had encouraging results with oral chemotherapy drugs when using the Gerson treatment. New treatments/drugs are being developed every year and it is important to keep abreast of new developments in this field. Generally the newer targeted treatments are much less toxic than chemotherapy regimes.

It is vital to remember the context in which you may seek to apply chemotherapy. A basic understanding of the nature of the cancer in relation to chemotherapy should be borne in mind by both the practitioner and patient when deciding upon this course of action. The stem cell model of tumour growth, set out below, will give you more insight into the limitations of chemotherapy.

## Stem Cell Model of Tumour Growth

The phenomenon of cancer is still not adequately explained. It is commonly agreed that extrinsic factors (epigenetic) such as chemicals, metabolites, viruses and radiation can act as carcinogens which mediate the genetic changes involved in neoplastic growth. What is not clearly understood is whether neoplastic growth arises from the reversion of a normal cell to its undifferentiated state, or from an aberrant pluri-potent stem cell that gives rise to cells that fail to fully differentiate to their determined state. This latter theory, the stem cell model of tumour growth, supports the statistical evidence that treatment by chemotherapy and radiotherapy tend to effect remission rather than cure, and that these therapies should only be viewed in this light.

The stem cell model of tumour growth has been extended from the stem cell system in the bone marrow and applied to the growth of non-haematopoietic tissues including tumours. Stem cells are unspecialised cells, incapable of performing any ultimate functions. However, they have an unlimited capacity for self-replication, and the potential to genetically program for different clonal expansions within a specific tissue, dependent upon their location in the body. For example, the stem cell of the bone marrow, can give rise to five specialized cell lines; the erythrocyte, granulocyte, monocyte, thrombocyte and lymphocyte. Extrinsic humoral controls, such as anaemia/blood loss or infection, will determine the specific cell line for clonal expansion.

The unspecialised, but determined cell, undergoes a process of differentiation during its various stages of maturation. This involves genetic adaptation of the cell to perform specialized functions according to the tissue type. The capacity for self-replication is a function that remains with the cell until it reaches maturity. Once fully differentiated and mature, it cannot replicate. The highest proliferative rate occurs amongst the immediate descendents of the stem cell, and progressively reduces as the cell becomes more differentiated and reaches maturity. The stem cell, itself, has an extremely low rate of proliferation.

It is interesting to note that most tumour cells have a very limited potential for self-renewal. The progressive nature of tumour formation is governed primarily by the equation that cell production is greater than cell loss. The growth of the tumour is determined by its resident stem cells. Stem cells number 1:1,000 to 1:10,000 cells in a tumour, and it is these cells that are capable of forming colonies of cancer cells. However, the low proliferation rate of the stem cell itself means that it can remain in its resting phase, $G_0$, for long periods of time. Both chemotherapy and radiotherapy exert their most destructive effects upon the cell once it has entered the mitotic phases leading to cell division. The DNA of the cell is most vulnerable to destruction during these phases of replication. Therefore, the highly aggressive, undifferentiated tumours, which have a higher level of cell proliferation, may appear to respond more dramatically to the effects of chemotherapy than the more differentiated, slower growing tumours. Hyperthermy (microwave treatment) applied prior to chemotherapy, is used as an adjunct to improve the effectiveness of chemotherapy. Hyperthermy synchronizes the mitotic cycle, i.e. it stimulates cells to enter $G_1$, the initial phase leading to mitosis. The greater the number of cells that enter this phase, the greater the level of destruction, and the more effective the treatment.

"A further impediment to effective chemotherapy is the conclusion that proliferating cells, those that should be most vulnerable to the toxic effects of chemotherapy, are not necessarily the cells that must be eliminated in order to eradicate a tumour. Instead the critical cell population - the one responsible for the persistence and growth of a tumour - is often largely in $G_0$. The reasons for this apparent paradox are found in the stem cell model of tissue growth."[5]

It becomes clear that while chemotherapy may appear to effect a remission by the destruction of large colonies of malignant cells, if the stem cell responsible for the malignancy remains refractory to treatment, then the cancer will recur. Furthermore, although chemotherapy may effect an immediate response (e.g. tumour shrinkage), these results may not indicate long-term survival rates. In most cancers there is little clinical evidence of prolonged survival (over 5 years), which makes the use of highly toxic drugs in the treatment of cancer ethically questionable.

It is also stated by some authors that chemotherapy fosters the growth of resistant cell lines. In a majority of cases, particularly where the cancer is widespread, the disease-free interval following chemotherapy may be comparatively short. This is because there is usually a proportion of drug resistant cells within a tumour, and the larger the amount of tumour tissue in the body, the greater the likelihood of having drug resistant cells. This is why multiple drugs, or a combination of chemotherapeutic agents are used in order to try and eradicate as many resistant cells as possible. It has been found that resistance to one agent often results in coincident development of resistance to others. When this occurs, although the tumours can respond to therapy and shrink, the drug-resistant cancer cells remain and often show an increased capacity for cell renewal and proliferation. The cancer may then return more aggressively than before. [6] These situations, compounded by the severely damaging effects of chemotherapy on the immune system, liver and kidneys, lead to the return of a more aggressive cancer in a more deeply compromised body.

# Hormones

In prostate and breast cancer drugs are often prescribed which either inhibit normal cyclical hormonal output (gonadotrophin-releasing hormone analogues), antagonize hormonal binding (hormonal antagonists such as Tamoxifen) or inhibit hormonal conversion (aromatase inhibitors) to their active form. If your patient is already receiving these treatments, do not discontinue suddenly as withdrawal can exacerbate the cancer. After assessing the benefits and risks of treatment, your patient will need to make their own decision as to ceasing these drugs, but in any event you will need to give your patients the time required to detoxify and see evidence of healing before you or the patient could consider weaning from medication. It is very important that you continue to monitor tumour markers and bone health throughout the therapy. The risks of Tamoxifen given as a sole treatment following surgery, chemotherapy or radiotherapy in the pre-menopausal woman should be weighed against any benefits. Tamoxifen acts as an oestrogen in the bones and there is a strong possibility that it could drive bone metastases, particularly if there were existing micro-metastases in the bone that were not picked up by the scan. Tamoxifen also increases oestrogen output by the ovaries and patients may then become vulnerable to other hormone driven cancers.[7]

# References

1. Gold, J.: *Hydrazine Sulfate: A Current Perspective*, Nutrition and Cancer 9: 59-66, 1987 This article is on-line at http://www.ncbi.nlm.nih.gov/pubmed/0003104888

2. Mcgrath, H. Jr and P. G. Rigby; *Hepcidin: inflammation's iron curtain* Oxford Journals Rheumatology Volume 43, Issue 11 Pp. 1323-1325

3. Murphy, G.P., Lawrence, W. Jr., Lenhard, R.E. Jr.: Clinical Oncology, 1995, pp 107

4. Alexander, K; *Sulphur, heavy metals and detoxification*; http://www.kathrynalexander.com.au/sulphur-heavy-metals-and-detoxification.html

5. Murphy, G.P., Lawrence, W. Jr., Lenhard, R.E. Jr.: Clinical Oncology, 1995, pp 114-116

6. Murphy, G.P., Lawrence, W. Jr., Lenhard, R.E. Jr.: Clinical Oncology, 1995, pp 117-120

7. Alexander, K; *Tamoxifen, targeting the worried well*; http://www.kathrynalexander.com.au/gerson-therapy/tamoxifen-targeting-the-worried-well

# Chapter 7

# THE DIET RATIONALE IN DETOXIFICATION

The cancer patient is nutritionally depleted and, as a consequence, usually suffers from poor digestive capacity. This poses a vicious cycle: the greater the chronic illness, the more the digestive capacity is impaired and the more nutritionally depleted the patient becomes. In order to heal, the patient needs maximum digestive capacity and absorption and a plentiful supply of nutrients. The amount of nutrients the patient requires involves copious amounts of organic vegetable produce, much more than even a healthy person with a vigorous digestion could cope with on a daily basis. For example, the bulk amounts a patient will need to consume on a weekly basis just for the juices will approximate 4 kg oranges, 30 lettuces (not iceberg), 4 bunches of Swiss Chard, 21kg apples, 20kg carrots, 8 green capsicums. The dietary amounts are also large including around 11kg potatoes, 4kg onions, 5kg tomatoes, plus all the salad vegetables and additional ingredients for the Hippocrates Soup.

On a daily basis this represents around 6kg of vegetables daily (this volume includes the 3kg of vegetables in the juicing):

## Juices:

2.5kg carrots
1kg mixed greens
3kg green apples

## Diet:

involves a wide selection of all vegetables: salad vegetables, root, leaf and stem vegetables, tomatoes, potatoes. Each vegetable has different nutrient ratios, therefore it is important to include as wide a variety as possible to ensure adequate intake of all the essential nutrients.

In addition to the vegetable content, generous amounts of fruit, oatmeal, 2 slices of rye sour dough bread daily are allowed. At 6-8 weeks soured milk products are introduced into the diet.

With this quantity of dietary intake the methods of preparation become paramount for the patient. The foods must be prepared in a way to increase their digestibility, without destroying the nutrients, or taxing the digestive organs.

# Juice Preparation

All fresh, raw foods are rich in enzymes (amylase, protease, lipase) which contribute to the digestive process. These enzymes are destroyed when heated. Cooking at "wet" temperatures higher than 117°F/45°C, or at dry temperatures higher than 150°F/85°C will effectively destroy the enzymes[1]. This does not pose a problem with the fresh juices, prepared with the appropriate type of masticating and pressing equipment, and because of the volume of juices taken, most of the diet is raw and therefore "live". In addition, by extracting only the nutrient and enzyme-rich juice, free of fibre which ordinarily taxes the digestive system and inhibits the direct absorption of nutrients/enzymes, we are ensuring maximum uptake of nutrients with minimum digestive effort. You will be surprised how much digestive difficulty a patient will suffer if they do not use the appropriate equipment or do not take their juices fresh. Centrifugal juicing machines destroy the enzymes and antioxidants (you can see how quickly the juice oxidizes after preparation), and even with the correct equipment, once the juice is pressed you will have a maximum of 30 minutes before the bulk of the enzymes are oxidized and you have lost all the antioxidant value of the juice. Patients will suffer bloating and gas, and complain of great discomfort under these circumstances because they need the live enzymes to support their own weakened digestive system[1]. It is also important to understand that the nutrient value of juices prepared without the pressing of the pulp can be at times less than half the nutrient value of juices prepared the correct way. The volume of juice from the given quantity of vegetables will also be significantly less. The cancer patient cannot afford these losses and will fail to heal adequately if the diet is deficient. You must remember to core (not peel) the apples as the seeds contain quantities of enzyme inhibitors which may affect the digestion adversely.

Popular dietary regimes, such as food combining,[2] have convinced many people that fruit and vegetables should not be consumed together. It is true that many patients will suffer much bloating when both are taken together and prefer to take fruit on an empty stomach or away from meals. However, when they come to do a detoxification therapy, this can be a stumbling block. It is important to explain to the patient that through the work of Dr. Gerson we know that the malic acid found in apples draws out more nutrients from the vegetables when the pulps are mixed together, than would be available if taken separately. Additionally, pectin, which is high in green apples, has a role in the stimulation of the immune system. It has been found in experiments (Raz, Pienta and co-workers: Michigan 1995) that rats injected with fast growing prostate adenocarcinoma cells had 5% average frequency of metastases, and of those 5%, there was a 40% reduction of metastases when fed with modified citrus pectin. The recent scientific findings have identified pectin as a signalling molecule for the white blood cells - in other words it assists in turning on the immune system.

I hardly need to emphasize the importance of organic produce, not just from the chemically toxic aspect of commercial farming, but from its nutritional value. Enough research exists which compares nutrient content of organic and conventionally grown vegetables. The ORGAA (Organic Retail Frowers Association of Australia) conducted a study where they compared the difference in mineral value between organic and conventionally farmed vegetables. Four vegetables were compared: tomatoes, beans, capsicums and silver beet and the results were astonishing. Calcium levels in some produce increased by eight times, potassium by ten times, magnesium by seven times and zinc by five times.[3]

# Food Preparation

The preparation of the diet is equally important. Raw foods are invariably a problem for the cancer patient. We need to give the patient "pre-digested" food, which means food cooked at low temperatures for a long period. This has a three-fold advantage: cooking starts the breakdown of long chain carbohydrates to single glucose molecules which are easily absorbed, it breaks down indigestible fibres so that nutrients are more readily accessed and the conversion of carbohydrates to glucose through cooking almost doubles the available energy value of the food from raw food.[4] In addition we also recommend additional supplemental enzymes to ensure maximum digestion for the cancer patient. By using these methods we can often alleviate the digestive discomfort from high carbohydrate diets that results when the digestion of sugars is incomplete, which then pass to the colon and under bacterial activity will start to ferment, causing bloating and gas.

Slow cooking at low temperatures is one method of increasing the digestibility of starch. In order to achieve this, the patient will need to use the waterless cooking system, using heavy-based saucepans with lids that have a lip that fit snugly inside the rim of the pan and prevent the escape of any steam. A heat diffusing pad may also be required to prevent the food from burning. A small amount of water (20ml) may be added, but by cooking very slowly at a gentle heat, you will enable the vegetable/fruit cells to gently burst, releasing their sugars and water without burning. The food will then cook in its own juices in this low temperature environment.

Cooking (heating) starts to break down the long carbohydrate chains into shorter chains and glucose. This is why cooked vegetables taste sweeter than uncooked, where a proportion of carbohydrate has been converted to glucose. In addition, the breakdown and removal of fibres in the Hippocrates Soup when passed through a food mill, will make the soup very easy to digest, particularly in the weakened or convalescing patient. Any cooked vegetables could be passed through a mill and indeed when the patient is very sick foods such as gruel, apple sauce, mashed potato and the Hippocrates soup may be the only dietary option for nourishment. Nowadays we have lost much of our common-sense when treating a convalescent patient.

Like the juices, food has to be prepared freshly for each meal (the Hippocrates soup is allowed to be prepared and kept refrigerated for two days). In spite of this, there could be some debate as to whether the cooked food has retained any of its enzymes. However, its nutrient value would remain and be nutritionally accessible to the patient. There is an additional factor to be taken into account when heating food, and that is the effect of cooking on protein. Although vegetables are low in protein, cooking any protein at high temperatures, such as frying, distorts the protein molecule to the point where it may become a "non-food", which means effectively that the body cannot recognize its structure and therefore cannot break it down. These partially broken down proteins can then enter the systemic circulation and become toxic residues. In certain individuals, particularly those with autoimmune disorders, these proteins can exacerbate the disease and/or cause allergic reactions. Therefore, heating at high temperatures is counter-productive when embarking on a detoxification and healing regime. The same is true for the high heating of carbohydrates which can form acrylamides, again toxic for the patient.

# A Broad Overview of the Detoxification Diet

## Carbohydrates

The energy value of the detoxification diet comes from the carbohydrate component. Carbohydrate is a clean fuel which oxidizes to carbon dioxide and water, unlike fats and proteins which will leave acidic residues within the body, provide an additional toxic burden and inhibit the elimination of sodium from the tissues and the re-filling of the cells with potassium. It is a low kilo-joule diet, which means that the recovering patient needs to take large amounts of the allowed foods. The carbohydrate quota is obtained mainly from the oatmeal, potatoes and vegetables/fruits. These foods will provide sufficient energy for healing, regeneration and meet daily energy requirements. The high vegetable component (particularly taken in juice form) ensures an alkalizing environment which draws out sodium, neutralizes the acidity (toxicity), and paves the way for the re-filling of the cells with potassium.

The high carbohydrate diet is going to ensure a good insulin response, which is imperative for the uptake of potassium by the cells. Those patients with a good insulin response or who are not insulin-resistant, may have a speedier journey to their first healing inflammation and eventual cure. Nowadays, this insulin/potassium/glucose pathway may be severely taxed where the reinstatement of potassium into the cell becomes more prejudiced.

Insulin is important for digestion at cell level. Without insulin the body will not heal. Many patients who have a weakened digestion will show varying degrees of carbohydrate intolerance within the body, not just within the gastrointestinal tract, such as symptoms of low-blood sugar and the "cotton-wool" brain immediately after taking carbohydrates. These patients may feel very ill on this program and it can take many months, particularly with patients suffering from chronic fatigue syndrome, to see any initial turn-around.

The problem lies at the level of cell digestion, where the cells are failing to absorb nutrients and discharge toxicity. In other words they become "locked-up". In today's health climate we are now seeing people being diagnosed with the metabolic syndrome, diabetes and hyper-insulinaemia. Many people, before they are diagnosed with diabetes, will have elevated insulin in the circulation. This means that the cells are unable to accept glucose, the blood glucose fails to fall and more insulin is secreted. In essence, this means that the insulin is not received at the cell membrane, where it normally acts as an unlocking device to allow the cellular uptake of glucose.

How can the body heal if the cell is deprived of its main source of energy? The body has to resort to dirty fuels, such as protein and fats, and the glucocorticoid hormones are mobilized to break down existing tissue for energy resources. Instead of regeneration, we are looking at degeneration.

## Proteins

Protein intake is restricted on the detoxification plan. In the initial 6-8 weeks, the only protein allowed comes primarily from the potatoes, oatmeal and carrots. After this period of time (dependent upon practitioner's advice) protein is added in the form of soured milk products which include no fat, unsalted yoghurt or pot cheese, cottage cheese or quark, and buttermilk. The amounts vary with each patient but the starting dose is usually is 200g (1 cup) yoghurt or 100g pot cheese (or a combination of both, say, 100g yoghurt and 50g pot cheese), which may be increased as the therapy progresses.

Many critics of this type of detoxification therapy complain that the protein in the diet is in fact quite high, if you factor into the equation the raw liver juice along with the soured milk products. However, these proteins are raw and alive with enzymes and therefore do not pose the problems caused by cooked proteins. They are digestible as the *raw*, soured milk products are pre-digested through bacterial conversion of lactose to lactic acid. You will note that I stress *raw* milk products, as the pasteurization [5] process distorts the protein and kills the natural enzymes. It is becoming increasingly difficult to find raw skimmed milk products and, unfortunately, this is yet another area where we have had to compromise and choose the best available. However, we cannot compromise on the fat content - it is imperative that the product is non-fat.

At the beginning of the diet, brown rice is also allowed once a week. Later into the diet you may prescribe lentils. The correct preparation of both grains and legumes/pulses is important. They are all seeds, which means they are capable of sprouting and producing a new crop. They contain a factor called the anti-trypsin factor, which inhibits the seed from sprouting until conditions permit. Hence you can store these seeds for many months/years. The anti-trypsin factor remains in the seed even when cooked, and will oppose your own trypsin enzymes secreted by the pancreas for the digestion of protein.[6] For the patient with a weakened digestion, this poses serious problems of digestibility and nutrient accessibility. Even those with a strong digestion will be short-changed on nutrients by failing to prepare these foods in the correct way.

In order to overcome the anti-trypsin factor, you will need to recommend that your patient semi-germinates the seeds. This is not the same as sprouting; it is the activation of the sprouting mechanism. Sprouts are immature vegetables, no longer grains nor legumes, and therefore will not have the protein value of the seed. Additionally, some sprouts such as alfalfa have been found to contain the immature amino acid L-canavanine, which can exacerbate an immune reaction and lower the general immune response in patients, particularly those with an autoimmune component to their illness.[7] In order to germinate, you will need to soak your grains and legumes for 12 hours, then rinse and drain and leave in a glass dish at room temperature, with a damp cloth covering the seeds for 12 hours. If it is hot or humid, you may need to rinse again during this process. Do not let your seeds go mouldy. The grain/legume can then be cooked as normal.

Soy beans and soy products are forbidden on the detoxification diet. The phytosterols in soy inhibit thyroid function and therefore overall metabolism; they are implicated in breast cancer and are high in anti-trypsin, the factor which inhibits the digestion of any protein consumed in the meal. They are also associated with brain atrophy (shrinkage). Soy is also high in phytates which bind zinc, calcium and iron.[8]

Similarly the leavening of bread (we prefer the sour dough method, as yeast can pose an additional digestive difficulty for cancer patients) will inactivate phytic acid found in many grains and seeds. Phytic acid, as mentioned above, will bind important nutrients, making them unavailable through digestion. The enzyme phytase, produced through the natural leavening process, destroys the phytic acid, overcoming this problem.

You will find that many traditional indigenous cultures had very precise methods of food preparation to enhance the nutritional value of the food by a) making it more digestible, and b) ensuring maximum availability of nutrients. Techniques such as natural souring through lacto-fermentation and pickling (not recommended on the detoxification therapy) not only preserve the food in a healthy way, but the additional enzymes contributed by the bacteria themselves and their action on pre-digesting many of the food sugars increased the value of the food to the person as a whole. Modern preserving techniques of salting most foods (traditionally only used in cheese and meat products) and the use of chemical preservatives are cheap methods employed by the food industry to improve shelf-life. These are not healthy options for food preservation and we should avoid these processed, refined products at all costs, as many of the preservatives are toxic and burden many of the liver detoxification pathways.

If you turn to the table *Percentage of CHOs, fats and proteins in foods (g/100g)* at the end of this chapter, you will gain an idea of the distribution of carbohydrates, fats and proteins in the dietary food groups. You will see that vegetables and fruits have the lowest value at 0.5-3%; raw grains, 12%; raw legumes, 25%; nuts, 20%; and in animal meat we are looking at around 20-25%.

The actual protein content of cooked weight grains and legumes, when they have absorbed water, is reduced by two-thirds: therefore legumes are 8% and grains between 4-8%. Furthermore, the protein value of these incomplete or second-class proteins, may be reduced by a further 50% as they are deficient in one or more of the essential amino acid which limits the protein availability for tissue regeneration. The combining of specific groups of second-class proteins, such as grains with legumes, or legumes with nuts/seeds, will overcome this problem as each group can make good the deficiencies of the other. In many vegetarian regimes cultured dairy products are added to the meal to raise its protein value. Dairy is not only a first-class protein but is rich in the missing amino acids found in the second-class proteins and can therefore supplement all the lacking essential amino acids and improve the protein availability of that meal. Dairy products, such as yoghurt, will give around 3g/100g, and a soft pot cheese around 10-11g/100g. So you will begin to appreciate that we start with the lowest protein concentration foods and gradually move up to grains and legumes. Nuts would be introduced much later into the equation, because they are high in both protein and fat. To ensure maximum food value for nuts, they should be soaked overnight. Soaking enables the protein and the fat to chemically combine, rendering the fat water-soluble and therefore easier to digest.

# Fats

No fats, other than a minimal amount of flaxseed oil, are allowed on this treatment or on any strict detoxification plan. It is vitally important that fats are not used as an energy resource as they are not only "dirty" fuels, but they will increase free radical production in the cell, reduce the antioxidant reserves which, by default, increases insulin-resistance and hence slows the refilling of the cells with potassium.

Dr. Gerson found that fat encouraged tumours to grow, and therefore at the beginning of his work with cancer patients he omitted all fat. It was later that he introduced flaxseed oil into the diet, cold-pressed and organic, at the dose of 20ml daily during the first month and then reduced to 10ml daily. He found that amounts higher than this caused tumoural growth.

I feel that it is worth exploring the question of fats, as we have come so much further in our understanding of the cell membrane and its critical part in cell-to-cell communication. The cell membrane is built primarily from fatty acids, forming a double layer (bi-lipid layer). The type of fatty acids integrated at the cell membrane depends upon their dietary intake. Hence a diet that is rich in biologically inert saturated fats or damaged poly-unsaturated fats, will give rise to cell membranes that are saturated and inert. The biologically active unsaturated oils (essential fatty acids), the seed oils, belong to either the w6 series (linoleic, 2 double bonds) or the w3 series (linolenic, 3 double bonds). Both these series give rise to the anti-inflammatory prostaglandins which are produced when the cell is threatened by inflammation. Diets that are high in saturated or damaged poly-unsaturated fats provoke the production of pro-inflammatory prostaglandins which stimulate and perpetuate local inflammation. Hence the recommendations for flaxseed oil or fish oils in the treatment of chronic inflammatory disease.

**Linoleic Acid (18:2 w6 series)**

CH3 /\/\/⎓\/⎓\/\/\/ COOH

**Linolenic Acid (18:2 w3 series)**

CH3 /⎓\/⎓\/⎓\/\/\ COOH

In their natural configuration the EFAs are found as the cis isomer, which is bent at the double bond. The partial positive charges on the hydrogen ions cause repulsion at the double bonds, so the more double bonds a fatty acid contains, the more bending of its shape. As a consequence of this conformation electrons tend to gather at the double bonds (these are covalent which means a sharing of electrons between atoms) and hover. Double bonds are formed relatively closely to each other, so the more double bonds, the higher the electrical potential or electrical field in that area.

**Cis isomer:**

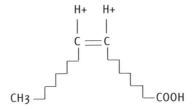

However, the natural form, or cis form, can easily be converted to the trans form, through heating, refining and oxidation, where the chain swivels at the double bond and straightens out. In this form they lose their biological activity and behave as saturated fats. They cannot be incorporated into structural lipids, but merely serve as an energy resource.

**Trans isomer:**

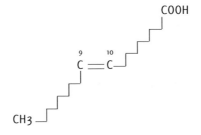

Flaxseed oil contains both the essential fatty acids linolenic acid and linoleic acid, but it is particularly rich in the omega 3 series, linolenic acid. It has been through the work of Dr. Johanna Budwig that we have begun to understand the role of linolenic acid and its involvement in energy transfer and oxidation at cell level. The essential fatty acids are incorporated into the outer cell membranes and the membranes of the intercellular organelles. These membranes cover a huge surface area, which act as a workbench for much of the cells' enzymatic activity. It is the molecular structure of the essential fatty acids which makes them biologically active. In its natural form, linolenic acid carries 18 carbon atoms, three double bonds with the first double bond at the third carbon atom.

Although the structure has no overall charge, by virtue of the grouping of these bonds, electrons hover at these double bonds, creating an electrical field and therefore, an electrical potential. This electrical field is stabilised by trans-membrane proteins which form weak hydrogen bonds with their sulphydryl groups (of the amino acids methionine and cysteine). The presence of these EFAs in the membrane means that the membrane is capable of storing charge or energy, which can be tapped into on demand. Additionally these electron fields will attract oxygen like a magnet and draw it into the cell.[8]

The entry of oxygen into the cell via the cell membrane becomes a crucial factor in cell metabolism and oxidation. Today's modern diet, high in saturated fats and destroyed unsaturated fats (processing, refining and heating destroys the natural configuration of the EFAs and they become biologically inactive and toxic to the system), leads to cell membranes which are inert, lacking full electrical potential. The cell is "shut off", fails to acknowledge hormonal/nervous signals and is deprived of oxygen. This leads to the onset of an array of chronic degenerative disease. Of critical importance is the availability of EFAs to the brain tissue, which requires a constant supply of oxygen. In 1926 Otto Warburg showed that it was a fatty substance that was required to restart oxidation, but it was through the work of Dr. Johanna Budwig that this factor was isolated. A deficiency of EFAs (particularly linolenic acid) leads to oxygen starvation by the cell.

Dr. Joanna Budwig goes further to state that the energy for metabolism is stored in the EFAs at the cell membrane and acts in a similar manner to the plant's seed oils, which absorb the sun's energy (photons) during photosynthesis. The electron-rich oils are set up to receive solar energy. They attract the electro-magnetic waves of the sun (photons) and store solar energy through resonance absorption. To simplify things, electrons vibrate continually on their own wavelength, they have their own frequency like radio receivers which are set at a certain wavelength. They love photons and attract them by means of their magnetic fields. The magnetic fields of both attract each other when the wavelengths are in tune. In the human being, the absorption of energy corresponds to one's own wavelength. The resonance in our biological substance is set to absorb the sun's energy, and the concentration of the sun's energy is improved when we eat foods which have electrons that in turn attract the electro-magnetic waves of photons. The electron-rich foods are found in the seed oils.

The issue here is not the sitting in full sun (Dr. Gerson was very clear on this point and did not recommend full sunlight to his patients) but having the capacity at the cell membrane to store energy. Electrons can store high energy like a battery in a stable, controlled environment, as Dr. Johanna Budwig so eloquently explains, provided by the association between the membrane fatty acids and protein. The higher this capacity, the greater the amount of energy available to the cell and the greater the attraction for oxygen into the cell.

This chapter serves merely to explain the rationale behind detoxification and healing, so that choices are informed and adhered to. You will need to refer to recommended source material for dietary specifics in detoxification and nutritional healing.[10, 11]

Healing, for many, can be a long process. What you eat today are your cells of tomorrow. In the healing process, it is not always a case of repairing existing tissue, but more a case of replacing old, damaged tissue. This takes time. Nowadays, in six months the patient may have replaced a small amount of tissue, but not enough to see an appreciable difference in health. However, in 18 months to 2 years of rigid application of the diet, we are going to see substantial differences in health. It is worth reminding your patient of this fact to inspire their strict adherence and additionally to ensure that when they have finished the therapy they don't fall into old eating patterns, but approach diet from an holistic point of view.

# Percentage of CHOs, Fats and Proteins in Foods (g/100g)

|  | Protein | CHOs | Fats |
|---|---|---|---|
| **Meat/fish** |  |  |  |
| Beef | 21-24 | 0 | 19-24 |
| Lamb | 18-24 | 0 | 19-35 |
| Chicken | 20 | 0 | 7-12 |
| Cod | 16.5 | 0 | 0.4 |
| Halibut | 18.6 | 0 | 5.2 |
| Herring | 17.3 | 0 | 18.8 |
| Mackerel | 18.7 | 0 | 12 |
| Salmon | 19.9 | 0 | 13.6 |
| Trout | 19.2 | 0 | 2.1 |
| Shell fish | 14-18 | 0-4 | 0.1-3 |
| **Nuts** |  |  |  |
| Almonds | 18.6 | 19.6 | 54.1 |
| Brazil nuts | 14.4 | 11 | 65.9 |
| Hazelnuts | 12.7 | 18 | 60.9 |
| Peanuts | 26.9 | 23.6 | 44.2 |
| Walnuts | 15.0 | 15.6 | 64.4 |
| **Cereals** |  |  |  |
| Barley | 9 | 76.5 | 1.4 |
| Buckwheat | 11.7 | 70 | 2.7 |
| Oats | 13.8 | 67.6 | 6.6 |
| Rice | 7.6 | 79.4 | 0.3 |
| Wheat (whole) | 12.1 | 71.5 | 2.1 |
| Wheat germ | 25.2 | 49.5 | 10.0 |
| **Dairy/eggs** |  |  |  |
| Cheese | 18-27 | 1.8-3.4 | 22-30 |
| Milk | 3.2 | 4.6 | 3.7 |
| Eggs (whole) | 12.8 | 0.7 | 11.5 |
| white | 10.8 | 0.8 | 0.2 |
| yolk | 16.3 | 0.7 | 31.9 |
| **Pulses** |  |  |  |
| Kidney | 21.3 | 61.6 | 1.6 |
| Lentils | 25.0 | 59.5 | 1.0 |
| Soya beans | 34.9 | 34.8 | 18.1 |
| **Vegetables** | 0.5 - 4.0 | 4-9.0 | 0.1-0.6 |
| Potatoes | 2.0 | 19.1 | 0.1 |
| **Fruits** | 0.5 - 3.0 | 9-16 | 0.1-0.4 |

# References

1. Fallon, S.: *Nourishing Traditions*, 1995, ISBN 1887314156 pp 43-44
2. Ibid., pp 55-56
3. *Food with Attitude*, Permaculture International Journal (March-May 2000, No. 74, ISSN 1037-8480), p.27.
4. Alexander, K.; *What's wrong with raw*; http://www.kathrynalexander.com.au/health-topics/whats-wrong-with-raw
5. Fallon, S.: *Nourishing Traditions*, 1995, pp 31-33
6. Ibid., p 468
7. Ibid., p 104
8. Ibid., pp 44, 185, 468.
9. Erasmus, Udo.: *Fats that Heal, Fats that Kill*, 1996, pp 46-48, 59
10. Gerson, C; Bishop, B; *Healing the Gerson Way* ISBN 9780976018605
11. Alexander, K.: *Dietary Healing, the complete detox program* ISBN 9780980376203

# Chapter 8

# PATIENT MANAGEMENT THROUGH THE HEALING CRISIS

Most patients will realise the importance of the healing crisis and will fret when nothing seems to be happening. Equally, when the crisis does occur, they may panic and think that the therapy isn't working or worse, that their disease is progressing. It is vitally important that you can manage your patient through this process and educate the patient, so that they learn how to self-manage and interpret accurately what exactly is happening. Many mistakes can be made by both the patient and practitioner around these periods, as the practitioner may be unsure of the type of reaction the patient is suffering from, and therefore not give appropriate advice, and the patient may interpret the symptoms negatively, changing or reducing parts of the therapy.

The healing process is dependent on the body building the momentum for detoxification and simultaneously restoring the oxidative potential at cellular level over a period of time. During this time detoxification reactions will be experienced as the waste is discharged. We may see symptoms in the eliminative organs (liver, genito-urinary tract, skin and mucous membranes), and symptoms will vary from mucus discharge (this may be inflammatory from toxic residues), spots/pimples/boils/dry skin, and most frequently in the digestive tract from the discharge of toxins via the bile system into the gastrointestinal tract, which can cause nausea, diarrhoea, muscle spasms/pain.

When the body is sufficiently detoxified and the cells reactivated then the patient will experience their first healing crisis. The time-frame for this will vary from individual to individual; some patients respond within the first month, while others, particularly if they have had chemotherapy, can take up to five months before a flare-up occurs. The nature of each flare-up will also vary from person to person, but the patient will learn to identify their own specific symptoms, which will usually follow their unique pattern. For example, before a flare-up a patient may become emotionally unstable. Having experienced this several times, the patient may then recognise that a flare-up is about to happen. The patient will also be able to determine how the flare-up will progress and will know what steps to take to alleviate any discomfort and allow the therapy to continue. The frequency and intensity of each flare-up will lessen as time goes on.

From my experience of the healing process there are three broad categories of symptoms that may occur during this time: toxic reactions, detoxification reactions and the healing crisis. Being able to differentiate between them enables the practitioner and patient to manage each set of symptoms appropriately. As the body builds a momentum for healing, the patient will start to experience greater amounts of toxic release within the body. The symptoms of toxic release fall into the two categories of toxic and detoxification reactions. It's important to remember that toxic and detoxification reactions/crises are not the healing crisis; they are not the same as the healing flare-up which is an indicator that the body is able to initiate and maintain a full-blown immune response. The healing flare-up is the first way point on the journey to cure as Dr. Gerson indicated that if he could bring a patient to this point, then he would almost certainly see cure. The healing flare-up (healing crisis) is marked by a spontaneous fever that is not a result of infection or tumoural progression.

# Toxic Reactions

Toxic reactions indicate toxins being pushed out of the cells where they have been "safely" harboured for many years and into the systemic circulation. The patient may feel foul and very toxic. They may experience headaches, nervous irritability (toxic residues of old drugs/nicotine/poisons will irritate the nerve endings), mental and emotional instability, depression, an inability to concentrate or think logically (very difficult for the carer), foul taste in the mouth with peculiar taints and odours, vivid memories from the past, possibly of traumatic situations which offer an opportunity to review a past event from a mature standpoint and so clear it; cravings for foods that are strictly forbidden (some authors suggest that these cravings are activated by the discharge of the toxins from that particular food into the system and as you discharge those toxic residues, so you crave it), and joint and muscle pains. Muscle pain and tension may be particularly severe around the neck/shoulder area and down the spine, as the shifting toxins can lodge in the muscle, creating a guarding of those muscles, a reduction of blood supply which traps the toxins further leading to inflammatory changes and pain.

Toxic symptoms are indicating to you that the liver needs additional help in filtering the toxicity from the circulation. There is only one remedy for the toxic reaction, and that is the coffee enema. The patient is quick to understand this from the experience of the relief of symptoms which follows an enema. You have to be aware also that a toxic crisis can occur when the patient is eliminating a great deal of necrotic tumour tissue into the systemic circulation. Never is it more important to keep the additional enemas going through these crises. The patient must be made aware that it is dangerous to do more than 9 enemas daily over a prolonged period of say more than a few days, without taking additional juices. There is a risk of dehydration and electrolyte imbalance if too many enemas are sustained over a long period. In times of extreme toxic crisis the coffee enema may be taken at two hourly intervals over a 24 hour period, but the patient must take some additional juices.

Muscle tension and pain can be alleviated by the warm castor oil pack, which will increase circulation to the area and help to shift the toxicity lodged in the muscles. The clay pack, which is a cool pack, will adsorb inflammatory oedema and is most beneficial over hot, swollen areas, or areas of fluid retention. It will draw the excess fluid and toxins out through the skin, alleviating the pain.

# Detoxification Reactions

Detoxification symptoms simply relate to the symptoms of discharge of toxicity to the outside. Most of the symptoms will arise in the digestive tract, as this is the main route of elimination from the liver through the bile system into the duodenum and out via the colon. However, other symptoms may be felt in the other organs of elimination; foul smelling mucus discharge, skin eruptions, foul-smelling and dark urine, and foul-smelling sweat. When these organs are carrying the additional burden, they may become prone to infection, and it is important that in the case of mucus discharge that this is facilitated by using the castor oil pack over the affected areas (sinus, chest, colon area) so that infection does not set in.

When detoxification symptoms occur in the digestive tract, it can become quite difficult for the patient to maintain the therapy, as the range of symptoms in the digestive tract, set out below, can inhibit both dietary intake and/ or enemas.

## Nausea, Vomiting, Diarrhoea & Inflammation of the Gastrointestinal Tract

### Nausea and vomiting

As the very alkaline toxic bile is discharged from the gallbladder, the patient may feel extremely nauseous, even suffering vomiting and be unable to eat or keep anything down. Drinking copious amounts of peppermint tea will increase stomach acidity, which will mechanically flush and neutralise toxic bile from the stomach, limiting irritation to the lining. Alternatively, gruel, which is also very nourishing, will buffer either excess acidity or alkalinity, while at the same time line and protect the gastrointestinal tract against any inflammatory reaction to the caustic nature of some chemicals/toxins released. If the patient is complaining of excess acidity, then chamomile tea can replace the peppermint tea. However, gruel is useful in both situations.

The patient may find that the nausea and vomiting worsen after an enema, and this is a prime area for a common mistake - that the enema is causing the bad reaction, and therefore they feel that they should stop the enemas for a while. The enema is actually causing the release of the toxic bile, it is assisting the liver in its role of elimination and therefore is acting in favour of the body and should not be stopped. However, you can recommend to your patient that they take a small glass of gruel before and after the enema. This will mop up the toxic bile and help any nausea and sickness. Fortunately these detoxification reactions are short-lived (a few days) and the patient feels much restored after they have passed. If these measures are not sufficient to relieve the severity of the symptoms, and the patient is vomiting bile, then you may have to reduce the coffee enemas and replace with chamomile tea enemas, while increasing the intake of herb teas (peppermint or chamomile) and gruel.

However, you may see extreme toxic eliminations in the weakened patient or in the patient who has had chemotherapy where nothing (gruel, peppermint tea) seems to work. The juices, especially the green juice, cannot be kept down, and the patient is in a serious crisis of potential dehydration and weakening of their condition. Under these circumstances you will be looking to alleviate the whole detoxification process and your first priority will be to ensure that the patient is still taking some food. You may reduce the juices, partially or completely, and replace with 1/2 juice:1/2 gruel, or just peppermint tea and gruel. Juices may also be taken by enema, brought to body heat and retained for as long as possible (usually they will be well-absorbed in 15 minutes). The diet will consist of apple sauce, thin oatmeal porridge, mashed potato and the Hippocrates soup. The enemas may be reduced, diluted with chamomile tea, or just consist of chamomile tea. You will need to use your common sense to do what is best for the patient and understand that pushing a debilitated patient to the point of damage and inability to undertake any of the therapy (even eating the modified diet) is bad patient management.

## Inflammation at the rectum

Toxins can cause caustic inflammation of the delicate mucous membranes which may be felt anywhere along the digestive tract, but particularly at the rectum, where it can directly interfere with the practice of the enemas. These caustic inflammations may worsen on the castor oil days, when greater amounts of toxic residue are being released. It is recommended that the patient either use a non-toxic suppository, such as Anusol, or liberally apply a baby barrier cream, such as Desitin, to the area to protect it from further insult and enable healing. It may be recommended to drink gruel if there are other areas of soreness along the tract.

## Diarrhoea

This frequently accompanies the nausea and is due to irritation of the intestinal tract by the toxic release, causing spasms and diarrhoea. It is the body's defence mechanism to flush out toxic, irritating bile. At the outset it may be quite useful to recommend 1/4 teaspoon of clay in peppermint tea along with 1/8th teaspoon of potassium gluconate (to replace potassium losses) every 4 hours. The use of gruel will reduce caustic irritation and buffer the toxicity. The patient may notice that the green juices often "pass straight through" and complain that the juices seem to exacerbate the condition. You may recommend mixing the juices with gruel. If the diarrhoea is prolonged, then it will have adverse affects on the patient's health and electrolyte balance. You must watch this carefully and remember that the diet remains the most important part of the therapy at this stage, even at the expense of the juices and enemas. Coffee enemas may be temporarily stopped (if the diarrhoea is excessive) or replaced by chamomile tea enemas, and the castor oil treatment will be put on hold. Oatmeal with apple sauce or raw, grated apple often helps to alleviate diarrhoea as the high levels of pectin found in apples acts as an astringent, and will mop up excess fluid in the colon.

# Problems in the administering of enemas

During periods of detoxification the patient may suffer additional bloating, gas and discomfort in the digestive system. This, once again, is the body's response to toxicity being eliminated through this channel. However, it can cause problems with either the administration or retention of the enema. The toxic irritation in the gut creates a greater sensitivity to the enema and the colon may become hyper-active, creating either counter-spasms, making it difficult to either accept the enema or retain it, or, on the contrary, the colon will clutch the enema and the patient will have difficulty in releasing it. These symptoms, if the patient has had no prior difficulties in holding and releasing the enema, will indicate that greater amounts of toxicity are being released at this time. Several other symptoms may confirm this, such as the patient may wake in the early hours feeling very toxic and bloated (this indicates that additional toxicity is building during the enema-free period), and the first enema is very difficult to hold. The patient would be well advised to consider doing an additional enema during the night (say at 2 am) or taking a 500ml chamomile enema immediately prior to the first coffee enema and adding 10ml of the potassium compound solution to it. This can be repeated for a few days, but the potassium can prove an irritant to the bowel, so it is not recommended for long-term application, only in crisis management. It is useful to remember not to hang or place the enema bucket too high, but to let the flow occur gently, which may alleviate some of the counter-spasms. If patients have taken medication in the past which would have directly affected the nervous system, then nervous symptoms in the gut may be more pronounced during these detoxification episodes.

# Haemorrhoids

Haemorrhoids are not caused by the enemas, but they may appear during the detoxification crisis. Traditionally, haemorrhoids are associated with back pressure from the liver, indicating liver stagnation/congestion. This seems a fair assessment when observing the exacerbation of haemorrhoids in certain patients during the detoxification crises. When the crisis is over, the haemorrhoids heal. For some patients this becomes one of their standard signs of the detoxification process. Many patients may make the mistake to stop the enemas, believing them to be the cause of the problem. The patient must be assured that this is not so and encouraged to use a soft catheter. If the haemorrhoids are painful, then Anusol suppositories may be used, and Desitin will alleviate any external haemorrhoidal pain and irritation from caustic burning.

# Dark Stools

This is a very favourable sign because it indicates increased efficiency in the bile system. The dark grey/green stool colour is caused by a high concentration of bile and the chemical changes it has undergone. If the stools are black, then the possibility of occult bleeding should not be overlooked.

# Cold sores and Fever Blisters

I have noticed that these are a common sign during detoxification, but may remain intermittent for many months during the healing process.

# Carotaemia

Carotaemia, or the orange tinge to the skin, soles of the feet and palms of the hand, is a common sign due to the high carotene levels in the juices. It is not a detoxification reaction, nor a toxic reaction, but can occur prior to a flare-up, in iron-deficiency anaemia, abnormal thyroid function (unlikely on the Gerson Therapy if supplementing with thyroid hormone) or zinc deficiencies. Both iron and zinc are required for the conversion of beta carotene to vitamin A by the liver, and deficiencies will result in carotene accumulating in the fat tissue. As vitamin A is involved in the uptake in dietary iron, a vitamin A deficiency can lead to an iron deficiency and an iron deficiency can lead to a vitamin A deficiency. A vicious cycle may then ensue where beta-carotene can accumulate due to iron deficiencies. It is interesting that Dr. Gerson used to supplement with vitamin A, vitamin D and iron prior to the introduction of the raw liver juice. Although liver is not that high in iron it has very high levels of vitamin A which could increase the bioavailability of the iron content even further.

.

# The Healing Inflammation

The symptoms of the healing inflammation are quite different from toxic and detoxification reactions. They relate to the symptoms dealing with the reactivation of the immune system and the regeneration of body tissue integrity. The symptoms can be *local* inflammatory reactions relating to the healing of old or new injuries, or *general* which will involve fever. Injury specifically refers to tissue trauma, whether it be physical (accident/fracture), bacterial (infection), the disease process or chemical insult - in short any insult which results in damaged tissue that has failed to heal completely. This includes scar tissue, old fractures or any area of damage that can be revisited and healed through the process of inflammation which results in redness and pain at the site before resolution.

The patient will remember old injuries or illnesses as they reappear, old scar tissue will inflame, previously broken bones will suddenly become sore with possible swelling as they heal. You cannot dictate which area is going to be healed next, the body will choose. In the cancer patient we are looking for healing reactions at the tumour site, so inflammation, redness, swelling and pain at the location is not necessarily a sign that the disease is progressing, but when experienced as part of the general healing process it can indicate immune activity and healing at that area. Subsequent reduction of tumour mass will confirm this.

In a full-blown healing crisis these reactions are usually accompanied by fever and general malaise, which is self-limiting. I have found that in many cases during the few days prior to a healing crisis the patient's general energy/vitality seems much higher than usual. The healing crisis can last from 3 –10 days. A word of warning: if you misread the symptoms and suppress the crisis, you may have difficulty from that point onwards in securing another healing crisis.

In general terms, for the cancer patient on a strong detoxification plan, the first crisis may occur between days 5-10 and last probably around 2-3 days. However, I have found that this is not always the case and the patient will not have a healing reaction until the sixth/seventh week, with the heaviest reaction in the third/fourth month. In chemotherapy patients you will not be looking for a reaction until the fifth/sixth month, and the flare-up may only comprise strong toxic and detoxification reactions rather than a healing inflammation. For the chemotherapy patient who comes through this period successfully, there may be an even stronger crisis at the 9th month. Many patients who have been very damaged with chemotherapy may slowly deteriorate from this point. This is not the cause of the detoxification therapy, but the inability of the body to respond. I have seen several patients with advanced cancer who have been given only 3-6 months to live by the medical profession, live up to 18 months, at home, doing the detoxification therapy and not requiring hospitalization until the very end. Even patients with severe bone metastases suffered no pain throughout the therapy.

Patient management during the healing inflammation is critical. The main areas of concern are fever and pain management.

# Fever

Fever often accompanies the healing inflammation. The practitioner must first rule out infection or tumoural growth, as both these conditions will give rise to fever.

## The Infectious Fever

In the case of infection, there will be accompanying symptoms to indicate a bacterial or viral component and, if possible, a culture should be taken to determine the cause.

### Treatment

It is important to treat infection appropriately:
- antibiotics if the infection is severe
- herbs such as Echinacea
- add hydrogen peroxide to the bath and rub the skin with a 2% solution after a hot bath
- add the juice of 6 lemons daily to the apple/carrot juice
- keep away from infectious people
- pay particular attention to the hygiene in the bathroom/kitchen

## The Tumoural Fever

A fever associated with tumoural activity is constant - day and night. The blood results may indicate tumoural progression (neutrophilia), but there is usually little doubt with the practitioner when a fever is tumoural. There is no natural treatment for fever in this instance other than tepid bathing, cool compresses on the forehead and nape of neck, or cool (not cold) enemas.

## The Healing Fever

Fever is an essential component of the total immune response. It activates and potentiates immune activity. It is standard medical text that if fever is suppressed, then the illness is prolonged. Without fever, the body may be unable to heal adequately. Fever helps destroy tumour tissue and therefore it is to be welcomed in any therapy whose aim is to enable healing.

The healing crisis fever will stay with the patient for several hours. A general pattern is for the fever to occur in the evening and break in the early hours of the morning. If the patient can tolerate the fever for around 5 hours, then it will be to his/her advantage. After this time the fever may be reduced by applying physical measures first, not medication.

### Treatment

Half hourly checks should be made on the patient's temperature. Do not allow the temperature to rise above 104°F (40°C). The following methods can be used to reduce the fever:
- Cool water enemas
- Cold compress/sponging; compress to the forehead and nape of neck
- Tepid bathing
- Cold drinks
- If these methods are not effective and the temperature remains high or intolerable, then an aspirin-based medication may be used. Dr. Gerson's Pain Triad works well in these circumstances (1 Aspirin, 1 niacin x 50mg, 500mg vitamin C).

# Pain

Pain can arise from inflammation of damaged or healing tissue, tumoural inflammation or tumoural pressure. The whole inflammatory process causes oedema, which presses on the nerves and surrounding structures, causing pain signals. In most cases any diseased or damaged area/joint of the body will inflame and after 2-3 reactions should be healed, so that joints enjoy normal movement. In the case of tumoural inflammation or growth, if this involves pressure on the spinal cord, brain or nervous system, then symptoms can worsen and medical intervention may have to be sought. However, if it can be established that the pain is not due to disease progression, then it is best to adopt natural, physical methods for alleviating pain, avoiding the anti-inflammatory drugs, which act by suppressing inflammation - the opposite of what the patient is trying to achieve.

## 1st line of treatment

- **The coffee enema.** The coffee enema will stimulate the liver to remove all inflammatory chemicals produced at the site of inflammation. These chemicals, if not removed, cause the formation of free radicals at the location, which sets up a vicious cycle inciting further inflammatory damage and perpetuating the cycle. Efficient removal of these toxins, facilitated by the coffee enema, relieves the pain dramatically. The coffee enema is also useful during an allergic reaction to clear excess histamine from the body.

- **Castor oil packs** may be used in cases of muscle tension, spasms/spastic spasms and bone pain. With bone pain, the muscles may contract around the area of pain and inflammation, due to both the release of toxins lodging in the muscles and as a defence by the body to protect the bone. The heated pack will assist in releasing the muscles and dispersing the toxins.

- **Clay packs** are used in hot inflammatory pain, arthritis, joint pain, tumour inflammation and in oedemas. They can be used around the head in brain tumours and for headaches.

- **Hydrotherapy/hot shower/tub.** This is very useful in bone pain and may be taken 2-3 x/week or more often for the control of pain. Hydrotherapy should never be done by the patient on his/her own. It must be remembered that it can reduce the blood pressure and, if fever is present, will increase it. Never bathe in fluoridated water.

- **Lymphasizing.** This is the method of increasing the flow of lymph and may either be achieved through gentle "stroking" of the body, the limbs and torso by a friend, or through gentle bouncing on a small trampoline. To have the patient gently bounced, like a baby, can bring relief from pain. Pain is often caused by fluid accumulation and just by moving the fluid, can alleviate the pain.

- **TENS machine** may be used to negate pain impulses. These units can be very useful and may be obtained through the doctor or hospital.

## 2nd line of treatment: The Pain Triad

The methods outlined above must not be disbanded when they appear to be ineffective. It is important that the patient understands their benefit and continues to support the body in these ways. If pain persists, the treatments above may be combined with a relatively non-toxic treatment, using aspirin based preparations (Aspirin, Ibuprofen, Nurofen). It is often more effective to take 1-2 aspirin with 500mg of Vitamin C and 1 x 50mg niacin. The patient should take this with gruel and never on an empty stomach. As the therapy progresses these treatments become more effective, and should work eventually.

## 3rd line of treatment

If pain cannot be controlled by the above methods, then the patient may have to resort to the stronger pain relievers. Many patients may have such severe pain that they cannot even eat or do any part of the therapy. Clearly, this is not in the patient's best interest. Similarly, if tumoural inflammation is creating severe pain, then the patient may have to resort to steroid treatment to resolve the inflammation. This often occurs with patients suffering from brain metastases.

- **Steroids:** used to reduce inflammation, swelling and pain. They inhibit the healing process and should only be used if there is no other alternative at that stage.

- **Narcotics:** morphine, or its derivatives, such as codeine, are often prescribed to alleviate severe pain. These drugs suppress the visceral nervous system (hence digestion is impaired), and reduce motility of the gastrointestinal tract, causing constipation.

- **Non-steroidal anti-inflammatory drugs (NSAIDs):** these may be more effective in the treatment of bone pain than the narcotics.

If a patient comes to you and is taking prescribed pain medication, do not discontinue this medication until you are into the detoxification therapy and then, if possible, under the guidance of the patient's doctor, reduce the dose gradually.

*Chapter 9*

---

# PATIENT EDUCATION
# RECOGNIZING THE PITFALLS

Throughout this manual I have made repeated references to the pitfalls of both patient and practitioner, usually due to failure in interpretation of the case or symptoms and consequently making inappropriate decisions regarding the therapy. These decisions can cause major setbacks to the patient's healing process. So it is really important to understand the detoxification and healing process inside-out, and how each individual is likely to respond during that process. Experience will teach you more than books, and you will be able to anticipate the nature of reactions and their effect on the individual. It is a very subtle art, modifications may be so slight that you feel they could not possibly have any effect, but we are bending the therapy to the patient's response, encouraging and enabling the detoxification and healing response. Detoxification is more than just a nutritional therapy, it is an exact process and science which obeys the laws of nature. We, too, have to obey those laws and we should always strive, through observation, to correctly assess the situation.

I have prepared a list of the common pitfalls that I have encountered in my practice. Sometimes you are taken completely by surprise at how the patient could have misinterpreted a medication or dietary procedure. The point is that people forget, they panic, or *think* they know, but unless you are practising as a practitioner every day, then it is easy to appreciate how the layperson can make mistakes. This list should prove useful as a pointer, so that you can be more aware of the type of mistakes patients, or you yourself, may make. Use this as a revision exercise on some basic aspects of a detoxification therapy.

With the best will in the world you will find that the biggest problems arise when the patient does not keep regular appointments and either self-medicates or fails to modify the treatment appropriately. It is then that the most mistakes are made. You must encourage regular check-ups with your patients, as this is critical for their successful progress.

## Enemas

- ◆ Reduction of the enemas too soon into the therapy. The number of enemas is dependent upon the tumoural mass and detoxification/toxic symptoms. It is not until the tumoural mass has started to shrink (or preferably gone) that the patient can afford to reduce the enemas and then must not be afraid to increase them in times of flare-up.

- ◆ Ceasing enemas:
    - o Toxic reactions, such as headaches, may be misinterpreted by the patient as being caused by the caffeine in the enema;
    - o Nausea after coffee enema. The patient thinks that the coffee enema is causing the nausea and therefore stops taking it;
    - o Tachycardia after the enema causes panic to the patient who may reduce the frequency or strength of the enemas;
    - o Fear of loss of bowel function; and
    - o Haemorrhoids/burning or pain in rectum/anus

- Too many enemas
  - The pretreated chemotherapy patient, or the patient with a very damaged liver, may decide to increase the amount of enemas to the amount recommended on the stronger therapy, thinking that they can accelerate their progress. This could ultimately be very damaging.
  - During flare-ups the patient may increase the number of enemas for too long a period without increasing the number of juices. This can lead to dehydration and electrolyte imbalance. Generally speaking, nine enemas in any 24 hour period is a safe number to take over a few days. If the patient needs to take more in a heavy crisis, then the number of juices would need to be increased (by three or more) accordingly.
  - The patient may increase the number of enemas, thinking that they are going to alleviate gas. Unless the gas is due to toxic release, then the enemas will have little effect. Poor digestive capacity is the usual cause of gas and the patient, if able, should be encouraged to increase the digestive enzymes and take exercise through gentle walking. Patients who tend to suffer the most from gas are usually those who are immobile.

- Enema preparation
  - Mistakes in the concentration/dilution of the enema. If the concentration is too strong (e.g. using the full 4 enema concentrate for 1 enema), or too weak, then the patient will either have too strong an effect from the caffeine or no effect at all.
  - Failure to brew the coffee using the recommended method - a coffee machine or percolator is not acceptable.
  - Failure to use organic ground coffee (mild roast); instant coffee is not acceptable.

- Colemas/colonic irrigation - these are high water enemas requiring around 10 litres of water, which washes in and out of the colon. Many patients feel that these will help alleviate a toxic colon. The colema does not fulfil the function of stimulating the liver and can cause serious electrolyte imbalance and dilution of body fluids in the sick patient. As a bowel wash, it may be ineffective as a treatment on its own as it does not address the causes of a stagnant bowel or inflammatory changes within the bowel. On the strict detoxification plan, much mucus and damaged bowel tissue will be released and the huge amount of pancreatic enzymes used will facilitate this softening, loosening and elimination process.

# Medications

- Inappropriate self-medicating, particularly if following text guidelines without referring to a practitioner.
- Failure to reduce the dose of thyroid, Lugol's and potassium compound solution after the initial 4 weeks of therapy. Overdoing the intensive phase will lead to weight loss and possible deterioration of the patient.
- Inappropriate reduction of thyroid in response to symptoms such as tachycardia. It is important to take all the symptoms into account, the temperature, pulse rate, taking the pulse after the enema, etc., in order to determine the cause. In many patients the cause will not be due to the high doses of thyroid, but you will find that the weakened patient with or without cardiac, respiratory and renal insufficiency, is more vulnerable to the thyroid medication. You will not see the effects of reducing the medication for around 7-10 days, so do not be tempted to lower the dose too drastically.
- Potassium compound solution: a common problem is that the patient may use the powder "neat" and not diluted as a 10%.
- Treat a fever/pain with inappropriate medications. Patients will usually forget and reach for whatever pain-killer is in the cupboard. Paracetamol is liver toxic.

# Diet

- The patient may use commercial vegetables/fruit when the selection is poor. It is wise to suggest to your patient to place a large order for carrots and apples before the growing season ends and ask the wholesaler/retailer if they could to store their produce in their cold room.
- Failure to use either distilled or reverse osmosis water. Many patients feel that filtered or spring water will do. It won't. Also the rinsing of vegetables/fruits must be done in either distilled or reverse osmosis water. Chlorine and fluoride both displace iodine and are therefore suppressive of thyroid function.
- Failure to restrict protein in a weak, thin patient, or failure to add protein at the appropriate time. Protein feeds the tumoural masses, but inadequate protein for too long a period of time will compromise the immune system.
- Adding extra protein too soon into the therapy which may lead to disease recurrence.
- Using a low-fat soured milk product as opposed to a skimmed-milk (non-fat) product.
- Cooking either the yoghurt or the pot cheese.
- Skipping meals, because the patient is too full on all the juices.
- Skipping the Hippocrates soup. The soup is a medicine and vitally important for renal detoxification.
- Skipping or not eating enough of the protein part of the diet (potatoes, oatmeal and carrots).
- Using inappropriate cooking utensils (lead-glazed ceramic casseroles, aluminium or iron pans, pressure cookers, etc.) and cooking techniques, such as baking at high temperatures, failing to cook at low temperatures in the vegetables' own juice, steaming, failure to germinate grains/legumes.

# Juices

- Many patients suffer candida/thrush at the outset of treatment and during flare-ups which may be alleviated by stopping the apple and carrot juice and replacing with green juices or reducing the amount of apple in the juices.
- Many patients substitute other varieties of green vegetables in their juices when some of the ingredients are unavailable. By adding too many of the dark greens or even celery, the juice may cease to become a medicine as the ratio of sodium to potassium becomes skewed in favour of sodium.
- Taking larger juices but at greater intervals to reduce time in the kitchen. It is not just the volume of juice that is important, but equally the incremental dosing of the juice and potassium at hourly intervals to achieve the effect of regular bombardment of the cells with potassium. When taken in large doses, the kidneys will simply remove the excess from the circulation before it can be of value to the tissues.

# Miscellaneous

- Hygiene and infection - tell your patient not to encourage visitors or helpers to come if they have an infection, particularly a gastrointestinal infection. Cleanliness is imperative in the bathroom and kitchen and particularly with the enema equipment.
- Failure to eliminate chemicals from the home (cleaning fluids, detergents, paint, bug sprays, etc.) and from daily products such as tooth paste, shampoo, soap, etc.
- The patient may not be careful enough about toxic fumes from the environment, electrical pollution (electromagnetic radiation).
- The patient may stop the therapy too soon.
- The patient may feel much better, with the cancer in remission, and start *doing too much* - this is a major cause of failure. Too much exercise/stress/worry will inhibit the healing process.
- If the patient has not discussed what dietary regime to follow after the therapy, then this can lead to relapse. Some patients need to stick close to the therapy for life.

# Chapter 10

# DETOXIFICATION & CHRONIC DEGENERATIVE DISEASE

We are seeing an escalation in chronic degenerative disease in Western societies of epidemic proportions - this means a higher percentage of the population being affected than would be considered normal. Currently up to 30% of our children now suffer from asthma; 1 in 68 children are identified with ASD (autism spectrum disorder) with the prevalence five times higher in boys (1 in 42); cancer is now predicted to affect 1 in 2; and dementia which has risen from nowhere since the late 1970s is now the fourth leading cause of death, only topped by cancer, heart disease and stroke. Diabetes, the most rapidly growing epidemic affects 10% of the US population, with a disturbing increase in childhood prevalence. And so the list goes on - autoimmune disease, conditions associated with infertility (PCOS and endometriosis) and depression, to name but a few, where drugs for mental illness and depression are the most widely prescribed, with a large percentage of our children prescribed amphetamine-type drugs for ADHD.

We are told not to worry - it's all in our genes and it can be fixed. We are now getting stuck into our genetic make-up and have discovered that carriers of specific gene codes predispose to certain diseases, particularly certain cancers and autoimmune disease. To the lay person this means that these genes, when they become aberrant, are the cause of the disease. So if we change the gene, or the expression of the gene, then the disease will not manifest. The truth is that our gene pool has been around for a very long time and does not radically change within a couple of generations; the truth is that a similar gene pool 50 years ago did not show the same prevalence of disease as now, which has led to questioning epigenetic factors, or what environmental stimuli make our genes turn on or off, or behave abnormally.

If we turn to the work of Pottenger and Price in the mid 20th century, we will find corroboration of the negative effects of dietary change on populations. Pottenger found that, within three generations, cats fed on a cooked meat and milk diet produced infertility, sexual dysfunction, joint problems, osteoporosis, allergies and low resistance to disease. When the diet was restored to a raw meat, raw milk diet then, depending which generation-deficiency level the cat belonged to (the lower the generation/deficiency, the deeper the health problems), the slower the reversal process. In the healthy generation, these cats could maintain health on their altered diet, but the offspring (first generation deficiency) could not sustain health on such a diet but only remained healthy on the raw diet. They had little constitutional resistance and needed to support their health with the diet. With subsequent generation-deficiency litters, the situation became more critical. It took several generations to reverse the damage in the constitution of each line.

Weston Price studied the dietary habits of many indigenous populations, comparing populations on their traditional diet living in close proximity with the same racial stock on a Westernised diet. His common findings among all the populations world-wide were: skeletal changes to the face and dental arch (narrowing and overcrowding of teeth), dental caries, lowered resistance to disease (TB affecting populations on Western food but unseen in neighbouring tribes on traditional food), changes in intellect and behaviour along with social and moral decay.

Weston Price could not find a common diet or even common elements in the varied diets that would give him a definitive "healthy diet". Some tribes in Africa only drank blood and milk (fresh); the Swiss ate bread and cheese and hardly any vegetables; some aboriginal tribes ate dried locusts for their protein; the Maori ate large amounts of sea food; the Melanesians shared produce with their warring neighbours (those living on the coast left sea food for the tribes of the interior who would bring fresh vegetables - no messenger carrying food ever got killed!); no tribe was purely vegetarian. The only common denominator was that food was fresh, and unpasteurized. Local preserving methods (such as drying/fermentation) were used that would not chemically interfere with the food but enhance its value, refined products were not used (whole grain/seed), and sugar was not available. Additionally, the animals were fed on appropriate food and rich pastures leading to animal products high in nutritional value.

The most fundamental changes in our society over the last 80 years, running parallel with the increase in disease, have been the devastation of the food chain and soil, toxic pollution from the environment and the onslaught of medical drugs. The true causes of disease are these environmental factors. An environmental factor is any external factor that enters the body, whether it be food, chemicals, drugs or bacterial/viral agents. Additionally, nutritional deficiencies and the toxic burden are handed down through each generation, with successive generations becoming constitutionally weaker. Hence diseases that were not even common amongst our old people, two generations ago, are now becoming common amongst our young. So disease is creeping forward by probably 20 years (or faster) in every generation.

I note that scientists in the UK are now blaming the rise in asthma and insulin-dependent diabetes on junk food diets which don't provide the nourishment to build resistance. The effect of vaccinations and antibiotics on the immune system are also being questioned - far from improving the immune system, there is a strong possibility that they may make it dysfunctional. A correlation has been found between vaccinated groups and the later onset of chronic degenerative disease and cancer. It would appear that the maturation of the immune system through natural exposure to the childhood illnesses generates a greater protective effect, critical for overall health. Likewise, antibiotics which may clear the bacterial burden do not absolve the requirement for a healthy immune response, and unless the patient restores their immune system, then their capacity to respond to antibiotic treatment may be inadequate. The activation and programming of the immune system requires both exposure to pathogens coupled with a competent response. As the immune system is most vulnerable to nutritional deficiencies, poor nutrition will lead to a dysfunctional immune response where opportunistic infections and viral attacks could trigger auto-immune disease.

We cannot isolate one environmental cause from another - it is multifactorial: but the one outstanding factor has to be that deficiencies in the food chain and toxicity in the environment break down human resistance. Science has always wanted to take up the challenge to do better and conquer nature. How far has science brought us, or should I re-phrase this - how far back has science taken us in terms of the general health of the population? We must not confuse the issue here: the task of science, or the interpretation of its discoveries, is not necessarily to point out the cause of ill-health and reverse it, but to deliver a scientifically-based remedy or a genetic solution. In industry, decision-making is based primarily on economic advantage, and it will not be until the balance shifts, when those decisions become uneconomical that the criteria will change.

I have been working with patients undergoing detoxification and nutritional healing for many years and I can confidently say that most diseases (other than genetically inherited disorders of metabolism), respond to dietary healing methods combined with detoxification, where you are using food as medicine.

The detoxification process will shift fatty and calcium deposits from the arteries, joints and soft tissues, enabling better function of the organs; it will reduce cholesterol, heavy metals (extraordinary results seen on heavy metals in hair analysis, probably due to the effect of pectin as a chelator of heavy metals), it will restore cell membrane integrity and the control of inflammatory responses. It is particularly effective with autoimmune disease, often taking the patient into complete remission. It will resolve skin diseases and breathing disorders such as asthma, and help resolve mental disorders and depression.

This simple approach of "one treatment for many diseases" flies in the face of exponents of a medical practice which advocates a myriad of drug treatments for the many and diverse ranges of symptoms/diseases. The difference between the simple approach and the sophisticated one is that in the former the patient is healed by the therapy (where the side-effect is the resolution of symptoms), and in the latter the medications suppress the symptoms (but produce more as side-effects of the treatment) which will return once the patient stops the medications.

As a society, we can either become locked into the complexities and variables of disease mechanisms which are infinite and can keep science busy for years; or we can address the one, unchangeable, inflexible law of nature, that healing cannot take place in a toxic, nutritionally deficient environment. If this is principle is ignored, which it usually is, then there can be no cure. One thing is certain, chronic degenerative disease can never be controlled, it always worsens and on a generational basis, disease will manifest earlier with each successive generation.

When we try to look at disease from the outside, we use remedies and treatments either to suppress the process or to try and stimulate healing. But if we look from the inside, we begin to recognise that even the best holistic treatments will be thwarted by a toxic environment, because it is the local environment that governs the cure. For example, in a toxic, polluted lake all the life forms die, but when the lake is cleansed, life starts to regenerate. As we become more toxic, the capacity of the healing mechanism to respond is dampened. When we detoxify and re-fill the cells with nutrients (from food), we change that internal environment to the point where we initiate and support the healing response.

There are many thousands of disease mechanisms, but only one healing mechanism. Every practitioner knows that regardless of the disease, the healing mechanism is the same - inflammation. Through inflammation we break down and remove dead/abnormal tissue and regenerate new healthy tissue. It is very simple, but its absolute requirement is a healthy, clean environment. Once we start to release toxicity at cell level (and this is dependent primarily on diet - not products) the cell vitality is restored and a process of healing inflammation occurs. Any previous tissue trauma will be revisited to establish a complete healing.

Infections, if they do present during this process, can be positive and assist healing if the vitality is strengthening. We do not create a healing inflammation to our own toxicity, but bacteria and viruses can act as a catalyst to a generalised immune response, which will create a fever, thin the lymph, and generate not only an attack against the infectious pathogen but, in the process, shift huge amounts of toxicity from the cells. When this occurs without suppressive treatment (which paralyses the movement of the toxic load to the outside), then overall vitality is increased.

As we know, the detoxification diet must meet specific criteria in order to release toxicity and replenish the cells. It is only when you have secured an environment that will support healing that the healing metabolism kicks in, and when the healing metabolism begins, the disease metabolism stops.

Scratching the surface with a sort of detoxification diet is not enough to make the significant changes required. The consequence of years of buffering acidity produces a hardening and weakening of the body. Many of the toxins from the environment are non-biodegradable, so the body packs these away (such as DDT) in fat cells; heavy metals migrate to the nerve cells (you've all heard of the Mad Hatter's tea party - this was caused by mercury poisoning from the felting industry), and the list goes on. Detoxification has to reach a point where the vitality of the tissues can overcome the forces which are holding the toxicity in the cells, and this requires time, momentum and absolute adherence to the diet. It is only then that you will start to release that toxicity.

You will receive many patients in your practice with chronic degenerative disease. It is important that the patient understands that their disease has not arrived out of the blue but has taken several generations to get there. You will both be working together to improve the constitution of the patient, but without an honest approach of what will work and what will not work (i.e. how many corners you are prepared to cut to pander to the patient) then you risk short-changing the patient and yourself. You must make the recommendations and give the patient the opportunity to decide for themselves whether they wish to embark on such a regime or, if not, how far they are prepared to accommodate it.

Unfortunately, it is usually only when the situation reaches either a life-threatening disease crisis, or an inability to have quality of life, that patients are willing to comply. The patient may also have lower objectives than you as their practitioner. For example, a patient with arthritis may only want to alleviate this condition but do nothing further or stronger to deal with another chronic disorder he or she may have. Ultimately the arthritis will return, because the patient was not healed; the healing achieved only alleviated some of the more pressing symptoms. Alternatively you may have a mother who brings her child with chronic asthma; the asthma may be corrected but give way to eczema, and the mother decides that she would rather deal with the asthma than see the eczema. The patient often fails to comprehend that there are levels of deepening chronic disease and that the healing process uncovers each level on its way to recovery.

A detoxification therapy will address most chronic degenerative diseases and it is for the practitioner to observe the criteria and dietary modifications required to stimulate healing. If the modifications are too little, then nothing will occur. Honest observation will give you your answer. If you adopt a hit and miss approach - "Oh, well, we'll try this new product that's just come on the market, it seems to have a good write up" and disregard the healing protocol:

- detoxify the body, as healing cannot occur in a toxic environment
- re-fill the cells with nutrients
- restore the immune system, so that the body can initiate a healing inflammation

then you are failing to obey the laws of healing; you will be offering a quick fix/alleviation of symptoms and healing will not occur.

# Some Absolutes

Many patients will be unprepared for the drastic changes required to ensure detoxification and healing. You may try and ease your patient into the regime, but you should be aware that there are some absolutes in detoxification. I can give you a few useful pointers:

## Diet

- A protein-restricted diet is essential to the healing process. You will not eliminate sodium or toxins on a high protein diet. The metabolic waste of protein is sulphuric acid and the kidneys will exchange this for sodium; so in the elimination of the acid, sodium is reabsorbed. It is impossible to restore the type of sodium/potassium balance we require for detoxification on a high protein diet. By low protein I mean restricted in that you must allow 0.7g of good quality protein/kg of body weight. The protein should be of a vegetable origin (grains, legumes - unless the patient has adverse reactions to any of these foods, as in many autoimmune disorders) and dairy, skimmed milk products only.
- A low fat diet is essential. One of the hardest parts of a detoxification plan for most people is giving up fat (this includes nuts, seeds and avocados), totally. Fats will perpetuate the cycle of acidity, free radical production and therefore prejudice cellular potassium uptake, and will tax the bile system and increase the metabolic burden of the liver. Unless we make maximum effort to reduce the burden and increase cellular uptake of potassium, then nothing will happen. Flaxseed oil is the only oil allowed in the therapy. I tend to keep my non-cancer patients away from fats for at least 6-8 months. One also has to be mindful of supplements, such as lecithin which are also not allowed.
- All food must be organic and unprocessed. Fresh food is best.
- No salt (added or "hidden").
- Ensure correct methods of food preparation and cooking.

## Juices

- Generally, depending upon the condition of the patient, no reversal or healing will occur on less than 1 litre of juice daily. 2 litres is the best recommendation and for the cancer patient, 3 litres. The more severe the disease, the greater the number of juices.
- The type of juices should include both the green juice and apple and carrot. If the patient is anaemic or suffering from blood deficiency, or has been on an inadequate diet for a long period of time, then at least 2-4 of the juices should be green. If the patient is only taking 1 litre of juice, then half this amount should be green.
- The juices must be made fresh whenever possible, particularly the green
- A good juicer is a must. The patient will not heal if using a centrifugal juicer and will fail to extract the nutrients from the more fibrous greens, unless using a machine that masticates and presses (Norwalk, Champion with Press, K&K grinder and press - essential for cancer patients) or the models which use trituration (Green Life/Green Power, Oscar, Samson – acceptable for non-cancer patients).

## Supplements

Never make the mistake of assuming that nutritional supplementation will take the place of dietary changes. For example, if you eat a processed beef-burger with a white bun and chips, then that is the physical food that your body transforms into your regenerating physical tissues. Taking supplements at the same meal, will not negate the effects of the poor quality food. What you eat today, becomes your cells of tomorrow.

## Enemas

All my patients on a detoxification program will take enemas. The rule of thumb is 1 enema/3 juices. On a litre of juice daily, if the patient is feeling toxic in the afternoon, they may take an additional half-strength coffee/chamomile tea enema. The criterion for increasing or reducing enemas does not change: you will increase in a toxic crisis and reduce as the patient heals.

All patients can heal to a greater or lesser extent if the therapy is appropriate and strong enough to secure a detoxification, while addressing the nutritional deficiencies. I have seen dramatic improvements in kidney disease, hypertension, breathing disorders, such as asthma, multiple sclerosis, auto-immune diseases such as myasthenia gravis and rheumatoid arthritis, coeliac disease, hyperactive disorders (ADHD), mental depression, infertility and irritable bowel syndrome. I have treated patients as young as 6 months (yes, with vegetable juices in the bottle - no enemas though!) to over 80 years. Failure is rare and usually due to non-compliance in one form or another. Some patients may have to be on the therapy for many months before seeing any improvement, such is the case in CFS. It is very hard for these patients to stay the course. But most patients, if they remain committed, do reap their rewards.

Detoxification will become a very important therapy in the not too distant future. Just as organic farmers are detoxifying their soil, so will human beings be looking to detoxify their bodies for greater health and resistance. Many detoxification plans will come onto the market - from the quick 10 day plans to the multilevel marketing strategies based on various products. Many of these detoxification plans will miss the key points, and consumers will fail to achieve their long-term expectations. Products will tend to dominate the market until the general awareness changes. At the present time, most people will agree that nutritional deficiencies play a major role in the onset of disease and believe that these deficiencies can be made good with nutritional supplements.

As we know, the picture is more complex than this. The organic farmer has to actively reduce the toxicity in his soil and replenish its nutrient status with organic matter. Once the ecosystem of his land is established (worms, bacteria, birds, etc.), then the soil has health and will produce healthy crops. The farmer who tries to replenish his soil primarily with commercial fertilizers and not through organic matter, will end up killing his soil. So it is with the human being who tries to rebuild their nutrient status (through human commercial fertilizers: supplements) without attending to the organic diet, with all its components, discovered and undiscovered, and additionally ensure the release of their toxicity.

It is for you to understand the philosophy of detoxification and educate your patients on these principles. There is no short-cut. The body cannot be forced into a healing, but the conditions can be prepared to support that healing. Your role is to ensure that this occurs, and the patient's role is to undertake and practise the therapy.

Healing is holistic. If we are not healing the soil and the planet, then we are not healing ourselves. Our work is very important at this moment. Educate your patients, build your reputation as a holistic practitioner and, most importantly, try to practise what you preach.

# Forms and Schedules

# Practitioner Forms

## PRACTITIONER CASE STUDY FORM

| Patient reference number (office use only) | Ethnic Origin | Sex | DoB |
|---|---|---|---|
| Date of consultation | Nationality | Blood Group | Current Age |
| Name | Address | Tel: | e-mail |
| Weight: | Height: | Occupation: | |

| Diagnosis | |
|---|---|
| Histology | Grade: |
| Dx date: | Stage |
| Recur | Stage at recur |
| Consultation date: | Stage at consultation |

| Date | Chronological history since diagnosis | Documents | Treatment |
|---|---|---|---|
| | | | |
| | | | |
| | | | |

**CURRENT MEDICATIONS** *(medical and alternative/nutritional supplements, alternative therapies, etc.)*

**FAMILY HISTORY**

**CASE HISTORY FROM BIRTH** (*include illnesses, medications, surgeries, exposure to chemicals, smoking, alcohol, recreational drugs*).

<u>Childhood:</u>
<u>Adolescence:</u>

<u>Adulthood:</u>

## Female History
**Details of menstruation:**
(Year of onset/menopause, irregularities, length of cycle/flow etc.)

**Have you taken the contraceptive pill or been prescribed any other type of hormonal treatment:** (Give details of medication, length of time prescribed, dates/year, side-effects etc.)

**Details of pregnancies and births with dates:** Was birth induced/forceps used/ Caesarian/ premature/ jaundice/ toxaemia or other complications during pregnancy?

**Health of any offspring (jaundice, colic, eczema, asthma, allergies, ADHD etc.)**

**Have you experienced any problems with the following and state the date/year and any treatment given:**

|  | date/year | Treatment |
|---|---|---|
| Miscarriages | | |
| Terminations | | |
| Complications | | |
| Infertility | | |
| Surgeries | | |

<u>Check list:</u>

| | |
|---|---|
| **Place of birth and upbringing** | |
| **Indicate if exposure to the following:**<br>agricultural or environmental chemicals/toxins<br>smoking (how long/how many/are you still smoking)<br>alcohol drinking (how much and how long for, are you still drinking). | |
| **Recreational drugs – which ones, how much and for how long?** | |

| | |
|---|---|
| **Medications –** <br> current medications (name of brand and dose and length of time prescribed) <br> Previous medications: | |
| **Allergies - drugs/foods etc.** | |
| **Mouth/throat/teeth /gum problems (ulcers, sore throats, condition of teeth and gums):** | |
| **Root canals, amalgam fillings, mouth abscesses? (state how many).** | |
| **Visual/eye disturbances (give details and medication):** | |
| **Ear problems (tinnitus, vertigo, earache, discharge):** | |
| **Lymph node swelling: neck/ armpit/ groin/ other:** | |
| **Catarrh/mucus discharge (give details of medication):** | |
| **Gastrointestinal - discomfort, inflammatory conditions, bowel habits:** | |
| **Current or past history of acute/chronic bleeding of the gastrointestinal tract:** | |
| Lungs - any pain, phlegm, fatigue, coughing? | |
| **Heart - irregularities, high blood pressure etc. Give details/ medications.** | |
| **Kidneys – history of renal function/infection, diabetes, medications:** | |
| **Fluid retention and where: ankles/ abdomen/ hands/ face/ other.** | |
| **Pain - current pain, indicate where and name any medication/treatment taken.** | |
| **Muscular system - mobility, bone/muscle/joint aches and pains: (give location, type of symptoms and occurrence plus medication taken/treatment given).** | |
| **Nervous disorders and state medication:** <br> **fainting/ blackout/ seizures/ weakness/ paralysis/ numbness/ pins and needles/ tremors/ involuntary movements.** | |
| **Implants, heart valves, hip replacements, breast implants, teeth, wires from surgery?** | |

| | |
|---|---|
| Blood transfusions (give reasons and dates)? | |
| Organ transplants (give dates) | |
| Bone marrow transplants (give dates) | |
| Accidents or injuries (give description, dates and treatment given): | |
| Sleep patterns: (insomnia, restless patterns) | |
| Give dates and any reaction to all vaccinations (if known): | |

## DIET

Diet as a child/adolescent: (including food habits)

Diet as an adult:

## Current diet:

| | |
|---|---|
| *How many meals per day* | |
| *How many cups of tea/coffee* | |
| *Food cravings (give details, type of, frequency, time of day/ month)* | |
| *Food allergies (give details and symptoms)* | |
| *Food intolerances or digestive difficulties (give details and symptoms)* | |
| *Daily intake of alcohol* | |
| *Daily fluid intake (other than alcohol)* | |
| *Lack/excess of appetite* | |
| *Give a detailed description of a normal daily eating plan for breakfast, lunch and evening meal. Include all foods, drinks, snacks etc.* | |

# Recommended treatment (detailing reasons for omissions/inclusions)

*Reference to blood results.*

| | |
|---|---|
| ___juices | |
| Potassium compound solution | |
| Niacin | |
| Lugols's      strength | |
| Thyroid | |
| Co Q10 | |
| Pancreatin | |
| Acidol/pepsin | |
| B12 0.1cc + crude liver 3.9cc – injection | |
| Liver capsules | |
| Coffee enemas | |
| castor oil treatment | |
| Tbs (mls) flaxseed oil daily. | |
| Packs | |
| Other: | |
| Diet: | |

# Practitioner Follow-up Form

**Name:**

**Date:**

**Blood work:**

**Comments:**

**Medication:**

Juices

potassium salts

Niacin

Lugols's 1/2 strength

Thyroid

Co Q10

Pancreatin

Inflazyme (or other enzymes)

Acidol/pepsin

B12 + crude liver

Liver capsules

Coffee enemas

Castor oil treatment

Tbs/mls flaxseed oil daily.

Clay packs

Non-fat yoghurt

Herbs

Other

- **Symptoms/flare-ups. (Treatment, drugs, surgeries)**

- general appetite
- energy levels
- Have you lost/gained weight since your last consultation? If so, how much?
- Have you introduced any other supplementation (homoeopathic, herbal etc.) or other treatment since your last consultation? If so which ones and why?
- What is your pulse rate before you rise in the morning?
- What is your temperature before you rise in the morning?
- General improvements

# Patient Initial Consultation Form

**Surname and Title**
**Fore names**
**Address**

**Postcode**
**Telephone no**
**e-mail address**
**Date of Birth**
**Place of Birth**

**Details of Birth:** Was birth induced/forceps used/Caesarian/premature/jaundice/toxaemia or other complications during pregnancy?

Were you breast-fed/how long?

**Occupation**
**Status (married/divorced/widowed/single)**
**Height**
**Weight**
**Children/ages**
**Recreational interests**

**Exercise activities.**

**When was the last time you had a fever?**

**How would you describe your energy levels? (please underline)**
high/medium/low/tired on waking/ variable.

**How would you describe your motivation/inspiration? (please underline)**
High/medium/low

**What do you personally wish to achieve from treatment?**

# Current symptoms/reason why seeking treatment:

(Give an account of your symptoms whether you are receiving treatment or not, any alleviating or aggravating factors or associated symptoms. Include your response to your illness and its effects on home, relationships, social activities, worries, and general self-esteem).

**NON-CANCER**
**If you have a diagnosis, what is your diagnosed condition? (please attach reports such as scans, blood results that confirm the diagnosis)**

**Date/year of onset**

**Medical opinion and treatment recommended:**

**Details of your treatment: (please give date for the start of each treatment)**

**What is the prognosis for your condition:**

**a)**     **if you undertake the recommended treatment; and**

**b)**     **If you decline treatment?**

**(Please ask your specialist how your disease is likely to progress, what symptoms you can expect and within what time frame both with and without medication.)**

**Please give details of any other medication you are currently taking (include herbs, nutritional supplementation, homeopathic etc.)**

**Medications –**
- **current medications (name of brand and dose and length of time prescribed)**

**Please give details of past medications you have taken for on-going complaints. Give approximate year, and the number of years for the prescribed treatment/s.**

- **Past medications (name of brand and dose and length of time prescribed)**

## CANCER
**Diagnosed condition** (state name of cancer, stage and grade, and if metastasized, to which tissues)

**Date of diagnosis/year of onset:**

**What is your medical prognosis in terms of overall survival and disease-free survival with the recommended medical treatment?**

**You will need to ask:**
What is the survival rate for my cancer with the treatment recommended? The answer to this question will be in two parts: the percentage of people who survived, and the length of time they survived.

What is the disease-free survival rate for my cancer with the treatment recommended? The answer to this question will be in two parts: the percentage of people who survived disease-free, and the length of time they survived disease-free.

**Or if there is no expected disease-free survival then you will need to ask:**
What is the response rate with the treatment recommended? The answer to this question will be in two parts: the percentage of people who responded and the percentage of shrinkage of the tumoural masses.

What is your medical prognosis in terms of overall survival if you do not take the recommended treatment/s?

**When did your symptoms first start and what were these symptoms? (Please give date of diagnosis).**

**What tests were undertaken? (enclose recent blood results for blood chemistry panel, liver function, complete blood count, thyroid function, details of tumour markers (if applicable), reports from all CT scans, MRI, ultrasound scans. Please give approximate dates).**

**What were the medical recommendations?**
Please indicate whether you followed medical recommendations at that time, or if not, what other treatment did you pursue. Please give the dates (or thereabouts) of treatments undertaken, how long, how many.

**Chemotherapy:**
**Radiation:**
**Hormonal treatment (drug type):**
**Surgery (type):**

**Other:**

Please give details of any other medication you are currently taking (include herbs, nutritional supplementation, homeopathic etc.)

---

## Do you have a history of: (please tick or underline)

Give the year of onset and/or frequency of the complaint. For example you may have suffered asthma as a child from the age of 7-14 in which case you would write 1960-67 or you may have ongoing arthritis from 1960 to present, or you may suffer regular bouts of sinusitis say twice yearly since 1985. Give details of treatment (medication, vaccines, operations).

|  | Year/ frequency | Treatment |
|---|---|---|
| Acne | | |
| Allergies | | |
| Anxiety | | |
| Arthritis | | |
| Asthma | | |
| Boils/abscesses | | |
| Bowel disorders | | |
| Bronchitis | | |
| Cancer (name type) | | |
| Candida | | |
| Chickenpox | | |
| Circulatory/heart | | |
| Coeliac | | |
| Colds/'flu | | |
| Colitis | | |
| Constipation | | |
| Crohn's | | |
| Cystitis | | |
| Depression | | |
| Dermatitis | | |
| Diabetes | | |
| Diarrhoea | | |
| Diphtheria | | |
| Diverticulitis | | |
| Dysentery | | |
| Eating disorders | | |
| Eczema | | |
| Epilepsy | | |
| Gall bladder | | |
| German measles | | |
| Glandular fever | | |

Haemorrhoids

Hay fever

Headaches

Hernia

Herpes

Hepatitis

Insomnia

Jaundice

Kidney infection/disease

Malaria

Measles

Meningitis

Migraine

Mumps

Peptic ulcer

Phobias

Pleurisy

Pneumonia

Psoriasis

Rheumatic fever

Scarlet fever

Sinusitis

Thrombosis/stroke

Thyroid (under/over-active)

Tonsillitis

Tuberculosis

Whooping cough

**Any other illnesses/operations:**


**Have you undergone any surgery or investigative procedures relating to the reproductive organs? (give dates/year, reason for treatment and results)**


# Is there a family history of: (please tick or underline)

Relationship (mother/father/sibling/grand-parent etc.)

Alcoholism

Allergies

Alzheimer's

Arthritis

Asthma

Bowel disorders

Cancer

Coeliac/Crohn's

Diabetes

Diphtheria

Eczema

Epilepsy

Gall bladder

Gout

Heart problems

Kidney problems

Neurosis

Mental problems

Multiple Sclerosis

Parkinson's

Polio

Rheumatism

Rheumatoid arthritis

SLE

Thrombosis/stroke

Thyroid

Tuberculosis

Ulcers

**Any other illnesses:**

# Female section only (* to be completed by all clients)

**Details of menstruation:**
(Year of onset/menopause, irregularities, length of cycle/flow etc.)

**Have you taken the contraceptive pill or been prescribed any other type of hormonal treatment:** (Give details of medication, length of time prescribed, dates/year, side-effects etc.)

**Details of pregnancies and births with dates:** Was birth induced/forceps used/Caesarian/premature/jaundice/toxaemia or other complications during pregnancy?

**\*Health of any offspring (jaundice, colic, eczema, asthma, allergies, ADHD etc.)**

**Have you experienced any problems with the following and state the date/year and any treatment given:**

| | date/year | Treatment |
|---|---|---|
| Miscarriages | | |
| Terminations | | |
| Complications | | |
| Infertility | | |

**Check List:**

| | |
|---|---|
| **Where were you born and where were you brought up?** | |
| **Indicate if exposed to the following:**<br>• agricultural or environmental chemicals/toxins<br>• smoking (how long/how many/are you still smoking)<br>• alcohol drinking (how much and how long for, are you still drinking). | |
| **Have you taken any recreational drugs – if so, which ones, how much and for how long?** | |
| **Medications –**<br>• current medications (name of brand and dose and length of time prescribed)<br>• Previous medications | |
| **When did your symptoms first start?**<br>What were your symptoms and what treatment/tests were undertaken? (enclose results and details of blood test markers, CT scan, MRI, ultrasound and recommendations at that time/if followed or not, or followed at that time. (Date) | |
| **Have you had chemotherapy, radiation or hormonal treatment? If so, how much and for how long? Give dates or thereabouts.** | |
| **Have you had any surgery? If so name type of surgery - dissection, excision of nodes, lumpectomy.** | |
| **Do you have any allergies - drugs/foods etc.** | |
| **Do you have any mouth/throat/teeth /gum problems (ulcers, sore throats, condition of teeth and gums):** | |
| **Do you have any root canals, amalgam fillings, mouth abscesses? (state how many).** | |

| | |
|---|---|
| Do you have any visual/eye disturbances (give details and medication): | |
| Do you have any ear problems (tinnitus, vertigo, earache, discharge): | |
| Do you have any lymph node swelling: neck/ armpit/ groin/ other | |
| Do you suffer catarrh (give details of medication): | |
| Gastrointestinal - can you eat and drink without discomfort? If not, give details. | |
| Do you or have you in the past suffered with any acute bleeding of the gastrointestinal tract? | |
| Lungs - any pain, phlegm, fatigue, coughing? | |
| Heart – do you suffer any heart irregularities, high blood pressure etc. Give details/medications. | |
| Kidneys – are your kidneys functioning normally? If not, give details. | |
| Do you suffer fluid retention and where: ankles/ abdomen/ hands/ face/other. | |
| Are you suffering any pain at the moment? If so, indicate where and name any medication/treatment taken. | |
| Muscular system – are you able to move around easily? Do you suffer bone/muscle/joint aches and pains: (give location, type of symptoms and occurrence plus medication taken/treatment given). | |
| Do you suffer any nervous disorders and state medication: fainting/ blackout/ seizures/ weakness/ paralysis/ numbness/ pins and needles/ tremors/ involuntary movements. | |
| Do you have any implants, heart valves, hip replacements, breast implants, teeth, wires from surgery? | |
| Have you had any blood transfusions (give reasons and dates)? | |
| Have you had any organ transplants? | |
| Have you had any bone marrow transplants? | |
| Have you had any accidents or injuries (give description, dates and treatment given): | |
| Sleep patterns: (insomnia, restless patterns) | |
| Give dates and any reaction to all vaccinations (if known): | |

**Diet as a child/adolescent: (including food habits)**

**Diet as an adult:**

**Current diet:**

| | |
|---|---|
| *How many meals do you have a day?* | |
| *How many cups of tea/coffee?* | |
| *Do you have food cravings (give details, type of, frequency, time of day/month)?* | |
| *Do you have food allergies (give details and symptoms)?* | |
| *Do you have food intolerances or digestive difficulties (give details and symptoms)?* | |
| *What is your daily intake of alcohol?* | |
| *What is your daily fluid intake (other than alcohol)?* | |
| *Do you experience a lack/excess of appetite? (please underline).* | |
| *Give a detailed description of a normal daily eating plan for breakfast, lunch and evening meal. Include all foods, drinks, snacks etc.* | Breakfast:<br><br>Lunch:<br><br>Evening meal:<br><br>Snacks: |

**State your blood group (if known):**

**Signature:**
**Date:**

# Patient Follow-up Consultation Form

Please provide results of blood tests (blood chemistry panel, complete blood count) thyroid function test and urinalysis prior to each appointment.

**Surname and Title**
**Fore names**
**e-mail address**

**Date:**

**Date of last consultation:**

- Are you experiencing any difficulties with the diet either with any specific foods or the routine? Please detail.

- How is your general appetite?

- Can you tell me what you are eating and drinking on a daily basis? (Include snacks).

Breakfast

Lunch

Evening meal

Snacks
Juices

- How would you describe your energy levels?

- How would you describe your energy on waking:  poor/medium/high

- How is your digestion on the diet? Is there any discomfort such as bloating or flatulence, indigestion, burning, nausea etc.? Please detail and medications recommended.

- Have you suffered any diarrhoea, or other abnormalities/discharges?

- How many coffee enemas and what strength/amount are you taking daily?

- Are you experiencing any problems with these?

- With what frequency are you taking castor oil treatments and what quantity of castor oil are you taking?

- Are you experiencing any difficulties with these?

- Have you lost/gained weight since your last consultation? If so, how much?

- Are  you experiencing any problems with the supplementation recommended?

- Have you introduced any other supplementation (homoeopathic, herbal etc.) or other treatment since your last consultation? If so which ones and why?

- What is your pulse rate before you rise in the morning?
- What is your temperature before you rise in the morning?
- How would you describe your mental state – mood, mental alertness/concentration, creativity/inspiration? Are there any obvious improvements?

- What was the date of your last period (if applicable)?
Was it early/late/on time? (If early or late by how many days/weeks?)

- Can you notice any improvements generally (PMT, pain, heavy/light flow, duration)? If so detail these.

- Have you suffered from any of the following since your last consultation? – (Please underline or circle)

Headaches, stuffiness of the head, catarrh, mucous congestion, earache, aching limbs, sore joints, poor skin/eruptions, exacerbation of any skin condition, salty or metallic taste in mouth, bad breath, bad body odour, sweats, pains in liver area, nausea, diarrhoea, old injuries flaring, any breathing difficulties, hair loss, dizziness, poor memory, worsening of eye conditions, thirst, frequent urination, infection or infectious illness, heart palpitations, discharge (mucous or infectious/fungal), tinea (athlete's foot), cold sores, genital herpes, mouth ulcers, tumour swelling, pain.

If you have underlined any of the above, or have had any other symptom, please elaborate and indicate the nature of the ailment, duration (date) and whether medication or treatment was required? Please state the name of any medications or treatment advised/taken.

- Are you suffering any fluid retention or oedemas? Please indicate location. When do you experience this and has any treatment/medication been recommended for this?

- Are you suffering any pain? If so state the location and treatment recommended.

- How many hours do you sleep at night?
- Are you sleeping well or do you suffer insomnia or difficulty getting off to sleep?

- Do you have any particular stress factors at this time? If so, can you outline these?

- Please list your general improvements.

- Please list any worsening of conditions.

- List any current medication as prescribed by a GP or specialist. Please give dosage.

- Have you undergone any medical procedures since your last appointment? If so, give the date, nature of the procedure and the results.

- Please detail your current medications

**Medications:**
Juices    (number and type)
Potassium salts  (ml/juice)
Niacin
Lugol's 1/2 strength (drops)
Thyroid (1/2 or 1 grain)
Co Q10 (total amount in mg)
Pancreatin
Inflazyme
Acidol Pepsin
B12 + crude liver
Liver capsules
Coffee enemas
Castor oil treatment

Tbs/ml flaxseed oil daily.
Clay packs
Non-fat yoghurt (amount)
Other

Additional dietary recommendations (if any).

- Do you have any major concerns or any questions? If so, please list them.

Signature:

Date:

# An Example of a Case Study

| Patient reference number (office use only) | Ethnic Origin | Sex<br>Female | DoB<br>1959 |
|---|---|---|---|
| Date of consultation | Nationality | Blood Group | Current Age<br>40 |
| Name | Address<br>Australia | Tel: | e-mail |
| Weight:<br>54kg | Height:<br>5'7" | Occupation: | |

| Diagnosis: Melanoma Stage 1V | |
|---|---|
| Histology | Grade: |
| Dx date: June 1999 | Stage 1V |
| Recur | Stage at recur |
| Consultation date: 05/12/00 | Stage at consultation |

| Date | Chronological history since diagnosis | Treatment |
|---|---|---|
| June 99 | Melanoma diagnosed.<br>Lump under R arm<br>Liver biopsy was clear | |
| 26/6/99 | FNA positive for melanoma<br>Right axillary dissection - microscopic report shows large malignant metastatic tumour cells in 2 of 18 lymph nodes.<br>Immunoperoxidase stains in progress. | |
| 17/5/00 | PET scan - whole body study<br>2, possibly 3 soft tissue metastases. Inferior medial aspect of L breast; over R greater trochanter (over R femur) and R upper anterior chest (near manubrium)<br>Excision of subcutaneous tumour on back<br>As soon as discovered the recurrence of cancer sought treatment from practitioner of Chinese medicine. Also felt lumps coming up under arm after the PET scan and felt that cancer was "exploding." The treatment really helped resolve these and it would appear arrested the progress of 2 of the mets. | Chinese herbs and acupuncture; veg diet with a few juices; MGM3 - mushroom extract; Green Barley powder |

| | | |
|---|---|---|
| 31/5/00 | Blood test:<br>Absolute lymphocyte count - 0.8<br>cell surface markers indicated that CD3, CD4, CD8 (T subsets) are low | |
| Aug 00 | Melanoma came up on shoulder - started juicing and coffee enemas and tumours started shrinking. | |
| 29/9/00 | PET scan<br>Lesion on R femur - less avid<br>Lesions to L of midline in upper anterior chest - not present<br>2 new lesions - one adjacent to the hilum and another in the L axilla. The other 2 soft tissue lesions have resolved spontaneously. | |
| 17/10/00 | MRI brain<br>MRI R thigh<br>Impression: L hilar mass; R lateral pelvis subcutaneous nodule (5x13x14mm); lesion in subhepatic region (? aetiology) | |
| 27/10/00 | Total body bone scan. OK<br>CT Abdomen and pelvis - clear. No lymphadenopathy; 2 x 2 x 4cm decreased density lesion in liver - thought to be a cyst.<br>CT chest - 1.7cm mass associated with L hilum - presumably relates to melanoma deposit. Mediastinum otherwise clear. Slight residual soft tissue in R axilla (possibly post surgical). Occasional tiny lymph nodes in L axilla - not of pathological size | No treatment recommended<br>Started to intensify efforts - 10 juices and coffee enemas. Visited Ian Gawler foundation and saw Professor O'Rourke re the vaccine program but tumour not large enough to excise for the program. |

**CURRENT MEDICATIONS** *(medical and alternative/nutritional supplements, alternative therapies etc.)*
Chinese herbs
B12 tablets
Chinese clay powder and ganoderma mushroom
Homoeopathic vaccines
Ascorbic acid (was having IV C)
CoQ10
Niacin with oat bran
Green Barley powder

**FAMILY HISTORY**
No details
Very healthy family - Scottish inheritance

**CASE HISTORY FROM BIRTH** *(include illnesses, medications, surgeries, exposure to chemicals, smoking, alcohol, recreational drugs).*

## Childhood:
Natural birth; BF 12 months. Mother 22 yrs.
4 - tonsillectomy - suffered badly as a toddler. Penicillin
5 - chickenpox, measles

## Adolescence:
Acne during teens - antibiotics - for 2 years

## Adulthood:
26 - 1st pregnancy - forceps; ADHD
28 - 2nd pregnancy - epidural
29 - 3rd pregnancy
Has always worked in office with lots of computers. High stress executive position- senior manager in public service
35 - acne recurred over last 5 yr
47 - severe viral infection - off work for 2 months. Never "picked up" - tiredness. The virus affected trachea and wheezing was initially misdiagnosed as asthma - prednisolone for 1 month - didn't work. Found that virus had damaged trachea

## Female History
**Details of menstruation:**
(Year of onset/menopause, irregularities, length of cycle/flow etc.)
Onset - 15 years; 21 day cycle
**Have you taken the contraceptive pill or been prescribed any other type of hormonal treatment:** (Give details of medication, length of time prescribed, dates/year, side-effects etc.)
8 yrs on the pill during 20s

**Health of any offspring (jaundice, colic, eczema, asthma, allergies, ADHD etc.)**
Son - ADHD

## Check list:
1.   **Where have you come from and where were you brought up?**
Melbourne, then moved to Canberra

2.   **Indicate if exposed to the following:**
agricultural or environmental chemicals/toxins -
smoking (how long/how many/are you still smoking) - 8 yrs 20/day
alcohol drinking (how much and how long for, are you still drinking).   Occasional glass of wine

3.   **Do you have any root canals, amalgam fillings, mouth abscesses? (state how many).** Amalgams
     **Do you have any mouth/throat/teeth/gum problems (ulcers, sore throats, condition of teeth and gums):**

4.   **Are you suffering any pain at the moment? If so, indicate where and name any medication/treatment taken.**
Pain in R thigh where tumour is located - no medication

5. **Have you had any accidents or injuries (give description, dates and treatment given):**
Fell as a child and damaged elbow

6. **Sleep patterns: (insomnia, restless patterns)**

7. **Give dates and any reaction to all vaccinations (if known):**

## DIET
**Diet as a child/adolescent:** *(including food habits)*
Meat and 3 veg, lots of fruit and veg.

**Diet as an adult:**
As above

## Current diet:
Has started the Gerson diet a few weeks ago.

## Recommended treatment - detail reasons for omissions/inclusions
*Reference to blood results.*
Currently suffering from sore chest and difficulty in breathing so have recommended an X-ray to rule out pleural effusion - will do modified juicing until X-ray tests are known.

7/12/00 - Xray clear - obviously a viral infection. Cannot give thyroid medications until thyroid tests are done. Has been taking Lugol's so have recommended to stop the Lugol's and have these tests in one week.

| | |
|---|---|
| **13 juices** | |
| **Potassium compound solution** | 10ml x 10 |
| **Niacin** | 6 |
| **Lugol's 1/2 strength** | nil |
| **Thyroid** | nil |
| **Co Q10** | 6 |
| **Pancreatin** | 12 |
| **Acidol Pepsin** | 6 |
| **B12 0.1cc + crude liver 3.9cc** – injection once daily. | |
| **Liver capsules** | 6 |
| **Coffee enemas** | 5 |
| **castor oil treatment** | nil |
| **Tbs flaxseed oil daily.** | 2 Tbs (20ml) |
| **Packs castor oil packs on chest** | |
| **Other:** | Imugen x 10 |
| **Diet:** | no milk protein |

# Follow-ups

**Date: 19/1/01**

**Blood work: Hb 13; RCC 4.1; WCC 5.8; lymphocytes 1.1**
**Comments:**
Improved blood work in all cell counts and immune function. The patient did not report the results of the thyroid function tests to me but started self-medicating with the Lugol's and thyroid on Dec 20th.

**Medication:**

| | |
|---|---|
| Juices | 13 |
| potassium salts | 20ml x 10 |
| Niacin | 6 |
| Lugol's 1/2 strength | 18 |
| Thyroid | 5 |
| Co Q10 | 600mg |
| Pancreatin | 12 |
| Inflazyme | |
| Acidol Pepsin | 6 |
| Imugen | 10 |
| B12 + crude liver | 0.1 + 3.9cc |
| Liver capsules | 6 |
| Coffee enemas | 5 |
| castor oil treatment | alt days |
| mls flaxseed oil daily. | 20ml |
| Clay packs | castor oil pack on chest |
| Non-fat yoghurt | nil |
| Herbs | essiac |
| Other | |

- **Symptoms/flare-ups. (Treatment, drugs, surgeries)**

Flare-ups in area of surgery (R axilla) extremely sore and inflamed

Tumor area in R hip worsened (pain) - oncologist could not feel any lumps in lymph area.

Headaches , mucous, aching limbs, sore joints. Nausea on one day.

Very low energy until beginning Jan. Chest was very painful and sore (viral infection - was taking Echinacea and lemons). Feels better now.

- general appetite. Good.
- energy levels.        Low - but better now
- Have you lost/gained weight since your last consultation? If so, how much? Stable
- Have you introduced any other supplementation (homoeopathic, herbal etc.) or other treatment since your last consultation? If so which ones and why? Echinacea
- What is your pulse rate before you rise in the morning?
- What is your temperature before you rise in the morning? 35.0
- General improvements. Haemorrhoids gone; energy rising. Chest is a lot better.

**Date: 20/02/01**

**Blood work:**

Good. Hb is slightly lower at 12.5 (13.0). There is blood in the urine but no growth - had her period at this time. Lymphocyte count still low 1.1

**Medication:**

| | |
|---|---|
| Juices | 13 |
| potassium salts | 10 x 10 |
| Niacin | 6 |
| Lugol's 1/2 strength | 6 |
| Thyroid | 2.5 |
| Co Q10 | 600mg |
| Pancreatin | 3 x 5 |
| Inflazyme | |
| Acidol Pepsin | 6 |
| Imugen | 10 |
| B12 + crude liver | 0.1 + 3.9cc |
| Liver capsules | 6 |
| Coffee enemas | 5 |
| castor oil treatment | alt days |
| Tbs/ml flaxseed oil daily. | 10ml |
| Clay packs | |
| Non-fat yoghurt | nil |
| Herbs | Essiac |
| Other | brown rice once/week. 5g spirulina |

- **Symptoms/flare-ups. (Treatment, drugs, surgeries)**

Tremendous amounts of pain in the muscles (back, down both sides of spine, shoulder blades) - used CO packs. Has been very acute; also above breasts and closer to underarm area. Pain for 1-2 days in right hip area where tumour was located. This has almost resolved now.

Cycle was only 19 days (she does have a short cycle) - flow light and for 2 days; in the past has been a lot heavier and longer.

Aching limbs - occasionally

Poor skin with eruptions before last period; lots of pimples on back with sore back and shoulder blades.

Nausea - occasionally.

Last enema - gets stuck (toxicity building up) - suggest 10ml K solution in the last enema. Also stomach bloats up at night. Few heart palpitations after the last enema.

Haemorrhoids since started the castor oil treatments.

- general appetite. Good
- energy levels. Better than last month.
- What is your temperature before you rise in the morning? 36C
- General improvements. More energy; skin less dry; less pain in R hip area.

# Lab Report

| | 11/05/00 | 19/06/00 | 10/11/00 | 04/01/01 | 09/02/01 |
|---|---|---|---|---|---|
| **General chemistry** | | | | | |
| Sodium (136-146 mmol/L) | | | 136 | 138 | 137 |
| Potassium (3.5-5.2 mmol/L) | | | 4.3 | 4.6 | 5.2 |
| Chloride (98-109 mmol/L) | | | 100 | 102 | 106 |
| Bicarb. (20-33 mmol/L) | | | 26 | 25 | 23 |
| Calcium (2.10-2.55 mmol/L) | | | | 2.34 | |
| Phosphate (0.75-1.35 mmol/L) | | | | 1.27 | |
| T. Protein (60-82 g/L) | 76 | 73 | 74 | 71 | 68 |
| Albumin (35-50 g/L) | 48 | 46 | 44 | 43 | 42 |
| Globulin (20-35 g/L) | 28 | | 30 | 28 | 26 |
| Urea (2.5-8.0 mmol/L) | | | 1.7 | 2.5 | 1.9 |
| Creatinine (0.05-0.11 mmol/L) | | | 0.09 | 0.06 | 0.07 |
| Urate (0.15-0.45 mmol/L) | | | | 0.34 | |
| Glucose (3.0-6.5 mmol/L) | | | | 4.6 | |
| Alk. Phos (30-120 U/L) | | 70 | 68 | 70 | 71 |
| Bilirubin (<25 umol/L) | 16 | 5 | 10 | 8 | 8 |
| GGTP (<50 U/L) | 6 | 11 | 11 | 15 | 13 |
| AST (<41 U/L) | 14 | 15 | 18 | 19 | 20 |
| ALT (0-50 U/L) | 13 | 17 | 19 | 24 | 33 |
| LD (50-280 U/L) | 259 | | | 153 | |
| Cholesterol (<5.5 mmol/L) | | | | 3.9 | |
| **Haematology** | | | | | |
| Haemoglobin (11.5-16.5g/dL) | 13.4 | 13.6 | 12.4 | 13.0 | 12.5 |
| RBC (3.8-5.5x10$^{12}$/L) | 4.6 | 4.51 | 3.9 | 4.1 | 4.1 |
| PCV (0.35-0.47) | 0.42 | 0.40 | 0.36 | 0.39 | 0.39 |
| MCV ((80-99 fL) | 91 | 87.9 | 92 | 95 | 94 |
| MCH ((27-32 pg) | 29 | 30.2 | 32 | 31.8 | 30 |
| **White cell count** (4-11x10$^9$/L) | 4.0 | 4.7 | **3.4** | 5.8 | 6.0 |
| Neutrophils (2.0-8.0x10$^9$/L) | 2.6 | 3.28 | 2.4 | 4.2 | 4.3 |
| Lymphocytes (1.0-4.0x10$^9$/L) | 1.2 | 1.03 | 0.7 | 1.1 | 1.1 |
| Monocytes (<1.1x10$^9$/L) | 0.2 | 0.19 | 0.2 | 0.4 | 0.5 |
| Eosinophils (<0.6x10$^9$/L) | 0.0 | 0.07 | 0.1 | 0.0 | 0.0 |
| Basophils (<0.2x10$^9$/L) | 0.0 | 0.03 | | 0.0 | |
| Platelets (150-450x10$^9$/L) | 224 | 257 | 223 | 257 | 225 |
| | | | | | |
| TSH (0.04-4.0 mIU/L) | | | 5.8 | 0.14 | |
| FT4 (10-25 pmol/L) | | | | 16.7 | |
| FT3 | | | | 6.2 | |
| | | | | | |
| **Urinalysis** | | | | | |
| culture | | | | | No growth |
| pH | | | 7.5 | | 7.0 |
| Protein | | | Nil | | |
| Glucose | | | Nil | | |
| Blood | | | +++ | | +++ |
| Specific gravity (1.015-1.025) | | | | | |

# Total Treatment Schedule

| Date | 05/12/00 | 07/12/00 | 19/01/01 | 21/02/01 |
|---|---|---|---|---|
| Juices | 8: 4 green, 4 carrot/apple | 13 | 13 | 13 |
| Diet | No cultured milk protein | No cultured milk protein | No cultured milk protein | No cultured milk protein. Add 5g spirulina |
| Flaxseed Oil | 20ml | 20ml | 20ml | 10ml |
| Acidol/pepsin caps | 6 | 6 | 6 | 6 |
| Potassium Compound Solution | 10ml x 8 | 10ml x 10 | 20ml x 10 | 10ml x 10 |
| Lugol's 1/2 strength Drops in juice | Nil | nil | 18 | 6 |
| Thyroid 1 gr tab | Nil | nil | 5 | 2.5 |
| Niacin 50mg | 6 | 6 | 6 | 6 |
| Pancreatin 325mg | 12 | 12 | 12 | 12 |
| Liver caps | 6 | 6 | 6 | 6 |
| CoQ10 90mg | 6 | 6 | 6 | 6 |
| Injection B12 0.1cc with crude liver 3.9cc | daily | daily | daily | daily |
| Coffee enemas | 5 | 5 | 5 | 5 |
| Castor oil treatment | nil | nil | Alternate days | Alternate days |
| Other | Imugen x 10 | Imugen x 10; juice of 6 lemons; castor oil pack on chest twice daily | Imugen x 10; juice of 6 lemons; castor oil pack on chest twice daily | Imugen x 10; spirulina x 5g; add 10ml of K compound solution to last enema to help release it. |
| Tests | TSH 5.8 Possible pleural effusion WCC 3.4 Lymphocytes 0.7 Na 136 | No pleural effusion; viral infection | Hb 13; WCC 5.8; Lymphocytes 1.1; Na 138 | Hb 12.5; WCC 6.0; Lymphocytes 1.1; Na 137; K 5.2 |

# Treatment Schedules

## TREATMENT SCHEDULE:    DATE: 7/12/00

| Time | Juices 240ml | Diet | Flaxseed oil | Acidol/ pepsin caps | K compound solution | Lugol's 1/2 strength; drops in juice | Thyroid 1/2 grain tab | Niacin 50mg | Pancreatin 325mg | Liver cap caps | CoQ10 90mg | Injection B12 0.1cc + 3.9cc crude liver | Coffee enema | Castor oil treatment |
|---|---|---|---|---|---|---|---|---|---|---|---|---|---|---|
| 8.00 | orange | breakfast | | 2 | 10ml | Nil | Nil | 1 | 3 | | 2 | daily | 6 am | nil |
| 9.00 | green | | | | 10ml | | | | | | | | | |
| 9.30 | Apple/ carrot | | | | 10ml | | | | | | | | | |
| 10.00 | Apple/ carrot | | | | 10ml | | | 1 | | | | | ✓ | |
| 11.00 | carrot | | | | | | | | | 2 | | | | |
| 12.00 | green | | | | 10ml | | | | | | | | | |
| 13.00 | Apple/ carrot | lunch | 10ml | 2 | 10ml | | | 1 | 3 | | 2 | | | |
| 14.00 | green | | | | 10ml | | | | | | | | ✓ | |
| 15.00 | carrot | | | | | | | | | 2 | | | | |
| 16.00 | carrot | | | | | | | | | 2 | | | | |
| 17.00 | Apple/ carrot | | | | 10ml | | | 1 | 3 | | | | | |
| 18.00 | Apple / carrot | Dinner | 10ml | 2 | 10ml | | | 1 | 3 | | 2 | | ✓ | |
| 19.00 | Green | | | | 10ml | | | 1 | | | | | 10 pm | |

Diet: No cultured milk products; otherwise diet as prescribed
Juices: 13
Enemas: 6am, 10am, 2pm, 6pm, 10pm
Other: Please order Imugen and take 10/day: 2 at 8am, 10am, 12 noon , 2pm , 4pm. Castor oil pack on chest area twice daily. Juice of 6 lemons daily for viral infection.
Tests: Have all blood tests done in one week's time – do not forget the thyroid function tests and urinalysis.

| Time | Juices 240ml | Diet | Flaxseed oil | Acidol/ pepsin caps | K compound solution | Lugol's 1/2 strength; drops in juice | Thyroid 1/2 grain tab | Niacin 50mg | Pancrea- tin 325mg | Liver caps | CoQ10 90mg | Injection B12 0.1cc + 3.9cc crude liver | Coffee enema | Castor oil treatment |
|---|---|---|---|---|---|---|---|---|---|---|---|---|---|---|
| 8.00 | orange | breakfast | | 2 | 20ml | 3 | 2 x 1/2 | 1 | 3 | | 2 | daily | 6 am | Alt days |
| 9.00 | green | | | | 20ml | | | | | | | | | |
| 9.30 | Apple/ carrot | | | | 20ml | 3 | | | | | | | | |
| 10.00 | Apple/ carrot | | | | 20ml | 3 | 2 x 1/2 | 1 | | | | | ✓ | |
| 11.00 | carrot | | | | | | | | | 2 | | | | |
| 12.00 | green | | | | 20ml | | | | | | | | | |
| 13.00 | Apple/ carrot | lunch | 10ml | 2 | 20ml | 3 | 2 x 1/2 | 1 | 3 | | 2 | | | |
| 14.00 | green | | | | 20ml | | | | | | | | ✓ | |
| 15.00 | carrot | | | | | | | | | 2 | | | | |
| 16.00 | carrot | | | | | | | | | 2 | | | | |
| 17.00 | Apple/ carrot | | | | 20ml | 3 | 2 x 1/2 | 1 | 3 | | | | | |
| 18.00 | Apple / carrot | Dinner | 10ml | 2 | 20ml | 3 | 2 x 1/2 | 1 | 3 | | 2 | | ✓ | |
| 19.00 | Green | | | | 20ml | | | 1 | | | | | 10 pm | |

Diet: No cultured milk products; otherwise diet as prescribed. Brown rice once/week (semi-germinated before cooking); 2 slices no-salt rye bread; don't forget your cooked vegetables
Medications: See schedule. The increased dose of potassium compound solution, Lugol's and thyroid is for 28 days only.
Juices: 13
Enemas: 6am, 10am, 2pm, 6pm, 10pm. If the last one is too last the bring back to 9.00pm. Castor oil treatment should be taken on alternate days.

## TREATMENT SCHEDULE:    DATE:    21/02/01

| Time | Juices 240mls | Diet | Flaxseed oil | Acidol/ pepsin caps | K compound solution | Lugol's 1/2 strength; drops in juice | Thyroid 1/2 grain tab | Niacin 50mg | Pancrea- tin 325mg | Liver caps | CoQ10 90mg | Injection B12 0.1cc + 3.9cc crude liver | Coffee enema | Castor oil treatment |
|---|---|---|---|---|---|---|---|---|---|---|---|---|---|---|
| 8.00 | orange | breakfast | | 2 | 10ml | 1 | 1 x 1/2 | 1 | 3 | | 2 | daily | 6am | Alt days |
| 9.00 | green | | | | 10ml | | | | | | | | | |
| 9.30 | Apple/ carrot | | | | 10ml | 1 | | | | | | | | |
| 10.00 | Apple/ carrot | | | | 10ml | 1 | 1 x 1/2 1/2 | 1 | | | | | ✓ | |
| 11.00 | carrot | | | | | | | | | 2 | | | | |
| 12.00 | green | | | | 10ml | | | | | | | | | |
| 13.00 | Apple/ carrot | lunch | 5ml | 2 | 10ml | 1 | 1 x 1/2 | 1 | 3 | | 2 | | | |
| 14.00 | green | | | | 10ml | | | | | | | | ✓ | |
| 15.00 | carrot | | | | | | | | | 2 | | | | |
| 16.00 | carrot | | | | | | | | | 2 | | | | |
| 17.00 | Apple/ carrot | | | | 10ml | 1 | 1 x 1/2 | 1 | 3 | | | | | |
| 18.00 | Apple / carrot | Dinner | 5ml | 2 | 10ml | 1 | 1 x 1/2 | 1 | 3 | | 2 | | ✓ | |
| 19.00 | Green | | | | 10ml | | | 1 | | | | | 10pm | |

Diet: No cultured milk products; otherwise diet as prescribed. Brown rice once/week (semi-germinated before cooking); 2 slices no-salt rye bread; Medications: See schedule. The reduce potas-sium compound solution to 10ml/10 juice, Lugol's to 6 drops and thyroid to2.5 grains daily. Please add 5g of Spirulina and take 10 Imugen daily.
Enemas: 6am, 10am, 2pm, 6pm, 10pm. Add 10ml of the potassium compound solution to the last enema to help release it. Castor oil treatment should be taken on alternate days.

# Dr. Gerson's General Schedule of Medications

| | 1-4 weeks | 4-8 weeks | 8-12 weeks | 12-16 weeks | 16-20 weeks | 20-24 weeks | 6-9 months | 9 months on |
|---|---|---|---|---|---|---|---|---|
| Acidol/pepsin | 2 before meals | Continued throughout | | | | | | |
| Potassium | 20ml x 10 | 10ml x 10 | 10ml x 10 | 10ml x 10 | 10ml x 10 | 10ml x 10 | 10ml x 10 | 10ml x 6-10 |
| Lugol's 1/2 strength | 6 x 3 drops | 6 x 1 drop | 6 x 1 drop | 3-6 x 1 drop. | Cont. on this dose | | | |
| Thyroid | 5 x 1 gr | 5 x 1/2 grain | 5 x 1/2 grain | 3 x 1/2 grain | Cont. this dose | | | |
| Niacin | 50mg x 6 for 6 month | | | | | | Possibly reduce | |
| Pancreatin 325 mg | 3 tabs x 4 | Continued throughout | | | | | | |
| Liver/extract B 12 injection | 4-6 months | | | | | | Alternate days | |
| Coffee enemas | 5 daily | Continue – dependent on tumoural mass | | | | | | |
| Castor oil treatment | Alternate days | 2/week | | | | | | |
| Flaxseed oil | 20ml daily | 10ml daily | Continue | | | | | |
| Cultured milk protein | None | Introduce at 6-8 weeks | 1 cup buttermilk + 1 cup non-fat, unsalted cottage cheese | | | | | |

# General Schedule of Medications - Current

## GENERAL SCHEDULE OF MEDICATIONS - CURRENT
*(For a patient who responds to and is progressing well on the therapy).*

| | 1-4 weeks | 4-12 weeks | 3-6 months | 6-9 months | 9-12 months | 12-15 months | 15-18 months | 18-21 months | 21-24 months |
|---|---|---|---|---|---|---|---|---|---|
| Acidol/ pepsin | 2 before meals | Continued | | | | 1 before meals | cont | | 2 daily |
| Potassium | 20ml x 10 | 10ml x 10 | 10ml x 10 | 10ml x 10 | 10ml x 10 | 10ml x 10 | 10ml x 10 | 10ml x 8 | 5ml x 6 |
| Lugol's 1/2 strength | 6 x 3 drops | 6 x 1 drop | 6 x 1 drop | 4 x 1 drop | 3 x 1 drop | 2 x 1 drop | 1 x 1 drop | cont | Cont |
| Thyroid | 5 x 1 gr | 5 x 1/2 grain | 5 x 1/2 grain | 5 x 1/2 grain | 5 x 1/2 grain | 3-4 x 1/2 gr | 3 x 1/2 gr | 2 x 1/2 gr | 1 x 1/2 gr |
| Niacin | 50mg x 6 | 50mg x 6 | 50mg x 6 | 50mg x 6 | 50mg x 6 | 50mg x 6 | 50mg x 4 | 50mg x 3 | 50mg x 1-2 |
| Pancreatin 325 mg | 3 tabs x 4 | 3 tabs x 4 | 3 tabs x 4 | 3 tabs x 3 | 3 tabs x 3 | 3 tabs x 3 | 3 tabs x 3 | 2 tabs x 3 | 1 tab x 3 |
| Liver Caps | 2 x 3 | 2 x 3 | 2 x 3 | 2 x 3 | 2 x 3 | 2 x 3 | 2 x 3 | 1 x 3 | 1 x 3 |
| Liver/extract B 12 injection | daily | Daily | Alternate days | Twice/week | Twice/week | Once/week | Once/week | Once every 2 weeks | Once/ month |
| Coffee enemas | 5 daily | 5 | 5 | 4 | 3-4 | 3 | 2 | 2 | 1 |
| Castor oil treatment | Alternate days | 2/week | 2/week | 3 every 2 weeks | 1/week | 1/week | 1 every 2 weeks | Nil | Nil |
| Flaxseed oil | 20ml daily | 10ml daily | Continue | | | | | | |
| Cultured milk pro- tein | None | Introduce at 6-8 weeks | | Add lentils once/fortnight | | Increase lentils once/ week | Add fish once/week | Fish twice weekly, few spices, nuts, all fruits | |

# Full Therapy – first four weeks only

## FULL THERAPY – 1ST FOUR WEEKS ONLY

| Time | Juices 240ml | Diet | Flaxseed oil | Acidol/ pepsin caps | K compound solution | Lugol's 1/2 strength; drops in juice | Thyroid 1 grain tab | Niacin 50mg | Pancrea- tin 325mg | Liver caps | CoQ10 90mg | Injection B12 0.1cc + 3.9cc crude liver | Coffee enema | Castor oil treatment |
|------|------|------|------|------|------|------|------|------|------|------|------|------|------|------|
| 8.00 | orange | breakfast | | 2 | 20ml | 3 | 1 | 1 | 3 | | 2 | daily | 6am | Alt days |
| 9.00 | green | | | | 20ml | | | | | | | | | |
| 9.30 | Apple/ carrot | | | | 20ml | 3 | | | | | | | | |
| 10.00 | Apple/ carrot | | | | 20ml | 3 | 1 | 1 | | | | | ✓ | |
| 11.00 | carrot | | | | | | | | | 2 | | | | |
| 12.00 | green | | | | 20ml | | | | | | | | | |
| 13.00 | Apple/ carrot | lunch | 10ml | 2 | 20ml | 3 | 1 | 1 | 3 | | 2 | | ✓ | |
| 14.00 | green | | | | 20ml | | | | | | | | | |
| 15.00 | carrot | | | | | | | | | 2 | | | | |
| 16.00 | carrot | | | | | | | | | 2 | | | | |
| 17.00 | Apple/ carrot | | | | 20ml | 3 | 1 | 1 | 3 | | | | | |
| 18.00 | Apple / carrot | Dinner | 10ml | 2 | 20ml | 3 | 1 | 1 | 3 | | 2 | | ✓ | |
| 19.00 | Green | | | | 20ml | | | 1 | | | | | 10pm | |

Diet: as prescribed. No cultured milk products for the first 6-8 weeks. Brown rice once weekly. 2 slices of Essene rye bread or unsalted sour dough rye bread daily.

# Full Therapy – after the first four weeks

## FULL THERAPY – AFTER THE FIRST FOUR WEEKS

| Time | Juices 240ml | Diet | Flaxseed oil | Acidol/pepsin caps | K compound solution | Lugol's 1/2 strength; drops | Thyroid 1/2 grain tab | Niacin 50mg | Pancreatin 325mg | Liver caps | CoQ10 90mg | Injection B12 0.1cc + 3.9cc crude | Coffee enema | Castor oil treatment | Castor oil treatment |
|---|---|---|---|---|---|---|---|---|---|---|---|---|---|---|---|
| 8.00 | orange | breakfast | | 2 | 10ml | 1 | 1x 1/2 | 1 | 3 | | 2 | daily | 6am | alt days | Alt days |
| 9.00 | green | | | | 10ml | | | | | | | | | | |
| 9.30 | Apple/carrot | | | | 10ml | 1 | | | | | | | | | |
| 10.00 | Apple/carrot | | | | 10ml | 1 | 1 x 1/2 | 1 | | | | | ✓ | | |
| 11.00 | carrot | | | | | | | | | 2 | | | | | |
| 12.00 | green | | | | 10ml | | | | | | | | | | |
| 13.00 | Apple/carrot | lunch | 5ml | 2 | 10ml | 1 | 1 x 1/2 | 1 | 3 | | 2 | | | | |
| 14.00 | green | | | | 10ml | | | | | | | | ✓ | | |
| 15.00 | carrot | | | | | | | | | 2 | | | | | |
| 16.00 | carrot | | | | | | | | | 2 | | | | | |
| 17.00 | Apple/carrot | | | | 10ml | 1 | 1 x 1/2 | 1 | 3 | | | | | | |
| 18.00 | Apple / carrot | Dinner | 5ml | 2 | 10ml | 1 | 1 x 1/2 | 1 | 3 | | 2 | | ✓ | | |
| 19.00 | Green | | | | 10ml | | | 1 | | | | | 10pm | | |

Diet: as prescribed. Add cultured milk products around 6-8 weeks from the start of the therapy.

# Modified Therapy: strong patients after chemotherapy

## MODIFIED THERAPY FOR STRONG PATIENTS WHO HAVE RECEIVED CHEMOTHERAPY

| Time | Juices 240ml | Diet | Flaxseed oil | Acidol/ pepsin caps | K compound solution | Lugol's 1/2 strength; drops in juice | Thyroid 1/2 grain tab | Niacin 50mg | Pancrea- tin 325mg | Liver caps | CoQ10 90mg | Injection B12 0.1cc + 3.9cc crude liver | Coffee enema | Castor oil treat- ment |
|---|---|---|---|---|---|---|---|---|---|---|---|---|---|---|
| 8.00 | or- ange | break- fast | | 2 | 10ml | 1 | 1 x 1/2 grain | 1 | 3 | | 2 | daily | 7am | Nil |
| 9.00 | green | | | | 10ml | | | | | | | | | |
| 9.30 | Apple/ carrot | | | | 10ml | 1 | | | | | | | | |
| 10.00 | Apple/ carrot | | | | 10ml | 1 | 1 x 1/2 grain | 1 | | | | | | |
| 11.00 | | | | | | | | | | 2 | | | | |
| 12.00 | green | | | | 10ml | | | | | | | | | |
| 13.00 | Apple/ carrot | lunch | 10ml | 2 | 10ml | 1 | 1 x 1/2 grain | 1 | 3 | | 2 | | ✓ | |
| 14.00 | green | | | | 10ml | | | | | | | | | |
| 15.00 | | | | | | | | | | 2 | | | | |
| 16.00 | | | | | | | | | | 2 | | | | |
| 17.00 | Apple/ carrot | | | | 10ml | 1 | 1 x 1/2 grain | 1 | 3 | | | | | |
| 18.00 | Apple / carrot | Dinner | 10ml | 2 | 10ml | 1 | 1 x 1/2 grain | 1 | 3 | | 2 | | ✓ | |
| 19.00 | Green | | | | 10ml | | | 1 | | | | | | |

Diet: as prescribed. Cultured milk products may be introduced between weeks 6-8. The flaxseed oil is reduced from 20ml daily to 10ml daily after 4 weeks. Continue on these medications for many months.

# Modified Therapy for the weakened patient

## MODIFIED THERAPY FOR THE WEAKENED PATIENT

| Time | Juices 240mls | Diet | Flaxseed oil | Acidol/ pepsin caps | K compound solution | Lugol's 1/2 strength; drops in juice | Thyroid 1/2 grain tab | Niacin 50mg | Pancrea- tin 325mg | Liver caps | CoQ10 90mg | Injection B12 0.1cc + 3.9cc crude liver | Coffee en- ema | Castor oil treatment |
|---|---|---|---|---|---|---|---|---|---|---|---|---|---|---|
| 8.00 | orange | breakfast | | 2 | 5- 10ml | 1 | 1 x 1/2 | 1 | 3 | | 1 | daily | 1 - 2 | Nil |
| 9.00 | green | | | | 5- 10ml | | | | | | | | | |
| 9.30 | Apple/ carrot | | | | 5- 10ml | | | | | | | | | |
| 10.00 | Apple/ carrot | | | | 5- 10ml | | | 1 | | | | | | |
| 11.00 | | | | | | | | | | 2 | | | | |
| 12.00 | green | | | | 5- 10ml | | | | | | | | | |
| 13.00 | Apple/ carrot | lunch | 10ml | 2 | 5- 10ml | 1 | 1x 1/2 | 1 | 3 | | 1 | | | |
| 14.00 | green | | | | 5- 10ml | | | | | | | | | |
| 15.00 | | | | | | | | | | 2 | | | | |
| 16.00 | | | | | | | | | | 2 | | | | |
| 17.00 | Apple/ carrot | | | | 5- 10ml | | | 1 | 3 | | | | | |
| 18.00 | Apple / carrot | Dinner | 10ml | 2 | 5- 10ml | | | 1 | 3 | | | | | |
| 19.00 | Green | | | | 5- 10ml | | | 1 | | | | | | |

Diet: as prescribed. Cultured milk products may be introduced between weeks 6-8, or earlier if blood protein levels are low. The flaxseed oil is reduced from 20ml daily to 10ml daily after 4 weeks. The medications will be at the discretion of the practitioner and the above table must only be used as a guide. Generally it is best to wean the weakened patient onto the therapy over a period of a few weeks so that you may determine the correct doses.

# APPENDIX

# Going Home

## Tips for Self-Management

*A transcript of a lecture given by Kathryn Alexander at the Meridien Hospital, 1999*

Suddenly, when it's time to go home, you feel at a loss - everything has been done for you, medications, diet and juices all prepared, there has been someone reassuring you and explaining all your reactions and flare-ups and applying the correct procedure - but what are you going to do when you are on your own? It's much like starting a new school or a new job - once you are there, you know you will learn the ropes pretty quickly and wonder why you had such trepidation - it is exactly like that with the Gerson Therapy.

And then many are put off by the length of time - two years or perhaps even more, how will you cope? Dr. Melendez once said at a training program to think of the new born baby: "You give the milk, change the nappy and let them sleep: the same is true for the Gerson patient - you give the juices, take the enemas and let them rest." Somehow putting it into the context of having a baby that you care for night and day, where everything revolves around that child, makes it seem that much easier. You willingly give that time to your baby - will you give yourselves that much time? Remember, at least you get your night's sleep!

## Medications

By the time you go home, you will all have your medications for the next few weeks. They will be different for each one of you. You will know that the purpose of the therapy is to create a healing and along with that comes an inflammation. In the first month the therapy is turned on full, or as Charlotte says - it's like getting into a car in winter, you put the heater on full blast until you reach a comfortable temperature, and then you turn it down to maintain a steady, comfortable heat. For each one of you, your maximum will be different. I like to see the body as a car - some people have Ferraris and you can accelerate really fast and maintain a high speed without the engine burning out; others have vehicles which are poorly serviced, the engine clanks, the brakes don't work very well, etc. - but you still have to make that journey in one piece. Those people have to go more slowly - they can still get there but at a gentler pace. Your medications will have been tailored to accommodate this, so that you can arrive at your destination in health.

### Thyroid/Lugol's/Potassium
The medications which turn the system on are the thyroid, Lugol's and potassium. You may have seen your dose being adjusted up and down during your first week, dependent on your blood results and how you are responding. These medications can remain the same for many months once you leave the clinic, but it's important that you keep your monthly appointments, as, very often, your doctor, depending on your progress/symptoms, will adjust the dose accordingly.

*Don't forget to dissolve your pot of potassium salts in one litre of distilled water and store in a glass bottle. Label the bottle - in case a youngster comes in and takes a swig - as happened in my home! The potassium compound solution dose is in 5ml teaspoons.*

## Niacin

Again, some of you may not be taking this medication, particularly if you have recently had surgery or any inflammatory disorders of the gastrointestinal tract/ulceration etc. We also discontinue it during menstruation. We use this vitamin to produce the famous "niacin flush" which is quite harmless, although some may find it extremely uncomfortable, and if it antagonizes the healing, it may be removed from the prescription for a while. Niacin promotes the irrigation of the tissues by the blood, taking nutrients to the site and removing toxicity.

*Tip - dissolve slowly under the tongue, after meals, to reduce flushing sensation.*
*Don't be tempted to substitute nicotinamide which is a derivative and produces no flushing effect.*

## Digestive enzymes

Some of you will be taking around 11 tablets/capsules around meal-times of various products. Most of these will be your enzymes which you take before and after meals. Some of you will be on pancreatin with additional enzymes, plus the acidol-pepsin. Gerson found that his patients had deficient digestive systems, which is a problem when the basis for the healing therapy is diet. If your digestion is impaired, you cannot liberate the nutrients from the foods, you do not absorb them and they will either pass straight through the digestive tract and cause terrible gas, or into the blood stream as partially digested foods placing a greater burden on the liver. So the acidol-pepsin prepares the stomach for the digestion of protein, while the digestive enzymes support the pancreas in its role by supplying the pancreatic enzymes required for the digestion of fats, proteins and carbohydrates.

These enzymes are not only valuable in digestion, but they also pass into the circulation and go on to digest tumour tissue and "debris". You may have spent time looking over your live blood analysis photographs and been explained the various foreign objects swimming around - from undigested foods, to liver toxins, dead cells and debris, bacteria and fungi. Well, our natural diet, if it is prepared according to the Gerson protocol, is high in raw foods (juices and salads), contains sufficient live enzymes in a healthy person to help with its digestion (thereby not taxing the pancreas), and with enough left over to enter the blood stream and keep the blood clean.

*Tip - at the beginning of the diet many experience a lot of gas which seems to get worse as the day progresses. It can be extremely uncomfortable. It's a good idea to take some charcoal tablets home with you and take 2, whenever you get the discomfort. You will find that as the digestion improves (a good sign of the healing process), then this will be less of a problem.*

## Other medications
*As prescribed by your Gerson doctor*

**Laetrile + hydrotherapy** (bone, breast and lung cancer). Some of you will have had laetrile by injection and then several times a week received hydrotherapy. Laetrile increases the temperature of the tumour, which causes the destruction of tumour tissue and stimulates the healing. The hydrotherapy will, of course, amplify this effect. When you go home, you will continue with the Laetrile but in tablet form, and you should take it as prescribed.

*Don't be tempted to take apricot kernels, as you would have to take too many to get a therapeutic dose and they are too high in fat.*

**Ozone** - you will have noticed the ozone generators in your rooms and most of you will be having ozone by rectal insufflation twice daily. It may be a good idea to invest in an *ozone generator (or ionizer)* for use in the home, as it will purify the air by destroying, through oxidation, indoor pollution from mildew, mould, air-borne bacteria/viruses, gases, chemicals, etc. The machine generates negative ions which will react with oxygen in the air to form ozone.

It is not always possible to continue with the application of ozone rectally, once you go home. I do know that some practitioners of colonic irrigation have these machines and will perform this for clients. You can buy these machines, but they are costly. They are easy to use, and many feel that the cost is well justified. Ozone in the blood stream will kill malignant tissue and viruses on contact, and mop up free radicals.

*Tip - apply either 30 minutes before the coffee enema or 60 minutes after.*

# Enemas

You all know by now the relevance of the enema. Removing toxicity from the cells is not the same as detoxifying. We have to help the liver release the toxicity by taking our regular coffee enemas and our castor oil treatment (castor oil by mouth followed five hours later by castor oil by enema). Most people have convinced themselves, by the time they check out, that the castor oil enema is not that relevant - even though they know to the contrary. In fact, as practitioners, we are more cautious in reducing the castor oil enema than the number of coffee enemas - so important is it to the release of toxicity. It is only if you have had chemotherapy, or if you suffer from any ulceration/bleeding of the gastrointestinal tract, that you may be advised not to take them during the initial stages of treatment. The castor oil treatment is contra-indicated for patients who have had chemotherapy.

## The castor oil treatment

Let's have a word about the castor oil treatment. Castor oil is not absorbed by the gastrointestinal tract but, taken on an empty stomach, it sends very strong messages to the liver to release a lot of bile at once for its digestion. Consequently the liver flushes the toxic bile into the digestive tract where it is trapped by the castor oil. Normally, bile reacts with dietary fat to emulsify it, preparing for its absorption, much like adding washing-up liquid and hot water to a fatty pan. In the absorption of dietary fat, a proportion of the bile is reabsorbed. However, as castor oil is not absorbed, it traps the bile and carries it out of the system. The coffee enema will keep the momentum going, but obviously a proportion of the bile is re-absorbed; the castor oil treatment gets around this problem and the subsequent castor oil enema ensures the rapid passage of all the toxic bile along the whole gastrointestinal tract to the outside.

Sometimes the castor oil treatment can precipitate a healing reaction and cause diarrhoea that may continue throughout the day. In these cases you may need to adjust your dose of castor oil. Excessive diarrhoea, particularly after the castor oil enema, will cause dehydration and unbalance your minerals, so this is self-defeating. It is best to adjust your dose to find the most tolerable amount. For example, you may try 10ml of castor oil instead of the 2 tablespoons or 20ml by mouth. The amount in the enema, 40ml, can remain the same.

*Tips - take on an empty stomach but do swill it down with black coffee and sugar so that it clears the stomach quickly, leading to less regurgitation. Sometimes you may need to drink peppermint tea to keep the bile flushing through. Warm the castor oil so that it is more fluid and mix with some of the black coffee or orange juice. One patient I know made a funnel so that it went straight to the back of the throat. I'm not quite sure how that worked, but he assured me it was a viable option.*

**General problems with enemas and tips for dealing with these:**
Most people, when they start the enemas, have a problem retaining them for the full 15 minutes. This occurs when the body is low in potassium and the muscles, which require potassium for healthy tone (contraction and relaxation), contract and spasm, either making retention impossible because of the strong peristaltic waves, or clutching the enema so that you can't release it. Neither of these symptoms are life-threatening. If you cannot release the enema, you will absorb it and urinate more frequently, and if you cannot retain it, then no harm done, providing you make it to the bathroom in time!

*Tips:*

- Take a 0.5L Chamomile tea enema before the coffee enema. Do not retain. Chamomile will soothe and relax the muscles prior to your coffee enema.
- Take a chamomile and coffee enema mixed (0.5L coffee:0.5L chamomile tea)
- Take the enema in two smaller doses (this will take twice the time, as each enema must be retained for the full 15 minutes).
- Make sure the enema bucket is not too high. If the enema feeds into the rectum too quickly, this can set up counter-spasms in the intestine.
- If you cannot release the enema, take another one back to back.
- Add 10ml of the potassium compound solution to the enema. This should not be done for longer than a few days, as the solution can be an irritant.
- Make your total day's coffee enema requirement at one go and keep as a concentrate in the refrigerator. Dilute before use.

# Flare-ups or healing reactions

The healing process is a combination of clearing out the rubbish and regenerating new tissues. This happens on both the physical and mental/emotional level. When you release toxins from the body you also release emotions. This can happen spontaneously when old memories are suddenly stirred up out of the blue, which are then mentally processed for their release from the body. So the healing reaction can involve bouts of irrational behaviour, depression and crying. Toxins in the tissues may also irritate the nerves and you may feel more irritable and short-tempered at these times. Of course, the coffee enema is excellent for flushing these toxins through.

## Clay and castor oil packs

Healing will also involve the inflammatory process. Many of you will have already experienced this. It can be from the simple shifting of toxins which go out into the muscle tissue, causing muscle stiffness and pain, particularly in the shoulder/neck area. For this type of pain the warm castor oil pack is wonderful, as it helps to improve the circulation to that area, relax the muscles and disperse the toxins. It is also useful for shifting mucous congestion in the lungs if you get a cold. You will all know by now how to prepare one of these packs and how to use it with your heat pad. Another idea is to use it with a wheat bag which can be heated in the microwave (the only useful purpose this gadget will have!). You can make these yourselves, any size and any shape, and they will curve to your body. Also, with bone pain, the muscles will tend to contract around the bone, exacerbating the pain, and the castor oil pack will prove invaluable. The main job of the castor oil pack is to alleviate spasms and cramping. This pack can be used again and again and kept on for as long as required - all night, if you wish. When you have finished using it just roll it up and store, adding more castor oil as required. The packs don't keep indefinitely and don't attempt to wash them in you washing machine unless you want all your washing to come out smelling of castor oil with a vague greasy "stiffness" to it.

The clay pack is used for "hot" inflammations around the joints, tumour swelling, and to reduce areas of fluid retention either through injury or general oedema. Clay packs are often administered twice daily over the liver area, where they actively draw out toxicity. It is really important to keep on with your clay packs if this is part of your prescription. They can be kept in place for 2-3 hours and should then be thrown away, as they are full of toxins.

You will experience these flare-ups: old injuries will be revisited, scar tissue and bones will inflame and then heal, old injuries may also reappear. Don't forget to use your clay and castor oil packs, as they will greatly alleviate any problems.

### Pain management

- In addition to the packs the coffee enema is the first line of treatment. Why should this work, you may wonder? Well, the body releases a lot of inflammatory chemicals during the reaction, which causes the formation of free radicals. All these compounds at the site of inflammation can create a vicious cycle and perpetuate the inflammation and the associated pain. By using the coffee enema, the liver is stimulated to clean the blood more efficiently of these toxic compounds, and therefore pain management can be achieved quite successfully. The coffee enema is also useful during an allergic reaction to clear excess histamine from the body.
- The pain triad - this should be the second line of treatment and it is well-outlined in your Gerson Handbook. Remember: 1 aspirin, 1 niacin and 500mg of viatmin C (not sodium ascorbate). Don't forget to take a little gruel before the medication.
- If this is insufficient there are minimally toxic medications on the market for pain relief, but you should check with your Gerson Doctor before using any of these.

### Nausea and Diarrhoea

Elimination of toxic bile will cause either or both nausea/vomiting and diarrhoea. Toxic bile will often reflux into the stomach and make you feel sick. This can also occur after eating, drinking or taking a coffee enema, because they all stimulate the release of bile (either for digestion or just due to the action of the enema on the bile ducts). If this occurs remember to:

- Take your gruel just before and just after the enema (the gruel will line the stomach, protecting it from toxic irritation, and also bind the bile acids).
- Take plenty of peppermint tea to flush the toxic bile through the system.
- If you don't feel like eating much, make sure that you don't skimp on your oatmeal in the morning, take your Hippocrates soup, some potato and apple sauce. The juices can be mixed with a little gruel until you feel better.
- If the problem is diarrhoea, then add 1/4 tsp clay to some peppermint tea after each bout of diarrhoea. You may also add 1/8 tsp of potassium gluconate powder. If the diarrhoea persists, consult your Gerson Doctor.

# Infection

For those of you who have had young children, you will remember that your doctor would ask you if your child was in good health or harbouring any infection before he gave immunization. If your child had a cold, he would send you away, to return when the child was better. This is because the child's natural immunity would be compromised if he gave the vaccination, as the body can only fight one infection adequately at a time. This is the danger of infection in the Gerson patient. If you get an infection, your body's defences will not only become dissipated but we will also see tumoural progression and you may suffer a relapse. So do, in the most diplomatic way, discourage well-wishers and even family, from coming to see you if they have an infection - in the same way as you would discourage those with infection from visiting your newborn baby.

If you do get an infection, it must be treated, probably with antibiotics, but make sure from proper laboratory investigation that you indeed do have an infection. You may also take a hot bath (those on chlorinated mains should run the bath water very hot, open the windows and let the steam evaporate as chlorine is volatile), to which you have added 200ml of 35% hydrogen peroxide, preferably food-grade. Soak in this and repeat twice daily for 3 days, and thereafter once daily for another 3 days. After each bath, while the skin pores are open, rub in a 2% solution of hydrogen peroxide, over the body. (To convert 35% hydrogen peroxide to a 2% solution use 16 parts distilled water to 1 part hydrogen peroxide). Hydrogen peroxide releases the oxygen radical which is a powerful disinfectant and killer of bacteria and viruses. You can also make a cloth poultice soaked in 2% hydrogen peroxide solution to place over a tumour site.

# The Diet

I am going to give you some tips on the basic practical management of the diet. Sometimes these tips may seem really obvious, but we don't always think of the obvious - rather look at climbing the mountain than go around the side.

- Order your food in bulk from a reputable organic distributor and get them to deliver to your door once a week. You can buy your carrots, potatoes and apples in bulk, plus other root vegetables like beetroot, sweet potato, pumpkin, etc. Salad stuff and greens will have to be bought probably twice weekly, as they can go slimy in the refrigerator.
- If you can, then grow your greens! It is even possible to grow them in the polystyrene boxes that your vegetables may be delivered in. There is nothing nicer than going to pick just enough fresh greens that you need for your juices. We often grumble about the price of organic produce and its quality when it reaches our door. Well, there's more land in all your back yards and gardens put together than the land that is used for agriculture. Perhaps we should go back to growing our produce like our parents did, and relieve some of the stress of our life-styles by pottering in the back yard!
- Either get someone in the household, or if you can afford it, employ someone to work 2 hours a day preparing all the vegetables for the meals and the juices. The soup can be kept for 2 days in the refrigerator. I have found some plastic vegetable bags with a lining approved by the organic industry as being non-toxic, which will enable you to weigh and prepare the vegetables for the day's juices in 12 bags and place in the refrigerator. All you have to do is to grab a bag and chop up the apple and carrots and put through the juicer.
- You may be able to commission a local baker to produce a number of loaves of bread for you according to the recipe in the Primer. You can then cut these loaves in half and freeze them, taking them out upon requirement.
- When you're allowed yoghurt (remember non-fat), you can also try making a soft cheese by hanging the yoghurt in a muslin cloth over the sink overnight. Discard the whey. You will then have a small amount of soft cheese to which you can add onions, chives and garlic and have on your baked potato or as a spread on your bread. Remember that you are allowed 200g of yoghurt/day or 100g soft cheese/a day or an equivalent amount combined.

- Adding protein - please don't be tempted to include this before you are allowed. The omission of protein for 6 weeks, or longer in some cases, has an important stimulating effect on the immune system. We have two main branches of fighter cells: the **T**-cells which fight **T**umour tissue and the **B**-cells which form anti-**B**odies. All our cells have a "bar code" which gets "swiped" by the immune system. If a cell has the wrong bar code, then this alerts the immune system to eradicate it. Tumour cells have the wrong bar code, but very often antibodies are produced which are not strong enough to destroy the cell, but end up attaching themselves to the tumour cell and cover up the bar codes (or antigenic sites, areas on the cell wall which stimulate the immune response) inhibiting the T cells from attacking the tissue. The omission of protein in the first 6 weeks changes the immune profile substantially: T-cell population is increased while the B-cell population is decreased. This gives the body an opportunity to attack the tumour tissue. In order not to compromise the immune system and keep it at an optimal level and balance between these two branches (T and B-cells), small amounts of protein in the form of non-fat, no salt yoghurt/cheese are then added at a later date. However, it is important to keep specifically to these amounts, as excess protein will cause tumour tissue to release toxins which increases the oedema around the tumour. This has the dual effect of protecting the tumour from destruction by the immune system and making the surrounding tissue toxic and more vulnerable to spreading of the tumour.

Good Luck, Good Health and bon appetite!


Kathryn Alexander.

# Protein and Healing - Part 1

## Why You Can't Heal on a High-Protein Diet

The high-protein diet is coming back into fashion. It has done the rounds of weight-loss diets, stabilizing blood sugar diets, and now for the next wave of controlling "hyperinsulinaemia." I would be the first to agree that yes, you can manipulate symptoms through diet, but I would qualify that manipulation is not the same as healing, and furthermore, it does not address the cause of the problem.

What is it about protein that has given it such a high profile? Take the overweight person who finds it difficult to go on a diet because of hunger pangs and cravings. The theory is that calories are not the be-all and end-all to a weight loss diet and that you can eat a high protein, high fat diet (therefore highly calorific) and still lose weight! It's true - you can. If the release of insulin isn't triggered by dietary intake of carbohydrates/sugars, then the cells cannot take up the excess sugar, and protein and fat synthesis is hindered. Insulin is an "anabolic" hormone, which means that it is required for body tissue synthesis. Hence the diabetic who has a malfunction with their insulin metabolism will lose weight and waste away, unless they medicate with insulin. Certain dietary regimes ask the client to maintain a specified acidic pH of their urine (they test the urine with pH indicator strips). On a high protein, high fat diet the body produces vast amounts of acids which are cleared in the urine (placing a great strain on the liver and kidneys). Within a narrow band of pH you will maintain your weight-losing state, but with the introduction of carbohydrate (any amount), these pH levels will change - so if you want to keep the weight loss up, you maintain your nil carbohydrate diet!

Let's take blood sugar control. We know that in certain individuals, when they eat carbohydrate, they experience a sudden drop in blood sugar (symptoms include lethargy and fatigue, poor concentration, mood swings, "foggy" brain, disperceptions, panic attacks, hot and cold sweats, heart palpitations), and we believe that the cause of this could be an inappropriate insulin response - too much insulin being secreted bringing the blood sugar levels down too much. So these sufferers are recommended to eat high protein/low carbohydrate diets. It works - the symptoms abate because protein doesn't stimulate such a strong insulin release as carbohydrate.

Next the new wave of "hyperinsulinaemia", where we have moved on from hypo-glycaemia (low blood sugar) to high amounts of insulin in the blood stream. The symptoms appear to be more or less the same, along with the discovery of excess insulin in the blood stream. What's the answer? Reduce the secretion of insulin by omitting carbohydrates and increasing your protein intake. Once again manipulation of symptoms with diet - but as soon as you go back on the carbohydrates, the symptoms return. Not only this, six months down the track on such a diet you start to experience new symptoms of a more chronic nature.

*A lady, aged 59 years, came to see me. She had been diagnosed with hyperinsulinaemia and been following a high protein diet for a year. Initially her symptoms of low energy, bloating, digestive difficulties and cravings did improve, but after six months on the high-protein plan the symptoms returned more aggressively, along with weight increase, fluid retention, a racing brain and insomnia. She still maintained the diet but took Chinese herbs to help the symptoms. This worked for a while, but then it seemed as though even the herbs would not help. When we looked over her case history, we could see that she was very toxic; from a very young age she had suffered from food allergies and candida, she had taken the contraceptive pill for 12 years (synthetic sex hormones inhibit the flushing of bile from the liver and therefore stop detoxification), and by the age of 36 years she had an abnormal smear, followed by a hysterectomy with cysts being identified on the ovaries. Later she took HRT (hormone replacement therapy) for a period of 4 years. By the time I saw her, she was extremely toxic, deficient, and the liver was stagnant. She assured me that there was no way she could go on the detoxification plan, as all the carbohydrates would make her worse. I did persuade her to try the high vegetable and fruit diet along with juicing and we worked out a diet where we omitted all the foods she was allergic to (gluten, tomatoes), removed all the oils including nuts and seeds (except for flaxseed oil), and reduced protein to a minimum (100g non-fat yoghurt daily, brown rice and legumes twice/week, and a little fish), and of course enemas were added to the regime. By the next month all the digestive difficulties had abated, she had lost 4 kg, was not suffering cravings or hunger, was sleeping better and had no hot flushes or mood swings. However, she did feel as though her body was "locked" up with toxicity, with pains and stiffness in the joints. I recommended warm baths and warm castor oil packs on the areas of stiffness and pain allowing the circulation to remove the toxicity. She continues to improve, step-by-step, as the body heals itself.*

Of course, good quality protein is essential for growth and tissue maintenance, particularly during infancy, childhood, adolescence and pregnancy. But the question arises - how much is enough and how much is too much? The average requirement is 1g of protein /kg of body weight which for the average 50-70kg person means the equivalent of say 200g meat or fish and 4 slices of bread per day - 64g. The body does not lay down excess protein. If you eat protein in excess of your requirements, then the surplus is either converted to carbohydrate or fat by the liver and the amine portion (the nitrogenous portion which makes it a protein) is converted to urea and eliminated by the kidneys. Excess protein creates acidity and puts a strain on the kidneys, which will later affect the heart.

Protein metabolism is under the control of our hormones - insulin, growth hormone and the sex hormones for the laying down of protein, and the corticosteroids for the breaking down of protein (cortisone is the natural stress hormone, which is why you cannot heal if you are under stress, as it opposes tissue synthesis and regeneration). The growth spurts from childhood through to adolescence are controlled by high levels of growth hormone and the sudden increase in sex hormones which, during puberty, rise to eight times the adult levels. Growth hormone and the sex hormones begin to fall after puberty, until they reflect the stable adult levels by the early 20s. Growth hormone becomes practically non-existent after reaching 30 years. So the health/sport professionals found that if they wanted to increase body muscle mass, then it was necessary to take anabolic steroids along with a high protein intake. High protein intake on its own will not increase muscle size. Muscles store a very limited supply of protein (4-6kg) and after this capacity is reached, excess dietary protein has to be broken down and discarded. Exercising increases muscle tone and size, because the more you "work" your muscles, the greater their capacity to store carbohydrate fuel (not protein - muscles do not use protein for energy). Beware of the high protein message if you are seeking fitness.

Let's leave the manipulation of symptoms and come back to healing, which deals with the cause or the "why" you have that imbalance - not the "how" or the mechanisms involved in that imbalance. Treatment often revolves around the "how", but in order to truly resolve imbalances, we must address the "why." For example, "why" should a person appear to have too much insulin - we can address "how" to reduce its secretion, but unless we address the why or the cause, then nothing is going to change, and on a high protein diet the situation will inevitably deteriorate.

In order for the body to heal, no matter what the imbalance, it has to release its toxic load and rebuild its nutrient status. When this occurs, the vitality rises and healing begins. The body's intelligence (not the brain) will determine which areas will be healed and in what order. You must imagine your body like a house which requires touch-up jobs, renovations, etc. from time to time. The workman you call in to do the job will only be as good as your vitality - in fact we could call him Mr. Vitality. In a toxic, deficient body, Mr. Vitality isn't very vital and does a bodged job. But maybe that's OK as long as it's covered over, until later down the track, when the toxicities and deficiencies are greater, Mr. Vitality can't do the job at all and you require on-going medication - not to do the job but to allow you to wear blinkers and ignore the area that needs attention. However, once you have started to detoxify and rebuild, Mr. Vitality returns unannounced to attend to those bodged jobs, to do the job properly, which often means chipping out the old stuff and reworking the area until it is as good a new (well, almost!). So here we come to the crux of the matter: what do we need to do to detoxify and rebuild?

Let's start at a point where 20th century science catches up with the old healing techniques of the preceding centuries. This brings us to the work of Dr. Max Gerson. For those of you unfamiliar with Dr. Gerson's work, he was a physician working, until the time of his death in 1959, with chronic degenerative disease and cancer, and he developed a specific regime of detoxification which remains unsurpassed to date. Dr. Gerson observed and recorded that on a low sodium/high potassium diet (vegetable juices, fruits) the kidneys eliminated high amounts of sodium and with this approach tissue oedemas reduced, tumours started shrinking and the patient started healing. (Sodium is always elevated in damaged/diseased tissues and is the most fundamental enzyme inhibitor. A damaged cell, swollen with sodium and water, cannot oxidize but sinks into fermentation, throwing out more toxins, which then damage adjacent cells and the condition perpetuates). In cancer, Dr. Gerson noted that supplementing with a specific mixture of potassium salts (potassium acetate, gluconate and mono-phosphate) in the vegetable juices, the elimination of sodium was increased and healing accelerated. However, he noted that the inclusion of protein in the diet reduced sodium elimination, retarded detoxification and slowed the process down. In fact, it is impossible to reduce sodium levels in the body on a high protein diet, as the more acidic waste you produce from a high protein diet, the greater the amount of sodium reabsorbed by the kidneys.

Dr. Gerson also found that in cancer dietary protein stimulated tumour growth and that patients with a higher protein intake could not be saved. We have more corroborating information on this through the work of Thomas Tallberg (M.D., Helsinki University) who has isolated certain amino acids (building blocks of protein) as growth factors for specific tumours. Of course, the suggested scientific answer to this is to amend the food through genetic modification, i.e. genetically modify non-pathogenic bacteria to induce them to consume these specific amino acids in foods.

Dr. Gerson also noticed that when he restricted dietary protein, the immune profile changed - the white T-cell count went up. This is the branch of the immune system which fights tumours, viruses and fungi, and generally reinforces the whole immune response. With the oedemas shrinking from around tumour sites (indeed any damaged tissue), the blood supply along with a heightened immune cell profile can access the damaged area and start the healing process. After 6-12 weeks Dr. Gerson recommended the addition of 1 cup of buttermilk and 1 cup of no-fat, unsalted cottage cheese (nowadays the recommendations are: 200g of non-fat yoghurt and/or 100g of no-fat/ unsalted pot cheese, as it is impossible to obtain naturally cultured buttermilk), to the diet, which was sufficient to keep the immune system intact. Severe dietary restriction of protein for a prolonged period can have an adverse effect on the immune system, so just enough had to be supplied to maintain the immune system and yet not inhibit detoxification.

We have also discovered that protein restriction in patients with auto-immune disease often leads to the complete remission of that disease. The work of Dr. Robert Good using dietary restriction of protein and calories in animals supports the fact that in genetically determined diseases (SLE - systemic lupus erythematosus) if such a diet is implemented at weaning, then the animals did not go on to get the disease; or those who were left to develop the disease went into regression upon the initiation of the restricted diet. Dr. Good went on to replicate these findings in mice which were genetically predisposed to mammary tumours.

So we come to the question of how much can a high protein diet be blamed for the rising incidence in chronic disease? Obviously this is only one factor in the whole toxicity/deficiency debate - but what is clear both from my own experience and through recorded data is that high protein diets inhibit detoxification and healing.

There is a further debate on "cooked" versus "uncooked" protein. There is some protein in most foods - in meat we are looking at around 20%; in raw grains 12%, raw legumes 25%, and nuts 20%; in vegetables around 2% and in fruits 0.5 - 3%. (The actual protein content of cooked weight grains and legumes when they have "swollen" with water is reduced by two-thirds: therefore legumes contain around 8% protein and grains between 4 - 8%). When protein is heated or when foods are preserved through pasteurisation or the addition of vinegars/acids, then the protein structure changes its shape. Observe what happens to an egg white when cooked, or to raw fish soaked in lemon juice - you can see the transformation. The protein has straightened out from its normal globular form. The digestion of altered protein does not pose too much of a problem for a person with a strong digestion (provided that it is taken in moderation); but as we get older or if we become sick or show symptoms of an impaired digestion (bloating, flatulence, heart-burn/indigestion, irritable bowel syndrome, allergies), then this altered protein may cause problems. The body's digestive enzymes can digest protein in its globular form because it has a recognisable shape, so the enzyme fits like a lock and key and "opens" the protein, breaking it into single amino acids. I describe the digestion of protein like the eating of a foreign language. The words need to be broken down into their single letters before the body can recombine them into your own language. If these proteins are only partially broken down, then you get foreign protein (or words) entering the system. These are toxic, they are foreign, and the liver has the job of mopping them up and dealing with them. If the liver cannot cope, they enter the systemic circulation and set up inflammatory reactions in the tissues and joints. Inflammatory diseases are often aggravated by cooked protein, which is why a raw food diet is advocated in so many of these cases.

So while we can promote protein-restricted diets, we can also say that protein taken in its raw form may not be a burden on the system. Dr. Gerson used the juice of raw veal liver (it had to be fresh, not frozen, no older than 48 hours, so that it was replete with living enzymes), 750g of raw liver juiced daily, and found that patients responded better to the therapy. Nowadays we cannot use the raw liver with safety because of the risk of cross contamination in the abattoir from camphylobacter, an infection which would be disastrous to the immune compromised patient.

Although a detoxification therapy is predominantly raw (the huge volume of juices consumed which must be prepared fresh, hourly), foods that are taken at meal times are cooked. On a diet therapy it is essential that the patient is able to digest their food and absorb the nutrients. It is very important to understand that a weakened digestion can be overpowered by raw foods; the patient will not digest such foods and not extract the nutrients, and the condition will worsen. Therefore the juicing of raw fruits and vegetables and the cooking of others becomes essential. The removal of all the fibre in juicing minimizes the digestive burden, and the nutrients from the juice can be absorbed easily. The patient can then consume vast quantities of minerals and enzymes without having to eat the whole amount. The slow cooking of vegetables and potatoes and oatmeal does not pose the problem of cooked proteins, as the protein molecule is less damaged by slow cooking, but also the protein content of required foods is minimal (only 2% in vegetables). The bonus of cooking is that the carbohydrates become partially digested. The long carbohydrate chains are reduced to shorter chains and glucose, thereby lifting the burden of digestion. You can tell this by the sweeter taste of most vegetables in their cooked state than in their raw state.

Many people who have an apparent digestive intolerance of carbohydrates (bloating, flatulence, diarrhoea) will opt for the high protein diet to manage their symptoms. It is worth remembering that the digestion only becomes impaired as a consequence of general nutritional deficiencies in the body, brought about by poor quality foods and poor eating habits over a long period of time. As the gut has one of the highest rates of tissue turnover/renewal, symptoms will usually manifest here before anywhere else in the body. Unfortunately this is a vicious cycle - the more compromised the digestion becomes, the lower the general integrity of the entire body, and over a long period of time the body will become weaker, giving way to chronic disease. The *local* symptoms manifest as carbohydrate intolerance (bloating, flatulence), as these are the specific symptoms of fermenting undigested sugars in the gut. However, poor digestion is not exclusive to carbohydrates as many believe. If you are not digesting your carbohydrates, then you are not digesting your proteins, but you will not have the uncomfortable local symptoms from the partial digestion of protein in the gut. Hence by removing carbohydrates and increasing protein your symptoms of discomfort will abate. But bear in mind that you may be setting yourself up for deeper problems associated with the high protein diet: excessive burden on the liver and kidneys, gradual accumulation of sodium and fluid in the tissues which "drowns" the cell and inhibits its activities, and the potential problem of "cooked" proteins and the onset of inflammatory disease.

# Protein and Healing - Part 2

## How much and what type of proteins

In the first of this series of articles on Protein and Healing, I mentioned that the recommended daily protein requirement is around 1g of protein/kg of body weight. To the average person this represents 50-70g protein daily. The best type of protein for healing is derived from vegetable sources; more specifically, protein in its least concentrated form as found in vegetables. You will obtain an average of 2% protein in most vegetables; an average of 8-14% in cereal grains (dry weight); 21-35% in legumes (dry weight); and 12-27% in nuts. Animal protein is more concentrated at 16-25% raw weight. Remember, as grains and legumes swell with water during cooking, the protein content of these foods, per cooked weight, will be reduced by two-thirds.

Many professional nutritionists often complain that patients on the Gerson Therapy, whether for cancer or chronic degenerative disease, cannot possibly be getting enough protein, as the diet seems to consist of only vegetables! However, not only do our patients heal, but also their bodies are regenerated and restored to full functioning capacity.

So it's time to get the calculator out. How much protein does a patient on the full Gerson Therapy actually get from their diet? Let's start with the 13 daily juices. Twelve of these are vegetable juices; 4 green and apple, 3 carrot only, and 5 carrot and apple. The vegetable content of these juices amounts to 3.6 kg daily. The juices alone would provide around 57.6g of protein daily (taking a conservative 1.6% estimate of protein content in vegetables). Potatoes are also on the menu (6g protein from this source); oatmeal (another 7g) and additional quantities of both cooked and raw vegetables.  I would say that an average Gerson patient, at the beginning of the therapy, is consuming between 75g and 80g of quality protein daily. When 200g of non-fat yoghurt is added to the regime, then we are looking at an additional 7g of protein daily.

Having satisfied traditional dietary recommendations, we come to a more pressing matter - that of digestibility. This concept is usually totally ignored. Scientists will refer to the gross amounts of nutrients found in foods with little reference to their true biological value to the human being. The biological value of a food depends on two criteria: the strength and efficiency of the patient's digestive system, and the accessibility of nutrients within a given food. The bottom-line remains: that no amount of "good" food is beneficial to the patient if they cannot adequately digest it, if the nutrients remain bound within the food and are unavailable, if the food contains enzyme inhibitors which render it indigestible, and if the cooking process has rendered it a "non-food".

By the time we become sick, our digestive system is already impaired. How can we then heal on a diet therapy if we are unable to digest our food? It was against this background that Dr. Gerson formulated a diet that would fulfil the nutritional requirements for healing and regeneration, even for the most compromised digestive system.

Assisting the digestion means that you take living foods, unprocessed, that come with their own quota of enzymes required for their digestion. The juicing of vegetables, taken fresh every hour, ensures maximum digestion and assimilation of a plentiful supply of nutrients. The removal of all the fibre ensures that the digestion does not have to work hard to release and absorb the nutrients. All natural foods contain living enzymes: it is the processing of foods which destroys their life force (enzymes), and taxes the pancreas to release greater quantities of digestive enzymes to complete the task. Additionally the food enzymes help in the assimilation of minerals. The slow cooking at low temperatures of vegetable dishes also ensures maximum breakdown of indigestible fibres, the conversion of starches to the more digestible sugars, and maintaining a greater integrity of the enzyme and protein structures.

As the healing proceeds we begin to add foods that have a higher protein value. This becomes important when patients are winding down the Gerson Therapy and they start to ask, "How much protein, and what type is safe for me to eat?" They immediately recognise that by cutting down their juices to perhaps only four daily, the nutritional and protein content of their diet is going to suffer considerably. They will be looking to foods that provide concentrates of nutrients, particularly the grains, legumes and dairy products.

As the patient is healing, so the digestion strengthens, and it becomes possible to include the more difficult to digest foods. However, what most people fail to realise is that grains, legumes and dairy produce are of little nutritional benefit, even to people with the strongest digestion, if they are not prepared correctly. These foods need to be "predigested" through various techniques that prepare the food for the best assimilation.

The easiest example of this is the natural souring of raw milk, where lactose is digested by the lactobacillus bacteria. Products such as buttermilk, natural whey and yoghurt are high in lactic acid which assists both in the digestion of the product itself and in the general digestion. Isolated protein powders, such as whey powders, are processed at high temperatures, which denatures the amino acids, and the product becomes useless as a food. Similarly, pasteurisation destroys all the natural enzymes, nutrients will not be absorbed, and the protein profile (lysine and tyrosine specifically) of the milk is damaged. It is now difficult to obtain raw milk products, but if you can, then this is obviously the way to go. The inclusion of predigested dairy products is important on the vegetarian diet as it supplies good amounts of tryptophan (an amino acid) that is lacking in many vegetarian foods.

This brings us to seeds, and by this I mean anything that sprouts - legumes, grains and nuts. There are two major problems with this group of foods: the amount of phytate they contain, and the presence of enzyme inhibitors. Phytate is particularly nasty in that it will bind to calcium, magnesium, iron and zinc and take it out of the body. Phytate is found in the outer covering, or bran, of the seed. Soy beans are particularly high in phytates. Traditional methods of soaking or fermenting seeds will neutralize the phytates in most seeds. It is a form of predigestion, and one that ensures maximum absorption of nutrients.

Soaking oats in warm water overnight before cooking the next morning will neutralise the phytic acid; similarly soaking any grains and legumes for 12-24 hours before cooking will decompose phytic acid; natural fermentation of grains or flour products through soaking in an acidic medium such as buttermilk (high in lactic acid), or in water, with whey or yoghurt added, will also predigest the food and neutralise the phytic acid. Many traditional cultures allow a natural fermentation of their grains for a 36 hour period before cooking. This allows lactobacilli and other useful organisms to break down and neutralise the phytic acid. Similarly if you soak grains for 7 hours in warm acidulated water, this too, will neutralise most phytic acid.

The traditional leavening process of bread using sour dough techniques also predigest the grain. These techniques have been largely been discarded in favour of the quicker fermentation methods using yeast. It is doubtful whether the phytic acid is destroyed with rapid yeast fermentation. It is known that yeast proving diminishes and destroys much of the grain's nutritional value. Fermentation using a sour dough starter is a much longer process, requiring a fermentation period of seven days for the starter alone, and seven hours for the bread proving. The nutritional value of sour dough bread is much greater than the traditionally yeast leavened breads.

Gluten, a protein found in wheat (also in rye, oats and barley), is very burdensome on the digestion. However, during the soaking and fermenting process, the natural microbes (lactobacilli) break down or predigest the gluten, and many people who suffer wheat intolerance/allergy are more able to digest the product when prepared by these methods.

Most traditional bread is not leavened but made from sprouted wheat or rye. The germinating or sprouting of seeds will also neutralise phytic acid. However, a word of caution: raw sprouted grains/seeds/legumes contain irritating substances in their shoots, so it is not a good idea to include too many in the diet. These substances are neutralized through cooking. Alfalfa seeds should not be included in any healing diet, as they contain an immature amino acid, L-canavanine, which is known to inhibit the immune system and contribute to inflammatory disorders.

There is another case for the germination of seeds. All seeds, in their dormant state, contain enzyme inhibitors. These compounds stop the seed from germinating until conditions become favourable. They also neutralize our own enzymes in the digestive tract. These enzymes are not de-activated by cooking, so if we eat grains or legumes that have not been adequately prepared before cooking, the digestion of all proteins taken at that meal will be impaired.

The correct preparation of both grains and legumes is to soak them for at least 12 hours at room temperature. Soaking will not only neutralize the phytic acid, but allow the proteases within the seed to neutralise the inhibiting factors and so activate the natural enzymes. If you then drain and rinse your seeds and place on a tray, or in a large jar, covered by a damp cloth, for at least 12 hours, you will notice germination tips appearing on your seeds. They are just beginning to germinate. It is at this stage that you can cook your grains and legumes as normal. Germination will increase the enzyme activity six-fold. Additionally, certain of the complex sugars are broken down, making them more digestible. You will find that if you have had digestive difficulties with legumes and cereal grains in the past (lots of gas), then these preparation techniques should be enough to alleviate the problem by increasing their digestibility.

Soy beans have the highest amount of phytic acid of all the seeds. Phytic acid is particularly high in tofu. They are also high in very potent enzyme inhibitor substances. Traditionally they were only planted for their nitrogen-fixing capacity, and not as a food. Unlike other seeds, even using preparation methods described above, the soy bean cannot be rendered edible. The process of precipitation during the manufacture of tofu or bean curd, will only remove a portion of the enzyme inhibitor substances but none of the phytate. It is only through the specific fermentation process during the making of soy sauce and miso, that these anti-nutrients are eradicated. Soy beans and soy products are therefore not recommended in any dietary regime, as they will cause chronic nutritional deficiencies both of minerals and protein by virtue of their high phytate and enzyme inhibitor content.

I have also mentioned how heating denatures proteins. By denaturing we mean changing the shape of the protein and rendering it biologically inactive. The higher the temperature, the greater the distortion of the protein molecule. Food, when cooked in water, will reach a maximum temperature of 100°C; fried food can reach 215°C; and certain processing techniques such as those used in puffing cereals apply a very high temperature and a pressure of 1500 pounds/square inch. The more damaged the protein becomes, the more toxic it becomes in the system, and may even act as a poison. A study using four groups of rats revealed just this. The first group was fed only water and nutrients, the second group was fed whole wheat, water and chemical nutrients, the third group was fed on sugar and water (no nutrients), and the fourth group was fed on puffed wheat, water and chemical nutrients. The first group fed on water and chemical nutrients lived 8 weeks; the second group fed on whole wheat, water and chemical nutrients lived for over a year; the third group fed on sugar and water only lived 4 weeks; while those fed on puffed wheat, water and chemical nutrients lived for only 2 weeks. These results indicate that the inclusion of puffed grains were acting in a morbid fashion, accelerating the mortality rate.

In order to keep your proteins digestible, it is important to cook using the lowest possible temperature. Simmering on the stove or baking in the oven are the preferred methods. Try to use the waterless cooking method where applicable, so that no nutrients are lost. Frying not only heats the food to very high temperatures but it destroys both the cooking oil and the natural oils found in the foods themselves. You will end up consuming both toxic oil and toxic protein products. It is interesting that traditional Asian cooking methods add water to the wok, then the vegetables and then the oil. The water and the vegetables keep the overall cooking temperature down so the proteins and the oils are not destroyed.

Many patients with chronic degenerative disease will start to improve after they have removed the bulk of protein from their diet. As Dr. Gerson so rightly stated, in chronic degenerative disease and cancer, the liver is damaged and toxic. It is the liver's responsibility to deal with abnormal, partially digested proteins. When the liver is unable to detoxify properly, these abnormal proteins may build up in the system and even affect the brain. Research has indicated that the build-up of a digestive end product of A1 beta casein, found in cows' milk, is implicated as a factor in the development of schizophrenia and autism. This same protein is known to have immunomodulatory properties, and it is suggested that early exposure to cow's milk in youngsters genetically predisposed to insulin-dependent diabetes mellitus, can be one environmental factor which triggers the autoimmune response. Additionally, research into Parkinson's and Alzheimer's diseases has shown a greater vulnerability to these diseases in those with measurable deficiencies in their liver detoxification capacity.

So how much protein can you eat? This obviously depends on your state of health. Many patients who have had cancer, or who suffer from a chronic degenerative disease, may find that they have to watch their protein intake for life. Many of my patients who have been chronically ill, can remain symptom-free taking up to 2 -3 servings of each of the rice and legumes weekly. They may also include 100-200g of yoghurt daily. Some patients include a little fish (1-2 times weekly) and some include a few nuts (always soak your nuts to increase their digestibility). To all may patients I recommend juicing daily, for the rest of their lives, along with a plentiful supply of vegetables and fruits, cooked and raw. We learn to monitor our own health and vitality. Do any of my patient's eat meat, you may ask? The answer is yes, some do. But for the purposes of detoxification, sodium elimination and reversal of the tissue damage syndrome - the Gerson Therapy, with its low-protein recommendations, remains the best.

# Protein and aging

O n any healing diet we are looking to create minimal burden on the system, and to deliver a plentiful supply of nutrients and living enzymes in order to restore the functional capacity of the body. Convalescent diets, through the ages, have abided by these principles, where highly nutritious and digestible vegetables, broths, soups and gruels have been the mainstay of treatment. High protein has never been a consideration of a healing diet; protein is difficult to digest, it not only taxes the digestive system but also depletes digestive enzyme activity, and it creates a tremendous toxic burden on the system. Dr. Gerson found that it was impossible to detoxify and rebuild the body on a diet that incorporated protein in excess of body requirements. His healing diet is high in the easily digestible carbohydrate foods and obeys all the rules of the traditional healing diet.

Nowadays we are seeing patients with very impaired digestive systems and it is very tempting to start removing foods, such as carbohydrates, that appear to aggravate the digestion. The mainstay of any healing therapy has to be to restore the digestive system, before the patient can truly recover. Removing carbohydrates while increasing dietary protein may resolve the symptoms of bloating and flatulence at gut level, but the overall condition will continue to deteriorate and manifest at a more chronic level further down the path.

# Protein and its Toxic Burden

Protein, when eaten in excess to requirements, creates tremendous acidity within the system and places a high metabolic burden on both the liver and kidneys. Although excess protein can be broken down and used for fuel, it is a laborious process for the liver, drawing on zinc and B6 reserves, and the two end-products, urea and sulphuric acid, are poisons which have to be eliminated by the kidneys. As we have seen, these metabolic acids are eliminated by the kidneys in exchange for sodium (which we are trying to eliminate), so the higher your protein intake, the higher your sodium re-loading.

### Protein as a diuretic
Urea is not only a poison, but also a diuretic. This means that a high protein diet leaches water and nutrients from the body. Calcium is particularly vulnerable as the kidneys have a most prominent role in overall calcium balance and retention. "Urinary excretion of calcium falls when dietary protein is reduced and rises when it is increased. The calcium loss is usually greater than any increased absorption on moderate and high protein intakes. This phenomenon helps to explain how people in developing countries have no more osteoporosis - possibly less than in Europe and North America, despite lower calcium intakes." (Davidson, S., Passmore, R.; Brock, J.F.; Truswell, A.S.: Human Nutrition and Dietetics, 1979 pp95-96).

### Protein, Dehydration and the Aging Process
The stress that a high protein diet creates on the body will ultimately accelerate the aging process. A healing diet must aim to reverse or slow down the degenerative process. Degeneration and aging go hand-in-hand, and as we know this process can be accelerated or reversed by the type of diet we consume.  If we introduce the concept of

dehydration into this framework, we can see that all three factors are synonymous. With aging, we gradually lose the capacity for hydration; in other words, our bodies lose their affinity for water. Our skin wrinkles; our joints lose their lubrication and stiffen; our mucous membranes dry and become prone to inflammation/ulceration; our bones become more brittle; our spinal discs, which separate and cushion the vertebrae, lose their sponginess and flatten, leading to backache; our digestion becomes impaired as we lose the quantity of digestive juices required for adequate digestion; and the inflammatory diseases, such as arthritis, become more prevalent. The list is endless, but each complaint shares a common denominator, dehydration. And with that dehydration comes a hardening which ultimately leads to a loss of functional capacity.

This process of dehydration is very much accelerated by the type of diet we eat. A diet high in refined foods, saturated fat and protein along with increased tea, coffee and alcohol consumption, will encourage dehydration. We have two aspects to consider: the simple diuretic action of protein, tea, coffee and alcohol, and the more chronic condition, where the body has lost its capacity to "hold" water, or its natural affinity for water, which is determined by the integrity of the hydrating structures of body tissues. This integrity is governed by the dietary amounts of complex carbohydrates and essential fatty acids.

We can see that over the last fifty years, nutritional deficiencies aside, the Western diet has swung in favour of the high protein, refined carbohydrate and saturated fat diet, while our consumption of whole cereals and legumes has dramatically declined. Parallel to this we are witnessing a rise in chronic disease in ever younger age-groups.

## Hydration and the role of soluble fibre

Hydration, contrary to popular belief, is not dependent upon the amount of water you drink but the body's capacity to hold it. Drinking water, on its own, will be to little avail. When you drink a volume of water, it is rapidly absorbed into the blood stream where it raises the blood volume and dilutes the blood. The kidneys respond by appropriately increasing urinary excretion to return the blood pressure and concentration values to normal.

It is the type of soluble fibre in the diet that determines your overall hydration. Soluble fibre, such as the pectins, gels and starches found in plant food, have physical properties that attract water. For example, a young, growing plant has a good hydration capacity due to the presence of pectin, a polysaccharide which attracts and binds water by virtue of its electrical forces. As the plant ages, the levels of pectin decrease and the lignin levels increase, which leads to the lack of flexibility and brittleness in the woody twig. Pectin acts as a gel. Similar gels are seen in the cactus family, notably in aloe, and in various herbs, which act as mucilages and demulcents through their capacity to attract water. These products, when taken medicinally, have the capacity to re-hydrate, sooth and heal affected tissues.

Similarly, our bodies are made up of structured polysaccharides known collectively as connective tissue, which gives the body shape and form. These tissues range from fluid (blood, lymph), to semi-solid (bone marrow, spleen, liver, muscles, ligaments, tendons), to solid (cartilage and bone). The capacity of each structure to hydrate is determined by the physical properties of its matrix. The body fluids, such as the blood, lymph and synovial fluids, obviously have a greater hydration capacity than the bones. So some structural networks can trap more water than others. If you imagine a three-dimensional string vest, where all the holes are filled with water, and now imagine a tightly woven fabric with very few spaces, you will be able to appreciate the difference between a well hydrated and a less hydrated structure.

When we digest these soluble fibres from complex carbohydrates (mainly through bacterial action in the colon), they are converted to sugar acids and amino-acid sugars (such as glucosamine), which form the structural polysaccharide templates for the different connective tissues found throughout the body. They confer the same water-loving properties in the body as they do in the plant, and it is through these foods that we restore our hydration capacity. The sugar acid found in pectin, D-galacturonic acid, is readily converted by the body to D-glucuronic acid, a principle component of all connective tissue. Glucosamine, a component of synovial fluid in joints, can also be converted from its parent, glucose, by the body. The body is capable of all the sugar interconversions, providing that there is sufficient unrefined dietary carbohydrate intake. Our connective tissue contains 95% polysaccharide and only 5% protein, and therefore the carbohydrate component of the diet will reflect our hydration capacity

These sugar complexes are also incorporated into the cell membrane as glycoproteins which have important immune stimulant properties. In particular the pectins, the beta glucans (found in oats and other cereal grains) and the glucomannans (found in aloe vera gel) have been found to have a specific function in "turning on" the cellular immune response leading to increased immune activity and subsequent healing.

## How "dry" am I?

When we assess our past diet, it is easy to see just how "drying" it has been when the balance hasn't favoured foods and beverages that encourage hydration. And if we look at the Yin/Yang concept of Chinese philosophy, it is easy to see how "dry" we have become. Yin and yang = water and fire, respectively. When the water is deficient, the fire burns out of control. This gives rise to the hot, inflammatory or "itis" diseases, such as arthritis, ulcerative colitis, diverticulitis, bronchitis, and includes allergies, auto-immune diseases, ulcers, burning digestion, hot flushes, along with an accelerated aging/dehydration pattern.

Some people, after a period of dehydration, may become "water-logged". This is not over-hydration, but incorrect hydration and occurs further down the line when the tissues are losing their integrity, and intra-cellular potassium levels have become vulnerable.

Many authors state that the easiest way to rehydrate the body is to drink salt water, and advocate at least 2 teaspoons of salt daily. Sodium chloride has a high affinity for water, it attracts and binds a great deal of water which leads to an increase in the volume of body fluids. However, the water is drawn to the sodium and not to the connective tissues. Furthermore, it can dehydrate the connective tissues by pulling water from their surfaces to accommodate the amount of sodium. This is a deeper form of dehydration. Perhaps the best example of this is seen in soil salinity. When the degree of salt in the soil exceeds 1.5%, it not only prevents the uptake of water by the plant, but also causes water to move out of the plant.

Correct hydration refers to a structured and finite binding of water governed by the electrical forces of the connective tissues and forces determined by the ionized potassium status within the cell. These electrical fields hold the water in structured layers where it becomes impossible to over-hydrate. Symptoms of water-logging within the body usually manifests at a critical point of degeneration, where sodium and water start to enter the cells, which then swell giving rise to fluid retention and oedemas. Once sodium has entered the cell, the cell is unable to oxidize or produce energy, and will slip into a fermentative phase. A high protein diet will obviously exacerbate this picture.

# How do I rehydrate?

## The Hydrating Carbohydrates

### Vegetables and Juicing

Protein intake must be reduced in favour of the carbohydrate foods. Vegetables, in their fresh, raw state are the most hydrating of all the food groups. Living foods, which are replete with enzyme systems and nutrients, have strong electrical fields, which not only attract the digestive fluids and enzymes in the process of digestion, but once digested, confer these hydrating qualities to the living tissues within the system.

Unfortunately, the digestive system can become impaired early on in the degenerative process and some patients may have difficulty in digesting raw foods. The juicing of vegetables then becomes the preferred option. This is an ideal way to deliver an abundance of nutrients and living enzymes to an impaired digestive system. Puréeing raw vegetables will not achieve the same results, as the digestion will still have to "fight" with the fibre before it will release its nutrients. Cooked vegetables, although they have lost many of their colloidal (water-attracting) properties, are more easily digestible than raw, and will still deliver a good supply of nutrients to the system. They should be cooked at low temperatures and in their own juice. The waterless method of cooking is ideal for this.

The process of rehydration can be speeded up by increasing the amount of mixed apple and vegetable juices. They not only deliver potassium to the cell, but are also rich in pectin (apples) and high in other nutrients. For rehydrating purposes, the drinking of vegetable juices is preferable to water. Water is not only devoid of nutrients, but a high intake will deplete the body's mineral status through its stimulus on urinary excretion.

### Cereal grains and legumes

You diet should contain some cereal grains and legumes which are very rich in soluble fibre. The capacity of a food to swell when soaked or cooked in water, and the glutenous or starchy, viscous fluids which arise following their cooking, is indicative of their high content of soluble fibre. Gruel, made from porridge, is an example of the high amount of soluble fibre found in oats. Gruel is one of the most nourishing and easily digested foods for the convalescent. It is invaluable for those suffering acidity and inflammation in the digestive tract and should form part of the dietary regime for people with these complaints. Never rinse your brown rice or legumes after cooking as you will be discarding many of their soluble fibres. It should be noted that many people find the protein part of the gluten molecule difficult to digest and they may need to avoid cereal grains such wheat, oats, barley and rye. However, unless there is a gluten-intolerance, such as in coeliac disease, most patients can tolerate gruel.

### Gels and Broths

Gels and broths made from the simmering of bones (organic), form the basis of many traditional convalescent diets. Gelatin, released from the bones during the stock-making process, has a strong rehydrating capacity and will build strength into bones, cartilage and nails. The unique property of gelatin is that it does not lose any of its colloidal properties upon cooking, it remains hydrophilic (water-loving) even after re-heating! It is very easy to digest and nutrient-rich. The adding of whey or vinegar to the stock during its preparation enhances the nutrient content by drawing out minerals such as potassium, magnesium and calcium from the bones into the stock. The whey or vinegar will also assist its digestibility by breaking down the gelatin carbohydrate chains, and releasing the nutrients. Broths have always been indicated for people suffering from chronic disorders. I often recommend using a de-fatted stock as the basis for soups, vegetable stews and as the cooking medium for cereal grains.

## The Hydrating Oils

### The Essential Fatty Acids

Fats and oils do not mix with water, they are hydrophobic; but some oils are more water-friendly than others. The type of dietary fats you eat will determine the type of fats that form the cell membrane. A cell membrane that is predominantly composed of saturated fats and cholesterol will be rigid and biologically inert (polyunsaturated fats that are processed and heated behave as saturated fats); it will not attract oxygen, and the transport of nutrients, in and out of the cell, will become compromised. Additionally, a membrane that is coated with cholesterol cannot respond to hormones or other such signals from the body which is why, with this pattern of accelerated dehydration, we start seeing the onset of hormonal problems and diabetes (insulin resistance at cell membrane).

The essential fatty acids found in unrefined foods, however, are biologically active. By virtue of their electronic fields, they attract oxygen and are more water-soluble than other fats. Unrefined, cold-pressed flaxseed oil is one of the best sources of these fatty acids. These fatty acids, at the cell membrane, can inhibit a local inflammatory and/ or allergic response. The hydrating role of the essential fatty acids fits so neatly with the Yin and Yang philosophy. As the cell membrane hardens and dehydrates, so the incidence of inflammatory disorders, allergies and asthma increases. The very oils that are required to moderate or inhibit these destructive responses are absent from the diet and hence the cell membrane. During the healing process, it is best to remove all the fats and oils, other than flaxseed oil, from the diet for a prolonged period of time while you rebuild new cells, which are composed of the correct balance of essential fatty acids.

What you digest today, are your cells of tomorrow - which is why restoration and healing is such a long process. There are no short answers, but with a prolonged adherence to a highly nutritious way of eating, the principles of which have sustained the human race for thousands of years, you will gradually reap the benefits and rewards that health brings. Beware of dietary protocols that promote the high protein diet. Protein, taken in excess to requirements, will increase the metabolic burden, inhibit detoxification by promoting the retention of sodium, erode the mineral status, and by virtue of all the above, will accelerate the dehydration and aging process.

# Managing Toxicity

I find that most health conscious people have tried various detoxification diets. In fact most of my patients will tell me that they have detoxed many times before. When I ask them if they had a discharge of their toxicity I am usually met with a blank stare. You see the idea of cleansing is so far removed from our understanding of health that when in fact the body does try to cleanse itself, or release toxins, we panic and perceive the symptoms as disease and take various preparations to "cure" ourselves. A healthy body with a high vitality has a natural capacity to throw out toxicity; much like a centrifugal force which flings toxicity to the outside. At these times, when the cleansing is active we may experience mucus discharge, fever and other symptoms including aching joints, nausea and diarrhoea. Have you noticed how easily a child can throw up a fever and yet 24 hours later be right as rain? A child with high vitality can release toxicity and heal himself.

The body does not create an immune response to its own toxicity. Instead it packages toxins away "safely". However, when you have worked on raising the vitality (through specific diet and juicing) this toxicity is released into the circulation creating systemic toxicity. If the liver cannot adequately clean the blood in a timely manner then we experience toxic symptoms.

So how do we manage the release of toxicity? We need to ensure that:

*the rate of release of toxicity from the cells must equal their rate of removal to the outside*

This is the first rule, because a toxic circulation poisons the body and can weaken the liver. You also need to know what toxins you are likely to release – whether from medical or recreational drugs, chemicals from the workplace/ agriculture/other, and you will need to have some idea of how "stuck" your body is – in other words over how many years and how much medication have you taken to inhibit the cleansing and healing response. A good question to ask yourself – "When was the last time I had a fever or an acute discharge (i.e. mucus release)?" If you have been on long-term medical drugs (particularly the corticosteroids), then the healing will be much slower and more difficult to attain.

Momentum also comes into the equation. As toxicity is reduced, the vitality rises and the body builds a momentum. It doesn't happen overnight, but after a process of what I call loosening and releasing. Dr Gerson refers to cycles of healing and detoxification that he observed in his patients. Each patient followed their own unique cycle of discharge and healing, as the vitality increased over the months and years, until eventually the body was totally cured. I have a good example to share with you.

*Sally, in her late 30s, was in good health and helping her partner on the Gerson Therapy. She decided to take some of the juices and adopt the vegetarian diet to keep him company. Although she was not absolutely strict (sneaking off for the odd cappuccino and the piece of chocolate cake), there was a definite improvement in overall vitality. 18 months later, still maintaining the change in life-style, around the equinox (21ˢᵗ September) she suffered the worst "flu" she had ever experienced. There was tremendous mucus elimination and in addition she was noticing "flare-ups" of previous old injuries dating back to childhood. Sally knew that she was experiencing a healing crisis.*

Momentum ebbs and flows like the tides and there are periods of greater release and greater healing, but the critical factor is the maintenance of that momentum through the diet over a long period of time. You have to be patient and allow the body the time that it needs to heal itself. It is interesting that in many traditional medicines the changes in the geomagnetic forces at the times of the autumn and spring equinox are factored into the health equation. It is known both in traditional and modern medicine that changes in symptoms occur around these times – in Western society it is called an exacerbation of the disease, but in other cultures it is observed to be a crisis which, depending on its management, can either worsen or improve the health picture. I have often wondered whether the term "spring cleaning" comes from our forgotten knowledge of the cleansing cycles.

Once the vitality is raised to a critical point, then detoxification will occur. You need to know what you can do to support this process. If you have observed specific patterns of illness in your own case, then it is likely that the healing/cleansing symptoms will occur in these areas, and it is wise to have in your medicine cupboard specific herbs that you know will support those organs/glands and the immune system through the crisis. This does not apply to Gerson patients who will need to seek the advice of a Gerson practitioner to assist them through the healing flare-up. It is also helpful to be able to differentiate between the different types of symptoms in order to know what to do.

## Toxic Symptoms

Toxic symptoms occur when you feel "poisoned". This indicates that elimination of toxicity from the cells is occurring more quickly than elimination to the outside. The symptoms include:
- Brain/mental level – headaches, foggy/heavy head, loss of concentration, disorientation
- Mood swings, extreme irritation
- Nervous irritation as old toxins/drugs return to the circulation and affect nerve endings
- Joint and muscle aches and pains/inflammation

*To do:* the coffee enema is the only method of effectively releasing this toxicity.

## Detoxification Symptoms

These occur most specifically at gut level and the symptoms are associated with huge amounts of toxicity being released from the liver into the duodenum. The strongly toxic and alkaline bile can make a patient feel extremely nauseous, vomit bile and be unable to eat or drink. It can also cause diarrhoea. Sometimes increased amounts of toxicity are released following an enema, as the coffee enema stimulates this release. This is a real tell-tale sign of increased liver activity and detoxification and is a positive sign.

*To do:*
- You may take an additional enema (Gerson patients must seek advice from their practitioner)
- Drink peppermint tea and gruel. Peppermint tea will increase stomach acidity and therefore help to neutralise the bile, and the gruel will "mop up" toxic bile and be soothing on the digestive tract. Gruel can be added to the vegetable juices at these times, as it will help to keep them down
- Also take gruel before and after the enema, as this will help to counteract the effects of the toxic bile
- You may need to reduce the concentration of the coffee enema to half-strength, or even replace with the chamomile tea enema if the detoxification reactions are severe enough to cause vomiting and prevent eating.

# Healing Reactions

At a certain point of the healing process the immune system will be reactivated sufficiently to produce a healing crisis or a spontaneous fever not associated with infection. Our normal reaction to fever or inflammation is to either go to the doctor for a prescription to stop the symptoms in the belief that it may be an infection, or to take natural medicines to alleviate the symptoms. In both cases the result of treatment may stop the cleansing and stop the immune response in its tracks. Over the years, if you throw enough spanners in the works, your machine will grind to a halt and you will experience fewer symptoms of fever, discharge or acute cleansing. At this point the body is holding so much toxicity that disease will manifest at the chronic degenerative stage. We tread a dangerous path in our "hygienic" society which prefers vaccination and indiscriminate use of antibiotics rather than enhancing the body's capacity to develop a healthy active immune system. Consequently disordered immune patterns are now emerging even in our young (10% of children world-wide now suffer with asthma with a doubling in the last 15 years) and we are fast becoming dormant to other conditions, such as cancer.

During the healing crisis the body will returning to old injuries/illnesses (bacterial/viral or physical trauma) or areas in the body where the pathology is abnormal (as in overgrowth of scar tissue in arthritis, or tumour tissue). An inflammatory response is generated by the immune system which increases the circulation of blood and immune cells to the area in order to start the destruction of pathological or scar tissue followed by the rebuilding of healthy tissue. In the process there is often a discharge of general toxicity. Each time these exacerbations occur, the vitality will keep increasing and over the months scar tissue will gradually be replaced by new tissue, old fractures will heal perfectly and more toxins will be eliminated through the skin, mucous membranes, liver, kidney and colon. Unlike toxic reactions and detoxification reactions these types of reactions are accompanied by inflammation, fever and general malaise which is self-limiting. Usually a few days prior to a healing crisis the general energy/vitality seems much higher and the crisis which follows can last from 3 –10 days.

## Fever

It is not a good idea to suppress a fever. Try to let it run its course, but keep a check by taking the temperature every half hour. Remember the saying, " If you suppress the fever, you prolong the illness." If the temperature rises above 40°C, then you will need to take an aspirin-based medication (not paracetamol, which is damaging to the liver). Drink a little warm gruel before taking the medication. Other ways of reducing the temperature (if it becomes too intolerable) are:

- Have a tepid bath
- Take a cool water enema
- Take cool drinks
- Sponge the forehead and nape of the neck with a cool, damp cloth (witch hazel can be used on the cloth – not with Gerson patients)
- General sponging down of the body with cool, damp cloths

## Hot and cold packs

The castor oil pack is a warm pack and will:
- release congestion from mucous membranes (respiratory, colon), so it is useful to place a pack over these areas to assist the elimination of catarrh and infected mucus
- increase elimination in the liver – particularly useful when you get liver "pangs" caused by spasms in the bile ducts
- release toxic accumulation in muscles (toxins often release into the muscles and cause contraction and

tension, with pain of the affected muscles). The castor oil pack will release any area of spastic pain and tension

You can keep the castor oil pack on the area until the pain is reduced. A minimum of 90 minutes is required to release congestion in the tissues. The pack can be re-used.

## The clay pack is a cool pack and will:
- reduce swellings from hot inflammations (tumour sites, swollen joints, fluid retention)
- adsorb toxins from the surrounding tissue

Clay accelerates healing on open and internal wounds through these methods of reduction and adsorption. You should not leave this pack on for longer than 2 hours and it should not be re-used, as it will be saturated with toxic by products.

Do not stop your juicing, diet or enemas through this process. Many people go "off the track" at these critical times through confusion about what is happening and why. I hope that I have given you a few useful pointers and the confidence to manage your own healing successfully.

# The Gerson Therapy® – A Concept of Totality

*The in-text page references are from Dr. Max Gerson's book "A Cancer Therapy, Results of Fifty Cases."*

"Science is built up of facts as a house is built up of stones; but an accumulation of facts is no more science that a heap of stones is a house." Poincare; Science and Hypothesis (xiii).

The task of a person diagnosed with cancer to find a total treatment for their cure, is daunting. There are no therapeutic approaches, either conventional or holistic, that can boast unanimous victory, and indeed many fail. Solving the cancer problem has remained elusive; this is partly due to our fragmented approach, where research and practice is divided into many specialities, observing the effects of single treatments on the symptoms of disease, with a clear disregard for the totality of natural biological rules in the human body. If the focus of research and clinical application remains symptomatic, and continues to ignore the underlying metabolism that supports the disease, then treatment will remain ineffective, offering little more than clutching at straws. What is required is an integrated approach that embraces the "concept of totality", a phrase coined by the late Dr. Gerson.

The concept of totality refers to the functioning of the whole body; the integrity of the organs, the level of defence and immunity, and the healing power - all governed by the metabolism. Dr. Gerson states "the onset of metabolic disturbance constitutes the beginning of disease…. the task is to bring the body back to that normal physiology… the next task is to keep the physiology of the metabolism in that natural equilibrium"(pp5-6). He went on to say that cancer develops when there is a general breakdown of the whole body. He maintained that malignancy is cell adaptation to local conditions, or an adjustment to the preceding pathologies. Dr. Gerson surmised, and went on to prove, that if you changed the internal environment, so that the malignancy could not survive, if the body was brought to a healing inflammation (digestion of the tumour), and if the body was able to eliminate toxicity including tumour products, then you would indeed see cure. "What is essential is not the growth itself or the visible symptoms; it is the damage of the whole metabolism, including the loss of defence, immunity and healing power" (p35).

The aim of the therapy is to restore and increase the oxidative metabolism of normal cells, reactivate the enzyme systems, restore the digestion and essential organs (especially the liver) and increase the detoxification of the entire system. It is an intense nutritional and detoxification program which restores total body integrity. Dr. Gerson found that in cancer patients nutritional deficiencies could not be restored as long as the essential organs remain poisoned, in other words, damaged organs lose their capacity to recycle, retain and utilize nutrients. By default, the sick body perpetuates this state of deficiency. Therefore, it became imperative on the therapy to ensure adequate detoxification and nourishment over a long period of time until all the tumours were absorbed and the essential organs restored sufficiently to take over their full function. Dr. Gerson found that the application of the therapy (diet and medications) encouraged the cells to take up the nutrients while simultaneously releasing their accumulated toxic burden into the blood stream where it would be delivered to the liver. He discovered that the liver of a cancer patient is not only damaged but toxic, and any increase in the toxic load had severely detrimental effects, in some cases resulting in "hepatic coma" and death. Cancer breakdown products added to the burden and the patient's condition was seen to deteriorate faster on the therapy than from the actual disease. Hence the introduction of the coffee enema which supported and facilitated the rate of liver detoxification required for effective treatment. (Research undertaken in the 1930s by Heuber and Meyer and later in the 1970s by Wattenberg confirmed the specific compounds in coffee which stimulate the detoxification pathways both in the liver and small intestine). So this combined approach of hyperalimentation and intensive detoxification became the basis of the treatment.

Dr. Gerson refers to the "secret" or end-effect of his treatment was to bring the body to a natural healing inflammation, where the body raises an immune response which destroys abnormal substances including cancer and scar tissue. Dr. Gerson says, "After I recognised the healing of cancer to be a parenteral digestion, the therapeutic endeavour was subordinated to this purpose" (p217). The von Bergmann school at that time stated that "Cancer metabolism takes place once the body is no longer capable of producing an active 'inflammation metabolism' …. the cancerous organism is anergic in respect to inflammation" (p120), and further "where the inflammation metabolism begins the cancer metabolism stops"(p43).

It was common practice during the 1900s to deliberately stimulate defence reactions by invoking fever through the administration of various toxins (Coley's toxins) and by inoculating the patient with cancerous tissue or extracts from cancer tissues. Coley's initial success was good; however, as time went on, the treatment proved less effective. Others partially succeeded in producing a defence reaction but no cure was obtained, only temporary improvement.

Similar practices are used today and we are faced with the same limitations of treatment. In the melanoma vaccine trials, where patients receive an autologous vaccine (prepared from their own tumour tissue) in order to activate an immune response to their cancer, the prognosis is improved if the patient has an inflammatory reaction at the site of the vaccine which indicates an active immune system. The vaccine can only stimulate an existing immune system; it will not rebuild or replenish it. This is where Dr. Gerson understood that the outcome such treatments was determined not by the degree or type of stimulus applied, but by the "energy-capacity of the healing apparatus" or the state of "inflammatory preparedness" (immune response) for any given patient. So raising the "energy capacity" of the body became fundamental to treatment. This underlines why the outcome of any adjuvant treatment ultimately depends on the fabric or integrity of the body, which in effect, indicates that it is the body which supports the treatment and not the treatment which supports the body. A curative diet, that rebuilds the system should therefore become the cornerstone of any therapeutic approach.

It was already established that cancer patients were "anergic" (unable to produce an inflammatory reaction) to a greater or lesser degree. Dr. Gerson believed, from his observations, that the "anergia" increased, the more advanced the disease became. In advanced cases, the differential count for lymphocytes often fell below 10% (p124-125), which, as Dr. Gerson points out, indicated that the body was no longer capable of producing the necessary amount of lymphocytes for defence and healing. However, he observed that after several months of detoxification the inflammatory response was restored, or in other words, the energy-capacity of the healing apparatus was increased. "It therefore appears that the body's capacity to produce an allergic inflammation (healing power) depends on a most complete detoxication and an equilibrium in the metabolism to near normal" (pp128-129).

Dr. Gerson acknowledged "that the idea of helping the organism through a strong inflammation is old but was correct from the beginning" (p128), and he was not averse to stimulating the immune system, in addition to his treatment. He remained cautious in this approach as he saw that the problem lay in finding "the surest and most effective way to do this." However, he differed from his colleagues in that he felt it was essential that the body was brought to a natural and spontaneous inflammation, achievable on his therapy and a positive indication of a reactivation of the healing power. He states, "It is not enough to introduce a temporary inflammation into the body. The body itself must be able to do it and do it continuously, because many cancer cells remain hidden in some areas where even the bloodstream cannot reach them. In order to maintain this healing process, it is, of course, necessary to apply the treatment for long enough to restore all vital organs to normal function to reproduce the same reactive processes as used by the body itself, for healing purposes" (p125). To his mind, this enabled cure; to merely induce an artificial fever while neglecting the fundamental cause of the disease was of no long-term benefit. It is interesting to note the work of Tallberg[1] who uses an integrated metabolic, hormonal and immunological approach, and who has had some good results in improving the disease-free interval in some patients. Part of his treatment involves autologous vaccination admixed with tuberculin PPD and/or repeated vaccinations against influenza A and B strains. However, it is necessary to keep giving the vaccinations in order to secure control of the cancer and this method is not seen as cure.

The Gerson Therapy is not a preventative therapy, it is a curative therapy, and through its specific application it restores the metabolism which alters the pathology as a consequence. We are dealing with two metabolisms which co-exist in the cancer patient; the fermentative or cancer metabolism (does not use oxygen), and the normal or oxidative metabolism. Each is nourished, grows and reproduces with the aid of the nutrition to its disposal. Malignant cells with their fermentative system cannot adapt to the oxidative metabolism, so the thrust of the therapy is to bring the body back to its full oxidative function which supports cell differentiation, maturation and a defence system that checks any abnormal cell formation.

In raising the resistance of the body, while lowering the resistance of the tumour we are feeding and increasing the capacity the healthy cells while starving the cancer cells. Dr. Gerson observed that the onset of any pathological change in the cell was marked by a loss of potassium and an uptake of sodium, chloride and water by the cell. Once this occurs the cell naturally starts to drop into fermentation, sodium being a potent inhibitor of oxidation. In the 1970s, specific studies undertaken by the physiologist Clarence Cone,[2] who generated substantial experimental data concerning changes in potassium and sodium levels in cancer cells, indicated that not only do cancer cells take up sodium, but this mineral has a mitotic regulating effect forcing cancer cells to continuously divide, producing tumours.

Dr. Gerson's X-ray studies revealed that sick or damaged tissues were characterized by an area of oedematous swelling, which in malignancy provides a protective layer. Malignancies secrete toxic cancer breakdown products, some from protein, which seep into the surrounding area weakening the tissues and reducing the natural barrier. On the high potassium/no salt therapy these internal oedemas reduced, the tumours started shrinking and the patient starts to heal. Dr. Gerson observed losses of up to 8g per day of sodium in the urine at the beginning of the therapy and at periodic intervals during flare-ups. Dr. Gerson understood, despite opposition from within the medical establishment, that potassium, as a key activator of the oxidative system, had to be re-instated within the cell. He found that the application of larger doses of supplemental potassium (equal parts of potassium acetate, gluconate and mono-phosphate, determined after 300 experiments over a 6 year period) to an already high potassium diet, not only facilitated the uptake of potassium by the cells, but accelerated the elimination of sodium and toxins from the system which led to increased healing.

It was not until the 1970s that we saw scientific validation of Dr. Gerson's methods. His therapy was reviewed by Freeman Cope, MD[3] (Chief of Biochemistry of the Naval Air Development Centre, Pennsylvania, USA) who predicted and tested, using NMRI technology, Dr. Gerson's theory, that large amounts of potassium could be added to a low sodium diet to reduce what he labelled the tissue damage syndrome. This technology reads tissue chemistry electronically, enabling us to record and interpret electrical fields within the body. Cope was in agreement with Gilbert Ling's[5] (biophysicist) "Association-Induction Theory" which was advanced in 1962. Ling approached the cell as an electrical model. He demonstrated that the latticework of microfilaments within the cell generates an electrical field which, through its force of attraction, causes water to polarise and form structured layers. In this electrical state, the cell is purified and will not accept sodium. This electrical field is governed by the association of potassium at the negatively charged sites along the microfilaments. When potassium is in place, the oxidation system is activated along with the production of energy (ATP) and normal metabolism occurs.  Cope verified that damaged tissues, whether from chemical, bacterial or traumatic insult, lose their electrostatic forces which hold the potassium in place, and start to swell with sodium and water. A vicious cycle is then set up as the cell metabolism becomes more and more impaired. Cope demonstrated that, unless the cell was irreversibly damaged, by bombarding the cells with potassium they are encouraged to regain their electrical state.

The application of thyroid and Lugol's (inorganic iodine) medication along with the potassium (in large doses at the beginning of the treatment) amplifies the cellular response to increase oxidative capacity and free energy. Thyroid and Lugol's stimulate the replication of cellular mitochondria (energy factories of the cell where oxygen in "burned" and ATP is formed) to meet the increased energy requirements. These medications also accelerate sodium and toxin elimination.

The cancer cell cannot adapt to these changes, and in effect are starved of their nutrition, while the oxidizing cells are revitalized. Additionally, all the other medications recommended by Dr. Gerson, were ones that only supported oxidative metabolism, such as niacin (and later we added CoQ10), and are not required by the cancer cell.  Dr. Gerson did try introducing various nutritional supplements but had negative results with the ones he tried, specifically calcium, magnesium, folic acid, and vitamins A and E, which he found had a stimulating rather than a replenishing effect. "Several times I observed that vitamins in good combinations, with or without minerals, produced a regrowth of cancer or new spreadings in a few days. The patient felt better for a shorter or longer period through what may be regarded as the stimulation of the entire metabolism. However, the cancer regrew, caused by what some other authors explained as the greater attraction power of the cancerous tissue"(p210). Tallberg [1] has also identified specific nutrients acting as growth factors for malignancies.

Cancer tissue is greedy for nutrients, especially protein. Excess dietary protein not only inhibits sodium elimination and the reversal of the tissue damage syndrome, but also promotes the growth of tumours. Experimental work carried out by Dr. Robert Good [5] on mice during the 1980s, confirmed Dr. Gerson's observations, that a restricted calorie and protein diet causes regression of tumours. When protein was added prematurely into the diet, Dr. Gerson's patients experienced regrowth of tumour tissue.

The nutrients as supplied in the food and the freshly prepared juices, however, did not have a stimulant effect on the tumour tissue. Dr. Gerson observed that while the nutrients were in their living state, as part of the living enzyme system of the plant, that they would be taken up and replenish the sick tissues. If the juices were not taken immediately after preparation (60% of enzymes die within 30 minutes of juice preparation), or if the enzymes were damaged in the juicing (as occurs when using centrifugal machines), then the patient failed to respond to the therapy. It would appear that nutrients, as part of the oxidizing system of the plant, will support the oxidizing cell, but when they fall out of this state, they are no longer as effective.

Due to Dr. Gerson's negative findings on nutritional supplements, he was opposed to their use as he regarded them as having stimulant value only, being chemical substances devoid of energy. He says, "We know that what we have inherited is not set of chemical substances but a pattern of dynamic energies"(p90), and that "the system needs animating energies besides the pure substances" (p99). He comments that by using organically grown foods, you bring both the discovered and undiscovered enzymes and nutrients (especially the unknown) together in the proper quantity, mixture and composition required for regeneration and healing.  It is important to understand that through the specific application of the Gerson Therapy (diet and medications) we bring  about a total change in cell metabolism, a shift of sodium and toxins and a re-instatement of potassium and the oxidative cycle, which cannot simply be achieved through nutritional supplementation. Dr. Gerson offers the following comment, "It is not necessary here to pay attention to the many proposals for applying one or more vitamins or enzymes or those mixed with minerals. It would be a primitive concept to propose that the administration of one or another enzyme, vitamin or mineral or their composition would change or counteract the enzymatic disturbance or intracellular nature" (p57).

If we approach the cancer problem from an holistic view point then the chances are that we will make informed and better choices rather than adopting a hit and miss approach. There are many adjunctive treatments available today, and clearly many have therapeutic value. Among the ones a Gerson patient may use are laetrile, ozone, hydrotherapy (hyperthermy) with laetrile or reduced chemotherapy/radiotherapy, and herbs. Choosing an integrated approach based on the concept of totality, means that any chosen treatment can be evaluated as to how far it can assist, or whether it undermines the healing process. According to the concept of totality the outcome of any treatment is dependent upon the existing energy-capacity of the body, as it is the body integrity that ultimately supports the treatment. The cornerstone of any treatment therefore must be diet-based.

With any proposed therapy I believe two questions need to be asked:
* am I releasing the accumulated, and the current, toxic burden?
* am I rebuilding my healthy cells and depriving my cancer cells?

Then you may ask how your chosen adjunct treatment fits into the overall plan.

I strongly agree with Dr. Gerson, that the fundamental cause of degenerative disease and cancer is unnatural nutrition (non-organic and processed) and the slow poisoning of the body due to the accumulation of environmental toxins. I believe that the time is critical and that we need to adopt more preventative measures by ensuring that we use only organic foods and refuse toxic chemicals in our environment. I quote Dr. Gerson, "I fear that it will not be possible, at least in the near future, to repair all the damage that modern agriculture and civilization have brought to our lives. I believe it is essential that people unite, in the old conservative manner, for the humanitarian purpose of producing nutrition for their families and future generations as natural and unrefined as possible" (pp3-4).

# References

1. Tallberg, Thomas: *"Cancer treatment, based on active nutritional biomodulation, hormonal therapy and specific autologous immunotherapy"*, Journal of Australasian College of Nutrition & Environmental Medicine, Vol. 15 No 1, April 1996, pp 5-23.

2. Cone, Clarence D. Jr.: *"Unified theory on the Basic Mechanism of Normal Mitotic Control and Oncogenesis."* Journal of Theoretical Biology 30: 151-181, 1971

3. Cope, Freeman W., "A Medical Application of the Ling Association-Induction Hypothesis: The High Potassium, Low Sodium diet of the Gerson Cancer Therapy", Physiological Chemistry and Physics 10: 456-467, 1978
   http://www.gerson-research.org/docs/CopeFW-1978-1/index.html

4. Ling, Gilbert: *A Revolution in the Physiology of the Living Cell*, 1992. www.gilbertling.org/

5. Good, Robert A., Fernandes, Gabriel, and Day, Noorbibi D., *"The Influence of Nutrition on Development of Cancer Immunity and Resistance to Mesenchymal Diseases"*, 1982, New York Raven Press, Molecular Interrelations of Nutrition and Cancer.

# Recommended Reading

A bsolutely essential reading is *A Cancer Therapy, Results of Fifty Cases* by Dr. Max Gerson. The articles *A History of the Gerson Therapy* by Patricia Spain Ward and the retrospective review, *Five-Year Survival Rates of Melanoma Patients Treated by Diet Therapy After the Manner of Gerson: A Retrospective Review* by Christine Hildenbrand and Gar Hildenbrand are both available on-line at www.gerson-research.org

I would also recommend *Our Stolen Future*, by Theo Colborn and *Secrets of the Soil*, by Tompkins and Bird. Both these books will give you a deep insight into the toxicity of our environment and its true impact on health. If these books don't convince you to go organic – then nothing will!

The lastest publication *Healing the Gerson Way*, by Charlotte Gerson and Beata Bishop, is a practical and clear explanation of the diet and medications, offering some instruction on management and includes Gerson recipes. As a general text, it does not fully cater for individual application of the program but is extremely useful for the beginner.

My own two publications, *Dietary Healing, the complete detox program* and my double audio CD, *The Principles of Detoxification*, are both worthwhile resources of information for the reader who is interested in the broader principles of nutritional healing and detoxification and the practical management of a detoxification regime. The book gives a detailed appraisal of how detoxification works, relates this process to case studies and offers the reader hands-on advice and recipes and is a must for those coming off the therapy or for those looking for not quite as rigorous approach as the Gerson Therapy. The audio CD offers much additional information, is more specific to the Gerson Therapy, giving a thorough overview of this therapy, and includes a session of questions and answers along with a 30 minute presentation on cancer.

Some texts on the scientific biological basis of a detoxification therapy are difficult to grasp and my video presentations Fundamentals of Cellular Cleansing Part 1 (sodium/potassium balance) and Part 2 (acid/alkaline balance) are a well worth addition to your resources.

## Courses

As a practitioner with 30 years experience and as a former Director of the Gerson Institute, with responsibilities for education and training, I have taught medical professionals world-wide in the methodology and framework of dietary healing and detoxification and offer various courses that are unsurpassed in content and training capacity, including a practitioner mentoring program.

For practitioners who wish to enrol on my mentoring program and learn advanced skills in patient case-taking and patient-management, then I offer the following:

- a 3 day practitioner course for those who wish to learn and adopt the principles of Dr. Gerson's treatment and its application in chronic disease and cancer;

- a 2 or 5 day course in Dietary Healing and Detoxification for those who wish to migrate the principles of Dr. Gerson's framework into programs for those with less serious conditions;

- an online practitioner course, *Managing the Patient's Journey*, using the Smart Patient® case management framework for case-taking, follow-up, interpretation, monitoring and fostering the practitioner/patient partnership to achieve better outcomes; and

- Practitioner mentoring program for those who have completed the online practitioner training course.

# Recommended Reading

Gerson, Max, M.D.: *A Cancer Therapy - Results of Fifty Cases*   ISBN 0-88268-105-2

Gerson, C; Bishop, B; *Healing the Gerson Way* ISBN 9780976018605

Alexander, K.: *Dietary Healing, the complete detox program* ISBN 9780980376203
Available from www.kathrynalexander.com.au

Alexander, K; *Smart Patient Journey Road Map, increasing your odds for success;* ISBN 9780980376296
Available from www.kathrynalexander.com.au

Alexander, K.: *Managing the Patient's Journey,* an online practitioner course
http://www.kathrynalexander.com.au/store/p38/Managing_the_Patient%27s_Journey_%28online_course%29.html

Bishop, B.: *A Time to Heal,*  ISBN 0-14-019517-3

Ward, Patricia Spain, Dr.: *A History of the Gerson Therapy.*
www.gerson-research.org/docs/WardPS-1988-1/index.html

Hildenbrand, G., Hildenbrand, L.C, Bradford, K.,  Cavin, S.W., MS: *Five-Year Survival Rates of Melanoma Patients Treated by Diet Therapy After the Manner of Gerson: A Retrospective Review:*
www.gerson-research.org/docs/HildenbrandGLG-1995-1/index.html

Hildenbrand, G.: *How the Gerson Therapy Heals.*
www.gerson-research.org/docs/HildenbrandGLG-1990-5/index.html

Cope F.W: "*A medical application of the Ling Association-Induction Hypothesis: the high potassium, low sodium diet of the Gerson cancer therapy*" http://www.gerson-research.org/docs/CopeFW-1978-1/index.html

Ling, G.N: *A Revolution in the Physiology of the Living Cell,*  Malabar, Florida; Kreiger Publishing Co 1992 (review the contents at http://bioparadigma.narod.ru/ling.htm)

Budwig, J.: *Flax Oil as a True Aid Against Arthritis, Heart Infarction, Cancer and Other Diseases,* Apple Publishing Co Vancouver, Canada 1992

Erasmus, U.: *Fats that Heal, Fats that Kill,* Alive: Vancouver 1986, ISBN 0-920470-38-6

Marshall, W.J.: *Clinical Chemistry,* Gower Medical Publishing, ISBN 0-39-44782-5

Murphy, G., M.D., Lawrence, W., Jr., M.D.,  Lenhard, R.E., Jr., M.D.: *Clinical Oncology,* American Cancer Society, Inc., Atlanta, ISBN 0-944235-10-7

Robinson, J. R.: *Fundamentals of Acid-Base Regulation,*  Blackwell Scientific Publications, ISBN 0-632-003472

Altman, N.: *Oxygen Healing Therapies,* Healing Arts Press, Rochester, Vermont USA  ISBN 0-89281-527-2

Brunt, P.W., Losowsky, M.S., Read, A.E.: *The Liver and Biliary System,* Heinemann ISBN 0-433-04560-4

Pottenger, F. M., Jr., M.D.: *Pottenger's Cats,* Price-Pottenger Nutrition Foundation, California, ISBN 0-916764-06-0

Price, W. A., D.D.S.: *Nutrition and Physical Degeneration,* Keats Publishing Inc, Price-Pottenger Nutrition Foundation, California. ISBN 0-87983-816-7

Dextreit, R.: *The Healing Power of Clay,* Editions Vivre en Harmonie, ISBN 2-7155-0013-9

Knishinsky, R.: *The Clay Cure,* Healing Arts Press, Rochester, Vermont, ISBN 0-89281-775-5

Tompkins, P., Bird, C.: *Secrets of the Soil,* Earthpulse Press Inc, 1998, ISBN 1-890693-24-3

Fallon, S.: *Nourishing Traditions,* ProMotion Publishing, 1995, ISBN 1-887314-15-6

Cameron, F.: Pauling, L., *Cancer and Vitamin C,* Warner Books Inc.

Colborn, T., Dumanoski, D., Myers, J. P.: *Our Stolen Future,* Abacus, 1997, ISBN 0 349 10878 1

## Gerson Support Group Publications
www.gersonsupportgroup.org.uk

- Healing at Home - a DVD containing essential practical information
- An Information Book for those beginning the Therapy
- Simply Gerson, a recipe book for beginners on the Therapy
- A Little Enema Book to help with the practical issue of taking enemas
- Gourmet Gerson giving recipes for those well into the Therapy and their carers & family

## Audio CD (digital download)
Alexander, K.: *The Principles of Detoxification*
Available from www.kathrynalexander.com.au

## DVD (digital download)
Alexander, K.: *Part 1 Fundamentals of Cellular Cleansing: the sodium/potassium balance*
Alexander, K.: *Part 2 Fundamentals of Cellular Cleansing: the acid/alkaline balance*
Available from www.kathrynalexander.com.au

# Index

Ling, Gilbert 7

Linoleic acid 138

Linolenic acid 138

Liver capacity, assessment of 35–36

Liver capsules
dosage 90

Liver detoxification
coffee enema, and 19–20
environmental toxins, and 22

Liver enzymes 55–57

Liver Extract Injections 24, 91

Liver function tests 53–59
reference ranges 53

Liver juice. See Juices

Lubile 24

Lugol's solution (see iodine also)
cardiovascular insufficiency, and 37
dosage and contra-indications to 85, 85–86, 85–86, 200
dosage for the weakened patient 121
dosage per drop 85
pleural effusion, and 38

Lymphocytes
calculating the differential 42
reference range 42, 49

Lymphocytosis
indications for 50
leukaemia, and 51

Lymphopenia 50
indications for 50

M

Malic acid, in apples 84, 133

Mannitol, brain oedema 126

Mean cell haemoglobin
calculation of 42
reference range 42

Mean cell haemoglobin concentration
reference range and calculation of 42

Mean cell volume
reference range 42

Medications 85–109, 200–201
bleeding, and 125
contra-indications 101
full therapy, and 101
general modifications, and 101
general schedule, and 114
long-term follow-up 114, 119–120, 193–194
mistakes in 152–153
modified therapy, and 102–103, 197
non-cancer patient, and 104, 104–105, 104–105
surgery, after 101
weakened patient, and 102, 121–123, 198

Megaloblastic anaemia 44–45

Metabolic complications in malignancy 124

Methylcobalamin
preferred form of B12 91

Microalbuminuria
urine test, and 77

Mitochondria 9

Modifications, diet 116–119
non-nancer patients 104–105

Modifications to the therapy 102–103
chemotherapy, pre-treated patient 102–103, 197
contra-indications to the full therapy 38
full therapy, and 101, 195–196
general modifications 193–194
non-cancer patients 104–107
weakened patient 102, 198

Morphine 39, 150

Multiple myeloma 59
case study 123
elevated calcium, and 74

Muscle pain
toxic reaction, and 143

Myeloid leukaemia 51

N

N-acetylcysteine
radiation therapy, and 129

Nausea
coffee enemas, and 125
gruel, and 204
management of 144
obstruction, and 125
peppermint tea, and 204

Nephrotic syndrome
dietary modifications, and 116
hypo-albuminaemia, and 58
plasma proteins, and 59

Neuron-Specific Enolase, tumour marker 80

Neutropenia 49

Neutrophils
calculating the differential 42
infection, and 49–50
reference range 42, 49
tumoural activity, and 49–50

Niacin
bleeding, and 38, 125
dosage and contra-indications 87, 101, 200
histamine release, and 10
oxidative metabolism 10, 27–29
surgery, and 125
ulcers. and 38, 125

Nightshades
allergy to 37

NMRI technology 4, 7–8

Non-Hodgkin's Lymphoma
LDH levels, and 57, 58

NPK 24

Nutrients
cooking, and 25
values in organic and non-organic foods 134

Nutritional supplements 25, 158–159, 228–229
regrowth of cancer. and 25

O

Obstruction
bile ducts 125
gastro-intestinal tract 38, 124–125
renal ureters 121, 125

Potassium gluconate, in diarrhoea  145

Pottenger  154

Price, Weston  154

Prostate-specific antigen (PSA), tumour marker  79

Prostatic acid phosphatase  80

Protein  135–136
  acidity, and  6, 216
  ascites, and  127
  autoimmune disease, and  13
  bee pollen  99, 117
  calcium losses, and  216
  cooked  134, 210, 214–215
  dietary intake, and  117–118, 135–136
  dietary protein and albumin levels  59
  fish, introduction of  117
  food values  140
  full therapy  101
  high protein diet  207
  immune profile, and  13–14
  legumes, introduction of  117
  metabolism, hormone control of  208
  modifications through the therapy, and  117
  modified therapy  102–103
  non-cancer patients  104
  oedema, and  14
  pasteurisation, and  210
  pleural effusions and ascites, and  126–127
  sodium retention, and  5, 209, 216
  spirulina  99, 117
  storage in muscles  208
  tumoural growth, and  14, 153, 209
  values in foods, table  140

Protein restriction  13–14, 14
  autoimmune disease, and  13
  healing, and  158
  immune profile, and  13, 206, 209

R

Radiotherapy  128
  bone marrow and immune recovery  39, 50, 128
  bone metastases, and  128
  breast cancer, and  128
  lymphopenia, and  50
  neutropenia, and  49
  vitamin C, and  95

Raw foods  134
  digestive capacity, and  210

Rectal inflammation  145

Renal failure
  contra-indications, and  39
  hyperkalaemia, and  72
  hypokalaemia, and  73
  potassium, and  85

Renin
  control of blood pressure, and  66

Rheumatoid arthritis
  chronic anaemia, and  127
  elevated inflammatory markers, and  58

Root canals  36

S

Saturated fats  137–139

Schedules, medications
  full therapy, after first four weeks  196
  full therapy, first 4 weeks  195
  general schedule, current  194
  general schedule, Dr. Gerson's  193
  modified therapy, post chemotherapy  197
  modified therapy, weakened patient  198

SIADH (see also Vasopressin and Paraneoplastic syndrome)
  hyponatraemia, and  67

Sick cell syndrome  68

Sick euthyroid syndrome  64

Silver  98

Sodi-Pallares, Dr  99

Sodium  66–69
  cancer cells, in  6
  daily losses in the urine  5
  dehydration, and  69
  depletion (see also hyponatraemia)  67–68
  elimination of  4–5, 8–9
  enzyme inhibition, and  5
  excess (see also hypernatraemia)  67
  fermentation, and  5
  high protein diet, and  158
  oedemas, and  4
  potassium balance, and  4
  protein, and  5
  reduction of enemas, and  116
  reference range  66
  serum sodium, control of  66–68
  sodium/potassium pump  7–8
  terminal disease, and (see also sick cell syndrome)  6

Soy products
  anti-nutrients, and  136–137, 214
  thyroid inhibition, and  136–137

Spirulina  99
  cobalamin analogues, and  99
  non-fat yoghurt, replacing  99

Sprouted seeds
  increasing digestibility  136, 214

Stem cell model of cancer  129–130

Stress
  reduction in digestive capacity, and  37
  thyroid function, and  60

Sunlight  139

Surgery  128
  niacin, and  101

T

Tallberg, Thomas, M.D.  12, 14, 209

Tamoxifen
  bone metastases, and  131

Thalassaemia  45

Thrombocytopenia  51
  hepatatis C, and  52

Thrombopoiesis  51

Thyroid
  chlorine and fluoride, inhibition  153
  hypothyroid, reference range  61

42659674R00144

Made in the USA
Charleston, SC
03 June 2015